Metabolic Regulation

A Human Perspective

Metabolic Regulation

A Human Perspective

Second Edition

Keith N. Frayn ScD, PhD, FRCPath
Professor of Human Metabolism
University of Oxford, Oxford, UK

Blackwell
Science

© Portland Press Ltd 1996
© Keith Frayn 2003

Blackwell Science Ltd, a Blackwell Publishing
Company
Editorial Offices:
Blackwell Science Ltd,
9600 Garsington Road, Oxford OX4 2DQ, UK
  Tel: +44 (0)1865 776868
Blackwell Publishing Inc., 350 Main Street,
Malden, MA 02148-5020, USA
  Tel: +1 781 388 8250
Blackwell Science Asia Pty Ltd,
550 Swanston Street, Carlton,
Victoria 3053, Australia
  Tel: +61 (0)3 8359 1011

Designations used by companies to
distinguish their product are often claimed
as trademarks. All brand names and product
names used in this book are trade names,
service marks, trademarks or registered
trademarks of their respective owner. The
Publisher is not associated with any product
or vendor mentioned in this book.

This publication is designed to provide
accurate and authoritative information in
regard to subject matter covered. It is sold on
the understanding that the Publisher is not
engaged in rendering professional services. If
professional advice or other expert assistance
is required, the services of a competent
professional should be sought.

First edition published 1996 by Portland
Press Ltd
Second edition published 2003 by Blackwell
Science Ltd

4   2008

Library of Congress
Cataloging-in-Publication Data
is available

ISBN 978-0-632-06384-0

A catalogue record for this title is available
from the British Library

Set in 10/13 pt Sabon
by Sparks Computer Solutions Ltd, Oxford
http://www.sparks.co.uk
Printed and bound in Singapore by
Markono Print Media Pte Ltd

For further information on
Blackwell Publishing, visit our website:
www.blackwellpublishing.com

Contents

Preface

I have been flattered, sometimes overwhelmed, by the kind comments I have received about the first edition of this book. Clearly I am not the only person who feels that there is a need to move onwards from a detailed understanding of molecules and cells, to see how they operate collectively in health and disease – what is now trendily called 'integrative physiology'. As I commented in the Preface to the first edition, concepts such as starvation, stress or exercise (and now I would add diabetes and obesity) apply essentially to the whole body and cannot be understood solely with reference to individual cells. A year or two after the first edition was published, J.-P. Flatt, Professor of Biochemistry in the University of Massachusetts, remarked to someone else in my presence that I had written a book that could be summarised in one sentence: 'The whole is greater than the sum of the parts.' How I wished that I had thought of that phrase as a way of introducing the book. I offer it now as a neat summary of what I believe integrative physiology is all about.

Why a new edition? Has metabolism changed that much? It is true that our understanding of the fundamental pathways of metabolism is still much as it was ten or twenty years ago. But our knowledge of how metabolism is regulated continues to develop. Indeed, at just the same time that I submitted the first edition to the publisher (early 1995), our understanding of the regulation of energy balance was being revolutionised by the discovery of the hormone leptin, a hormone with major effects on metabolic balance in rodents, later shown to have powerful effects also in humans. In addition, the last few years have seen great strides made in understanding the control of gene expression, particularly factors that interact with the DNA to control mRNA production. I am also very willing to admit that my own knowledge of this field was relatively rudimentary in 1995 and that my own understanding of the field of gene expression has increased considerably. In rewriting this book, I have taken the opportunity to restructure it somewhat, bringing in a new chapter (Chapter 2) that gives some details of the multiple means by which metabolic regulation is achieved. At the same time I have, of course, updated many other sections where knowledge (either that of the biochemical community generally, or just my own) has advanced over the intervening years.

Several people have read drafts of individual chapters and made helpful comments. I would like to thank Germán Cameo, Björn Carlsson, Geoff Gibbons, Fredrik Karpe, Jonathan Levy, Denise Robertson, Len Storlien and Garry Tan for their help in this respect. Dick Denton, Hilary Powers and Parveen Yaqoob kindly commented on the contents and made helpful suggestions. Any errors that remain are my own responsibility.

I would like also to record my gratitude to, and fond memories of, two metabolic biochemists who had a major influence on my own views of metabolism: Derek Williamson and Denis McGarry. Both have sadly died, far too young, since the first edition was published. Their influence on the field of metabolism is immeasurable and they are sorely missed.

Finally, I wish to redress a major omission from the first edition: thanks to my wife Theresa for her patience during the many long evenings and weekends that I spent glued to my computer in preparing this book.

Keith Frayn
Oxford
July 2002

Abbreviations

Note: some abbreviations for compounds that are used just once within a figure or box are defined in the corresponding legend and not listed here.

ABC	ATP-binding cassette (defines a family of proteins)
ACAT	acyl-coA : cholesterol acyltransferase
ACC	acetyl-CoA carboxylase
ACS	acyl-CoA synthase
ACTH	adrenocorticotrophic hormone
ADH	antidiuretic hormone
ADP	adenosine 5′-diphosphate
AGE	advanced glycation end-product
AIB	α-amino-isobutyric acid
AMP	adenosine 5′-monophosphate
ASP	acylation stimulating protein
ATP	adenosine 5′-trisphosphate
ATPase	enzyme hydrolysing ATP
BCAA	branched-chain amino acids
BFE	bifunctional enzyme (6-phosphofructo-2-kinase/ fructose-2,6-bisphosphatase)
BMI	body mass index
BMR	basal metabolic rate
cAMP	cyclic adenosine 3′,5′-monophosphate (cyclic AMP)
CCK	cholecystokinin
CE	cholesteryl ester
CETP	cholesteryl ester transfer protein
cGMP	cyclic guanosine 3′,5′-monophosphate (cyclic GMP)
ChRE(BP)	carbohydrate responsive element (binding protein)

CNS	central nervous system
CoA	coenzyme A (esterified form)
CoASH	coenzyme A (free form)
CPT	carnitine O-palmitoyltransferase
CRE	cyclic AMP response element
DAG	diacylglycerol
DHA	docosahexaenoic acid (22:6 n-3)
DIT	diet-induced thermogenesis
DNA	deoxyribonucleic acid
eNOS	endothelial nitric oxide synthase
F 1,6-P_2	fructose 1,6-bisphosphate
F 2,6-P_2	fructose 2,6-bisphosphate
F 6-P	fructose 6-phosphate
FABP	fatty acid binding protein
FAT	fatty acid translocase
FATP	fatty acid transport protein
FBPase	fructose-1,6-bisphosphatase
FC	free (unesterified) cholesterol
FH	familial hypercholesterolaemia
FQ	food quotient
FSH	follicle-stimulating hormone
G 6-P	glucose 6-phosphate
G-6-Pase	glucose-6-phosphatase
GDP	guanosine 5′-diphosphate
GH	growth hormone
GIP	gastric inhibitory polypeptide (also known as glucose-dependent insulinotrophic polypeptide)
GK	glucokinase
GLP(-1,2)	glucagon-like peptide(-1,2)
GLUT	glucose transporter
glycerol 3-P	glycerol 3-phosphate
G-proteins (G_i, G_s, G_q)	GTP-binding proteins (inhibitory and stimulatory forms with respect to adenylyl cyclase; stimulatory form with respect to phospholipase C)
GSK	glycogen synthase kinase
GTP	guanosine 5′-trisphosphate
HDL	high-density lipoprotein
HIF	hypoxia-inducible factor
HMG-CoA	3-hydroxy-3-methylglutaryl-CoA
HSL	hormone-sensitive lipase
IDDM	insulin-dependent diabetes mellitus (Type 1 diabetes mellitus)
IGF	insulin-like growth factor
IMP	inosine 5′-monophosphate

IP_3	inositol (1′,4′,5′)-trisphosphate
IRS	insulin receptor substrate
K_a	dissociation constant for an acid
$LCAT$	lecithin-cholesterol acyltransferase
LDH	lactate dehydrogenase
LDL	low-density lipoprotein
LH	luteinising hormone
LPL	lipoprotein lipase
MAG	monoacyglycerol
MET	multiple of resting metabolic rate (unit for whole-body energy expenditure)
M_r	relative molecular mass (molecular weight)
$mRNA$	messenger-RNA (ribonucleic acid)
$NAD^+, NADH$	nicotinamide adenine dinucleotide ($^+$, oxidised form; H, reduced form
$NADP^+, NADPH$	nicotinamide adenine dinucleotide phosphate ($^+$, oxidised form; H, reduced form)
$NEFA$	non-esterified fatty acid(s) (also called free fatty acids)
$NIDDM$	non-insulin-dependent diabetes mellitus (Type 2 diabetes mellitus)
PCr	phosphocreatinine
PDH	pyruvate dehydrogenase
$PDX1$	pancreatic-duodenal homeobox factor-1 (a transcription factor controlling expression of the preproinsulin gene)
$PEPT$	peptide transporter
PFK	phosphofructokinase
P_i	inorganic phosphate
$PI3K$	phosphatidylinositol-3-kinase
PIP_2	phosphatidylinositol (4′,5′)-bisphosphate
PIP_3	phosphatidylinositol (3′,4′,5′)-trisphosphate
PKA,B,C,G	protein kinase A,B,C,G
PL	phospholipid
PLC	phospholipase C
$POMC$	pro-opiomelanocortin
$PPAR$	peroxisome proliferator-activated receptor
PP_i	inorganic pyrophosphate
$RAGE$	receptor for advanced glycation end-products
RER	respiratory exchange ratio
RQ	respiratory quotient
$SCAP$	SREBP cleavage activating protein
$SGLT$	sodium-glucose co-transporter
$SR(-BI)$	scavenger receptor(-BI)

SREBP	sterol regulatory element binding protein
T_3	triiodothyronine
T_4	thyroxine
TAG or TG	triacylglycerol (triglyceride in some literature)
TCA cycle	tricarboxylic acid cycle
TRL	triacylglycerol-rich lipoprotein
TSH	thyroid-stimulating hormone
TZD	thiazolidinedione
UCP	uncoupling protein
UTP	uridine 5'-trisphosphate
VLDL	very-low-density lipoprotein
$\dot{V}O_2max$	maximal rate of oxygen consumption for an individual

1

Important Concepts

1.1   Metabolic regulation in perspective

To many students, metabolism sounds a dull subject. It involves learning pathways with intermediates with difficult names and even more difficult formulae. Metabolic regulation may sound even worse. It involves not just remembering the pathways, but remembering what the enzymes are called, what affects them and how. This book is not simply a repetition of the molecular details of metabolic pathways. Rather, it is an attempt to put metabolism and metabolic regulation into a physiological context, to help the reader to see the relevance of these subjects. Once their relevance to everyday life becomes apparent, then the details will become easier, and more interesting, to grasp.

This book is written from a human perspective because, as humans, it is natural for us to find our own metabolism interesting – and very important for understanding human health and disease. Nevertheless, many of the principal regulatory mechanisms to be discussed are common to other mammals. Some mammals, such as ruminants, have rather specialised patterns of digestion and absorption of energy; such aspects will not be covered in this book.

A consideration of metabolic regulation might begin with the question: why is it necessary? An analogy here is with mechanical devices, which require an input of energy, and convert this energy to a different and more useful form. The waterwheel is a simple example. This device takes the potential energy of water in a reservoir – the mill-pond – and converts it into mechanical energy which can be used for turning machinery, for instance, to grind corn. As long as the water flows, its energy is extracted, and useful work is done. If the water stops, the wheel stops. A motor vehicle has a different pattern of energy intake and energy output (Fig. 1.1). Energy is taken in very spasmodically – only when the driver stops at a filling station. Energy is converted into useful work (ac-

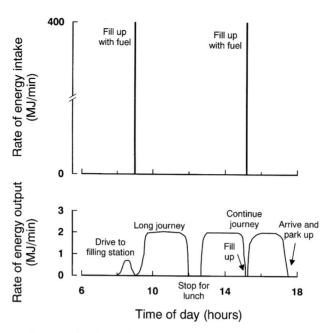

Fig. 1.1 Rates of energy intake and output for a motor vehicle. The rate of intake (top panel) is zero except for periods in a filling station, when it is suddenly very high. (Notice that the scales are different for intake and output.) The rate of output is zero whilst the car is parked with the engine off; it increases as the car is driven to the filling station, and is relatively high during a journey. When totalled up over a long period, the areas under the two curves must be equal (energy intake = energy output) – except for any difference in the amounts of fuel in the tank before and after.

celeration and motion) with an entirely different pattern. A long journey might be undertaken without any energy intake. Clearly, the difference from the waterwheel lies in the presence of a storage device – the fuel tank. But the fuel tank alone is not sufficient: there must also be a control mechanism to regulate the flow of energy from the store to the useful-work-producing device (i.e. the engine). In this case, the regulator is in part a human brain deciding when to move, and in part a mechanical system controlling the flow of fuel.

What does this have to do with metabolism? The human body is also a device for taking in energy (chemical energy, in the form of food) and converting it to other forms. Most obviously, this is in the form of physical work, such as lifting heavy objects. However, it can also be in more subtle forms such as producing and nurturing offspring. Any activity requires energy. Again, this is most obvious if we think about performing mechanical work: lifting a heavy object from the floor onto a shelf requires conversion of chemical energy (ultimately derived from food) into potential energy of the object. But even maintaining life involves work: the work of breathing, of pumping blood around the vascular system, of chewing food and digesting it. At a cellular level, there is constant work performed in the pumping of ions across membranes, and the synthesis and breakdown of the chemical constituents of cells.

What is your pattern of energy intake in relation to energy output? For most of us, the majority of energy intake occurs in three relatively short periods during each 24 hours, whereas energy expenditure is largely continuous (the *resting metabolism*) with occasional extra bursts of external work (Fig. 1.2). It is clear that we, like the motor vehicle, must have some way of storing food energy and releasing it when required. As with the motor vehicle, the human brain may also be at the beginning of the regulatory mechanism, although it is not the conscious part of the brain: we do not have to think when we need to release some energy from our fat stores, for instance. Some of the important regulatory systems which will be covered in this book lie outside the brain, in organs which secrete hormones, particularly the pancreas. But whatever the internal means for achieving this regulation, we manage to store our excess food energy and to release it just as we need.

This applies to the normal 24-hour period in which we eat meals and go about our daily life. But the body also has to cope with less well-organised situ-

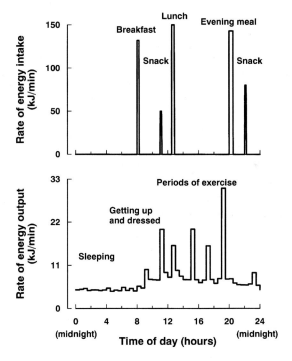

Fig. 1.2 Rates of energy intake and output for a person during a typical day. The rate of energy intake (top panel) is zero except when eating or drinking, when it may be very high. The rate of energy output (heat + physical work) (lower panel) is at its lowest during sleep; it increases on waking and even more during physical activity. As with the car, the pattern of energy intake may not resemble that of energy expenditure, but over a long period the areas under the curves will balance – except for any difference in the amounts of energy stored (mainly as body fat) before and after. Data for energy expenditure are for a person measured in a calorimetry chamber and were kindly supplied by Dr Susan Jebb of MRC Human Nutrition Research, Cambridge.

ations. In many parts of the world, there are times when food is not that easily available, and yet people are able to continue relatively normal lives. Clearly, the body's regulatory mechanisms must recognise that food is not coming in, and allow an appropriate rate of release of energy from the internal stores. In other situations, the need for energy may be suddenly increased. Strenuous physical exercise may increase the total rate of metabolism in the body to twenty times its resting level. Something must recognise the fact that there is a sudden need to release energy at a high rate from the body's stores. During severe illness, such as infections, the rate of metabolism may also be increased; this is manifested in part by the rise in body temperature. Often the sufferer will not feel like eating normally. Once again, the body must have a way of recognising the situation, and regulating the necessary release of stored energy.

What we are now discussing is, indeed, *metabolic regulation*. Metabolic regulation in human terms covers the means by which we take in nutrients in discrete meals, and deliver energy as required, varying from moment to moment and from tissue to tissue, in a pattern which may have no relationship at all to the pattern of intake. Metabolic regulation works ultimately at a molecular level, mainly by modulation of the activities of enzymes. But one should not lose sight of the fact that these molecular mechanisms are there to enable us to lead normal lives despite fluctuations in our intake and our expenditure of energy. In this book, the emphasis will be on the systems within the human body which sense the balance of energy coming in and energy required, particularly the *endocrine* (hormonal) and the *nervous* systems, and which regulate the distribution and storage of nutrients after meals, and their release from stores and delivery to individual tissues as required.

The intention of this preamble is to illustrate that, underlying our everyday lives, there are precise and beautifully coordinated regulatory systems controlling the flow of energy within our bodies. Metabolic regulation is not a dry, academic subject thought up just to make biochemistry examinations difficult; it is at the centre of human life and affects each one of us every moment of our daily lives.

1.2   The chemistry of food – and of bodies

Energy is taken into the body in the form of food. The components of food may be classified as *macronutrients* and *micronutrients*. Macronutrients are those components present in a typical serving in amounts of grams rather than milligrams or less. They are the well-known carbohydrate, fat and protein. Water is another important component of many foods although it is not usually considered a nutrient. Micronutrients are vitamins, minerals and nucleic acids. Although these micronutrients play vital roles in the metabolism of the macronutrients, they will not be discussed in any detail in this book, which is concerned with the broader aspects of what is often called *energy metabolism*.

The links between nutrition and energy metabolism are very close. We eat carbohydrates, fats and proteins. Within the body these are broken down to smaller components, rearranged, stored, released from stores and further metabolised, but essentially whether we are discussing food or metabolism the same categories of carbohydrate, fat and protein can be distinguished. This is not surprising since our food itself is of organic origin, whether plant or animal.

In order to understand metabolism and metabolic regulation, it is useful to have a clear idea of some of the major chemical properties of these components. This is not intended as a treatise in physical or organic chemistry but as a starting point for understanding some of the underlying principles of metabolism. The discussion assumes a basic understanding of the meaning of atoms and molecules, of chemical reactions and catalysis, and some understanding of chemical bonds (particularly the distinction between ionic and covalent bonding).

1.2.1   Some important chemical concepts

1.2.1.1   Polarity

Some aspects of metabolism are more easily understood through an appreciation of the nature of polarity of molecules. *Polarity* refers to the distribution of electrical charge over the molecule. A non-polar molecule has a very even distribution of electrical charge over its surface and is electrically neutral overall (the negative charge on the electrons is balanced by the positive charge of the nucleus). A polar molecule has an overall charge, or at least an uneven distribution of charge. The most polar small particles are ions – i.e. atoms or molecules which have entirely lost or gained one or more electrons. However, even completely covalently bonded organic molecules may have a sufficiently uneven distribution of electrical charge to affect their behaviour. Polarity is not an all-or-none phenomenon; there are gradations, from the polar to the completely non-polar.

Polarity is not difficult to predict in the molecules which are important in biochemistry. We will contrast two simple molecules: water and methane. Their relative molecular masses are similar – 18 for water, 16 for methane – yet their physical properties are very different. Water is a liquid at room temperature, not boiling until 100°C, whereas methane is a gas ('natural gas') which only liquifies when cooled to – 161°C. We might imagine that similar molecules of similar size would have the same tendency to move from the liquid to the gas phase, and that they would have similar boiling points. The reason for their different behaviours lies in their relative polarity. The molecule of methane has the three-dimensional structure shown in Fig. 1.3(a). The outer electron 'cloud' has a very even distribution over the four hydrogen atoms, all of which have an equal tendency to pull electrons their way. The molecule has no distinct electrical poles – it is non-polar. Because of this very even distribution of electrons, molecules near each other have little tendency to interact. In contrast, in the

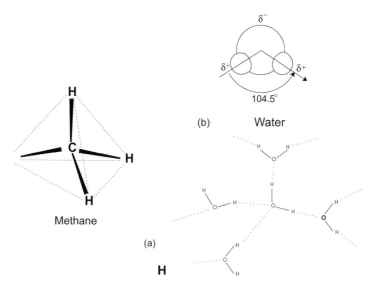

Fig. 1.3 (a) Three-dimensional structure of the methane molecule and (b) the molecular structure of water. (a) The hydrogen atoms of methane (CH_4) are arranged symmetrically in space, at the corners of a tetrahedron. (b) The molecular structure of water. Top: view of the 'electron cloud' surrounding the molecule; bottom, interactions between water molecules. The molecule has a degree of *polarity*, and this leads to electrical interactions between neighbouring molecules by the formation of *hydrogen bonds*. These bonds are not strong compared with covalent bonds, and are constantly being formed and broken. Nevertheless, they provide sufficient attraction between the molecules to account for the fact that water is a liquid at room temperature whereas the non-polar methane is a gas.

water molecule (Fig. 1.3(b)) the oxygen atom has a distinct tendency to pull electrons its way, shifting the distribution of the outer electron cloud so that it is more dense over the oxygen atom, and correspondingly less dense elsewhere. Therefore the molecule has a rather negatively charged region around the central oxygen atom, and correspondingly positively charged regions around the hydrogen atoms. Thus, it has distinct electrical poles – it is a relatively polar molecule. It is easy to imagine that water molecules near to each other will interact. Like electrical charges repel each other, unlike charges attract. This gives water molecules a tendency to line up so that the positive regions of one attract the negative region of an adjacent molecule (Fig. 1.3(b)). So water molecules, unlike those of methane, tend to 'stick together': the energy needed to break them apart and form a gas is much greater than for methane, and hence water is a liquid whilst methane is a gas. The latent heat of evaporation of water is 2.5 kJ/g, whereas that of methane is 0.6 kJ/g. Note that the polarity of the water molecule is not as extreme as that of an ion – it is merely a rather uneven distribution of electrons, but enough to affect its properties considerably.

The contrast between water and methane may be extended to larger molecules. Organic compounds composed solely of carbon and hydrogen – for instance, the alkanes or 'paraffins' – all have the property of extreme non-polarity: the chemical (covalent) bond between carbon and hydrogen atoms leads to a very even distribution of electrons, and the molecules have little interaction with each other. A result is that polar molecules such as those of water, and non-polar molecules such as those of alkanes, do not mix well: the water molecules tend to bond to each other and to exclude the non-polar molecules, which can themselves pack together very closely because of the lack of interaction between them. In fact, there is an additional form of direct attraction between non-polar molecules, the *van der Waals* forces. Random fluctuations in the density of the electron cloud surrounding a molecule lead to minor, transient degrees of polarity; these induce an opposite change in a neighbouring molecule, with the result that there is a transient attraction between them. These are very weak attractions, however, and the effect of the exclusion by water is considerably stronger. The non-polar molecules are said to be *hydrophobic* (water-fearing or water-hating).

A strong contrast is provided by an inorganic ionic compound such as sodium chloride. The sodium and chlorine atoms in sodium chloride are completely ionised under almost all conditions. They pack very regularly in crystals in a cubic form. The strength of their attraction for each other means that considerable energy is needed to disrupt this regular packing – sodium chloride does not melt until heated above 800°C. And yet it dissolves very readily in water – that is, the individual ions become separated from their close packing arrangement rather as they would on melting. Why? Because the water molecules, by virtue of their polarity, are able to come between the ions and reduce their attraction for each other. In fact, each of the charged sodium and chloride ions will become surrounded by a 'shell' of water molecules, shielding it from the attraction or repulsion of other ions. Sodium chloride is said to be *hydrophilic* – water loving. The terms *polar* and *hydrophilic* are for the most part interchangeable. Similarly, the terms *non-polar* and *hydrophobic* are virtually synonymous.

Ionic compounds, the extreme examples of polarity, are not confined to inorganic chemistry. Organic molecules may include ionised groups. These may be almost entirely ionised under normal conditions – for instance, the esters of orthophosphoric acid ('phosphate groups') as in the compounds AMP, ADP and ATP, in metabolites such as glucose 6-phosphate, and in phospholipids. Most of the organic acids involved in intermediary metabolism, such as lactic acid, pyruvic acid and the long-chain carboxylic acids (fatty acids), are also largely ionised at physiological hydrogen ion concentrations (Box 1.1). Thus, generation of lactic acid during exercise raises the hydrogen ion concentration (the acidity) both within the cells where it is produced, and generally within the body, since it is released into the bloodstream.

As stated earlier, polarity is not difficult to predict in organic molecules. It relies upon the fact that certain atoms always have *electronegative* (electron-withdrawing) properties in comparison with hydrogen. The most important of these atoms biochemically are those of oxygen, phosphorus and nitrogen. Therefore, certain functional groups based around these atoms have polar properties. These include the hydroxyl group (-OH), the amino group ($-NH_2$),

Box 1.1   Ionisation state of some acids at normal hydrogen ion concentrations

The normal pH in blood plasma is around 7.4. (It may be somewhat lower within cells, down to about 6.8.) This corresponds to a hydrogen ion concentration of 3.98×10^{-8} mol/l (since $- \log_{10}$ of 3.98×10^{-8} is 7.4).

The equation for ionisation of an acid HA is:

$$HA \Leftrightarrow H^+ + A^-;$$

this equilibrium is described by the equation:

$$\frac{[H^+][A^-]}{[HA]} = K_i$$

where K_i is the dissociation or ionisation constant, and is a measure of the strength of the acid: the higher the value of K_i the stronger (i.e. the more dissociated) the acid.

K_i in the equation above relates the concentrations expressed in molar terms (e.g. mol/l). (Strictly, it is not the concentrations but the 'effective ion concentrations' or ion *activities* which are related; these are not quite the same as concentrations because of inter-ion attractions. In most biological systems, however, in which the concentrations are relatively low, it is a close approximation to use concentrations. If activities are used, then the symbol K_a is used for the dissociation constant of an acid.)

Some biological acids and their K_a values are listed below, together with a calculation of the proportion ionised at typical pH (7.4).

The calculation is done as follows (using acetic acid as an example).

$$K_a = 1.75 \times 10^{-5} = \frac{[H^+][Ac^-]}{[HAc]}$$

(where HAc represents undissociated acetic acid, Ac$^-$ represents the acetate ion).

At pH 7.4, $[H^+] = 3.98 \times 10^{-8}$ mol/l. Therefore,

$$\frac{[Ac^-]}{[HAc]} = \frac{1.75 \times 10^{-5}}{3.98 \times 10^{-8}} = 440$$

(i.e. the ratio of ionised to undissociated acid is 440 : 1; it is almost entirely ionised).

The percentage in the ionised form $= \frac{440 \times 100\%}{441} = 99.8\%$.

☞

Table 1.1.1

Acid	K_a	% ionised at pH 7.4
Acetic, CH_3COOH	1.75×10^{-5}	99.8
Lactic, $CH_3CHOHCOOH$	0.38×10^{-4}	99.9
Palmitic acid, $CH_3(CH_2)_{14}COOH$	1.58×10^{-5}	99.8
Glycine, CH_2NH_2COOH (carboxyl group)	3.98×10^{-3}	100

and the orthophosphate group ($-OPO_3^{2-}$). Compounds containing these groups will have polar properties, whereas those containing just carbon and hydrogen will have much less polarity. The presence of an electronegative atom does not always give polarity to a molecule – if it is part of a chain and balanced by a similar atom this property may be lost. For instance, the ester link in a triacylglycerol molecule (discussed below) contains two oxygen atoms but has no polar properties.

Examples of relatively polar (and thus water-soluble) compounds which will be frequent in this book are sugars (with many -OH groups), organic acids such as lactic acid (with a COO^- group) and most other small metabolites. Most amino acids also fall into this category (with their amino and carboxyl groups), although some fall into the *amphipathic* ('mixed') category discussed below.

Another important point about polarity in organic molecules is that within one molecule there may be both polar and non-polar regions. They are called amphipathic compounds. This category includes phospholipids and long-chain fatty acids (Fig. 1.4). Cell membranes are made up of a double layer of phospholipids, interspersed with specific proteins such as transporter molecules, ion channels and hormone receptors, and molecules of the sterol, cholesterol (Fig. 1.5). The phospholipid bilayer presents its polar faces – the polar 'heads' of the phospholipid molecules – to the aqueous external environment and to the aqueous internal environment; within the thickness of the membrane is a non-polar, hydrophobic region. The physico-chemical nature of such a membrane means that, in general, molecules cannot diffuse freely across it: non-polar molecules would not cross the outer, polar face and polar molecules would not cross the inner, hydrophobic region. Means by which molecules move through membranes are discussed in Chapter 2 (Box 2.1).

The long-chain fatty acids fall into the amphipathic category – they have a long, non-polar hydrocarbon tail but a more polar carboxylic group head ($-COO^-$). Another compound with mixed properties is cholesterol (Fig. 1.6); its ring system is very non-polar, but its hydroxyl group gives it some polar properties. However, the long-chain fatty acids and cholesterol may lose their polar aspects completely when they join in ester links. An ester is a compound formed by the condensation (elimination of a molecule of water) of an alcohol (-OH) and an acid (e.g. a carboxylic acid, $-COO^-$). Cholesterol (through

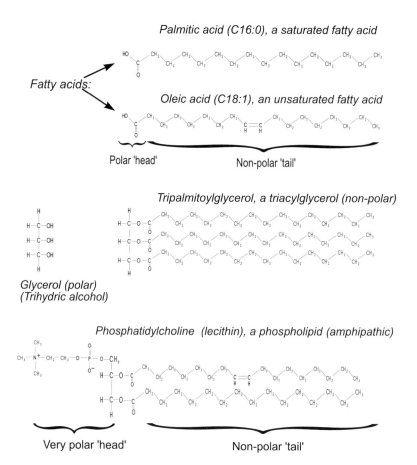

Fig. 1.4 Chemical structures of some lipids. A typical saturated fatty acid (palmitic acid) is shown with its polar carboxylic group and non-polar hydrocarbon tail. *Glycerol* is a hydrophilic alcohol. However, it is a component of many lipids as its hydroxyl groups may form ester links with up to three fatty acids, as shown. The resultant *triacylglycerol* has almost no polar qualities. The *phospholipids* are derived from phosphatidic acid (diacylglycerol phosphate) with an additional polar group, usually a nitrogen-containing base such as choline (as shown) or a poly-alcohol derivative such as phosphoinositol. Phospholipids commonly have long-chain unsaturated fatty acids on the 2-position; oleic acid (18:1n-9) is shown.

its -OH group) may become esterified to a long-chain fatty acid, forming a *cholesteryl ester* (e.g. cholesteryl oleate, see Fig. 1.6). The cholesteryl esters are extremely non-polar compounds. This fact will be important when we consider the metabolism of cholesterol in Chapter 9. The long-chain fatty acids may also become esterified with glycerol, forming triacylglycerols (Fig. 1.4). Again, the polar properties of both partners are lost, and a very non-polar molecule is formed. This fact underlies one of the most fundamental aspects of mammalian metabolism – the use of triacylglycerol as the major form for storage of excess energy.

Amongst amino acids, the branched-chain amino acids, leucine, isoleucine and valine, have non-polar side-chains and are thus amphipathic. The aromatic

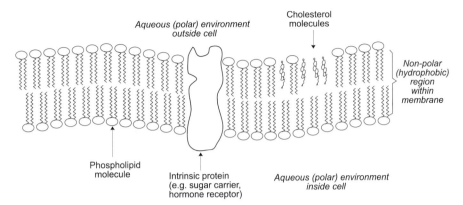

Fig. 1.5 Structure of biological membranes in mammalian cells. Cell membranes and intracellular membranes such as the endoplasmic reticulum are composed of bilayers of phospholipid molecules with their polar head-groups facing the aqueous environment on either side and their non-polar 'tails' facing inwards, forming a hydrophobic centre to the membrane. The membrane also contains *intrinsic proteins* such as hormone receptors, ion channels and sugar transporters, and molecules of cholesterol, in domains known as 'rafts', which stabilise the membrane and regulate its fluidity.

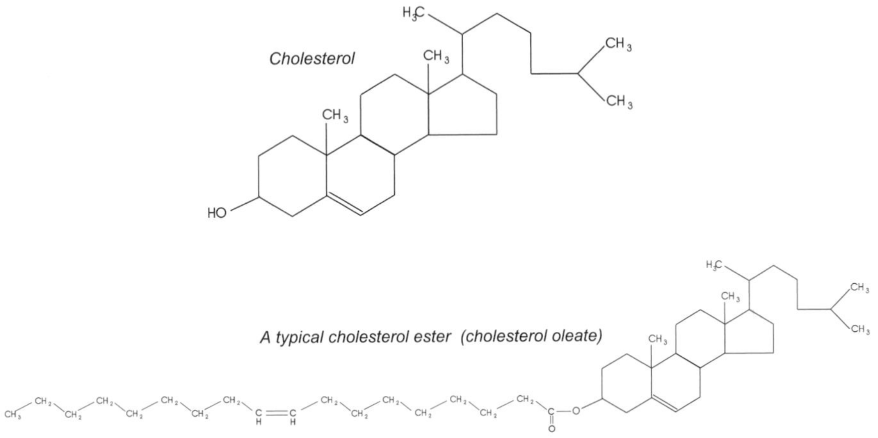

Fig. 1.6 Cholesterol and a typical cholesteryl ester (cholesteryl oleate). In the structure of cholesterol, not all atoms are shown (for simplicity); each 'corner' represents a carbon atom, or else -CH or -CH$_2$. Cholesterol itself has amphipathic properties because of its hydroxyl group, but when esterified to a long-chain fatty acid the molecule is very non-polar.

amino acids phenylalanine and tyrosine are relatively hydrophobic, and the amino acid tryptophan is so non-polar that it is not carried free in solution in the plasma.

The concept of the polarity or non-polarity of molecules thus has a number of direct consequences for the aspects of metabolism to be considered in later chapters. Some of these consequences are the following.

(1) Lipid fuels – fatty acids and triacylglycerols – are largely hydrophobic and are not soluble in the blood plasma. There are specific routes for their absorption from the intestine and specific mechanisms by which they are transported in blood.
(2) Carbohydrates are hydrophilic. When carbohydrate is stored in cells it is stored in a hydrated form, in association with water. In contrast, fat is stored as a lipid droplet from which water is excluded. Mainly because of this lack of water, fat stores contain considerably more energy per unit weight of store than do carbohydrate stores.
(3) The entry of fats into the circulation must be coordinated with the availability of the specific carrier mechanisms. In the rare situations in which it arises, uncomplexed fat in the bloodstream may have very adverse consequences.

1.2.1.2 Osmosis

The phenomenon of *osmosis* underlies some aspects of metabolic strategy – it can be seen as one reason why certain aspects of metabolism and metabolic regulation have evolved in the way that they have. It is outlined only briefly here to highlight its relevance.

Osmosis is the way in which solutions of different concentrations tend to even out when they are in contact with one another via a *semipermeable membrane*. In solutions, the *solvent* is the substance in which things dissolve (e.g. water) and the *solute* the substance which dissolves. A semipermeable membrane allows molecules of solvent to pass through, but not those of solute. Thus, it may allow molecules of water but not those of sugar to pass through. Cell membranes have specific protein channels ('pores') to allow water molecules to pass through, and they are close approximations to semipermeable membranes.

If solutions of unequal concentration – for instance, a dilute and a concentrated solution of sugar – are separated by a semipermeable membrane, then molecules of solvent (in this case, water) will tend to pass through the membrane until the concentrations of the solutions have become equal. In order to understand this intuitively, it is necessary to remember that the particles (molecules or ions) of solute are not just moving about freely in the solvent: each is surrounded by molecules of solvent, attracted by virtue of the polarity of the solute particles. (In the case of a non-polar solute in a non-polar solvent, we would have to say that the attraction is by virtue of the non-polarity; it occurs through weaker forces such as the van der Waals.) In the more concentrated solution, the proportion of solvent molecules engaged in such attachment to the solute particles is larger, and there is a net attraction for further solvent molecules to join them, in comparison with the more dilute solution. Solvent molecules will tend to move from one solution to the other until the proportion involved in such interactions with the solute particles is equal.

The consequence of this in real situations is not usually simply the dilution of a more concentrated solution, and the concentration of a more dilute one, until their concentrations are equal. Usually there are physical constraints. This is simply seen if we imagine a single cell, which has accumulated within it, for instance, amino acid molecules taken up from the outside fluid by a transport mechanism which has made them more concentrated inside than outside. Water will then tend to move into the cell to even out this concentration difference. If water moves into the cell, the cell will increase in volume. Cells can swell so much that they burst under some conditions (usually not encountered in the body, fortunately). For instance, red blood cells placed in water will burst (*lyse*) from just this effect: the relatively concentrated mixture of dissolved organic molecules within the cell will attract water from outside the cell, increasing the volume of the cell until its membrane can stretch no further and ruptures.

In the laboratory, we can avoid this by handling cells in solutions which contain solute – usually sodium chloride – at a total concentration of solute particles which matches that found within cells. This total concentration of particles is usually measured in mmol per kg of water, and is referred to as the *osmolality*. Solutions which match this osmolality are referred to as *isotonic*; a common laboratory example is *isotonic saline* containing 9 g of NaCl per litre of water, with a molar concentration of 154 mmol/l. Since this will be fully ionised into Na^+ and Cl^- ions, its particle concentration is 308 'milliparticles' – sometimes called milliosmoles – per litre. We refer to this as an osmolarity of 308 mmol/l, but it is not 308 mmol NaCl per litre. (Sometimes you may see the term *osmolality*, which is similar to osmolarity, but measured in mmol per kg solvent.)

The phenomenon of osmosis has a number of repercussions in metabolism. Most cells have a number of different 'pumps' or active transporters in their cell membranes which can be used to regulate intracellular osmolarity, and hence cell size. This process requires energy and is one of the components of basal energy expenditure. It may also be important in metabolic regulation; there is increasing evidence that changes in cell volume are part of a signalling mechanism which brings about changes in the activity of intracellular metabolic pathways. The osmolarity of the plasma is maintained within narrow limits by specific mechanisms within the kidney, regulating the loss of water from the body via changes in the concentration of urine. Most importantly, potential problems posed by osmosis can be seen to underlie the metabolic strategy of fuel storage, as will become apparent in later sections.

1.2.2   The chemical characteristics of macronutrients

1.2.2.1   Carbohydrates

Simple carbohydrates have the empirical formula $C_n(H_2O)_n$; complex carbohydrates have an empirical formula which is similar to this (e.g. $C_n(H_2O)_{0.8n}$). The name carbohydrate reflects the idea, based on this empirical formula, that these compounds are hydrates of carbon. It is not strictly correct, but illustrates an important point about this group of compounds – the relative abundance of hydrogen and oxygen, in proportions similar to those in water, in their molecules. From the discussion above, it will be apparent that carbohydrates are mostly relatively polar molecules, miscible with, or soluble in, water. Carbohydrates in nature include the plant products starch and cellulose and the mammalian storage carbohydrate glycogen, as well as various simple sugars, of which glucose is the most important from the point of view of human metabolism. The main source of carbohydrate we eat is the starch in vegetables such as potatoes, rice and grains.

The chemical definition of a sugar is that its molecules consist of carbon atoms, each bearing one hydroxyl group (-OH), except that one carbon bears a carbonyl group (=O) rather than a hydroxyl. In solution, the molecule exists in equilibrium between a 'straight chain' form and a ring structure, but as the ring structure predominates sugars are usually shown in this form (Fig. 1.7). Nev-

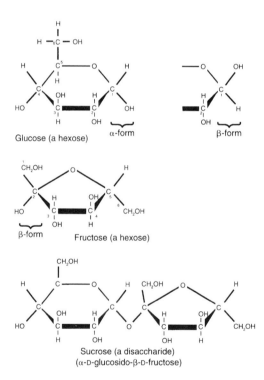

Fig. 1.7 Some simple sugars and disaccharides. Glucose and fructose are shown in their 'ring' form. Even this representation ignores the true three-dimensional structure, which is 'chair'-shaped: if the middle part of the glucose ring is imagined flat, the left-hand end slopes down and the right-hand end up. Glucose forms a six-membered ring and is described as a pyranose; fructose forms a five-membered ring and is described as a furanose. In solution the α- and β- forms are in equilibrium with each other and with a smaller amount of the straight-chain form. The orientation of the oxygen on carbon atom 1 becomes fixed when glucose forms links via this carbon to another sugar, as in sucrose; α- and β-links then have quite different properties (e.g. cellulose vs starch or glycogen).

ertheless, some of the chemical properties of sugars can only be understood by remembering that the straight chain form exists. The basic carbohydrate unit is known as a monosaccharide. Monosaccharides may have different numbers of carbon atoms, and the terminology reflects this: thus, a hexose has six carbon atoms in its molecule, a pentose five, etc. Pentoses and hexoses are the most important in terms of mammalian metabolism. These sugars also have 'common names' which often reflect their natural occurrence. The most abundant in our diet and in our bodies are the hexoses *glucose* (grape sugar, named from the Greek *glykys* sweet), *fructose* (fruit sugar, from the Latin *fructus* for fruit) and *galactose* (derived from lactose, milk sugar; from the Greek *galaktos*, milk), and the pentose *ribose*, a constituent of nucleic acids (the name comes from the related sugar arabinose, named from *Gum arabic*).

Complex carbohydrates are built up from the monosaccharides by covalent links between sugar molecules. The term *disaccharide* is used for a molecule composed of two monosaccharides (which may or may not be the same), *oligosaccharide* for a short chain of sugar units, and *polysaccharide* for longer chains (> 10 units), as found in starch and glycogen. Disaccharides are abundant in the diet, and again their common names often denote their origin: *sucrose* (table sugar, named from the French, *sucre*) which contains glucose and fructose (Fig. 1.7); *maltose* (two glucose molecules) from malt; *lactose* (galactose and glucose) from milk. The bonds between individual sugar units are relatively strong at normal hydrogen ion concentrations, and sucrose (for instance) does not break down when it is boiled, although it is steadily broken down in acidic solutions such as cola drinks; but there are specific enzymes in the intestine (described in Chapter 3) which hydrolyse these bonds to liberate the individual monosaccharides.

Polysaccharides differ from one another in a number of respects: their chain length, and the nature (α- or β-) and position (e.g. ring carbons 1–4, 1–6) of the links between individual sugar units. Cellulose consists mostly of β-1,4 linked glucosyl units; these links give the compound a close-packed structure which is not attacked by mammalian enzymes. In humans, therefore, cellulose largely passes intact through the small intestine where other carbohydrates are digested and absorbed. It is broken down by some bacterial enzymes. Ruminants have complex alimentary tracts in which large quantities of bacteria reside, enabling the host to obtain energy from cellulose, the main constituent of its diet of grass. In humans there is some bacterial digestion in the large intestine (see Chapter 3). Starch and the small amount of glycogen in the diet are readily digested (Chapter 3).

The structure of glycogen is illustrated in Fig. 1.8. It is a branched polysaccharide. Most of the links between sugar units are of the α-1,4 variety but after every 9–10 residues there is an α-1,6 link, creating a branch. Branching makes the molecules more soluble, and also creates more 'ends' where the enzymes of glycogen synthesis and breakdown operate. Glycogen is stored within cells, not simply free in solution but in organised structures which may be seen as gran-

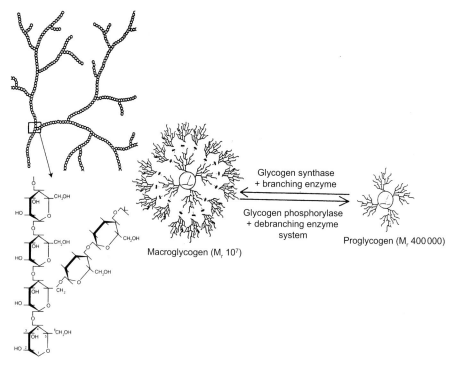

Fig. 1.8 Structure of glycogen. Left-hand side: each circle in the upper diagram represents a glucosyl residue. Most of the links are of the α-1,4 variety. One of the branch points, an α-1,6 link, is enlarged below. Amylopectin, a component of starch, has a similar structure. Amylose, the other component of starch, has a linear α-1,4 structure. Right-hand side: glycogen is built upon a protein backbone, glycogenin. The first layer of glycogen chains forms proglycogen, which is enlarged by addition of further glucosyl residues (by glycogen synthase and a specific branching enzyme, that creates the α-1,6 branch-points), to form macroglycogen. When glycogen is referred to in this book, it is the macroglycogen form that is involved. Pictures of proglycogen and macroglycogen taken from Alonso, M.D., Lomako, J., Lomako, W.M. & Whelan, W.J. (1995) A new look at the biogenesis of glycogen *FASEB J* 9; 1126–1137. With permission of the publisher.

ules on electron microscopy. Each glycogen molecule is synthesised on a protein backbone, or primer, glycogenin. Carbohydrate chains branch out from glycogenin to give a relatively compact molecule called proglycogen. The glycogen molecules that participate in normal cellular metabolism are considerably bigger (see Fig. 1.8), typically with molecular weights of several million. The enzymes of glycogen metabolism are intimately linked with the glycogen granules.

The carbohydrates share the property of relatively high polarity. Cellulose is not strictly water-soluble because of the tight packing between its chains, but even cellulose can be made to mix with water (as in paper pulp or wallpaper paste). The polysaccharides tend to make 'pasty' mixtures with water whereas the small oligo-, di- and monosaccharides are completely soluble. These characteristics have important consequences for the metabolism of carbohydrates, some of which are as follows.

(1) Glucose and other monosaccharides circulate freely in the blood and interstitial fluid, but their entry into cells is facilitated by specific carrier proteins.

(2) Perhaps because of the need for a specific transporter for glucose to cross cell membranes (thus making its entry into cells susceptible to regulation), glucose is an important fuel for many tissues, and an obligatory fuel for some. Carbohydrate cannot be synthesised from the more abundant store of fat within the body. The body must therefore maintain a store of carbohydrate.

(3) Because of the water-soluble nature of sugars, this store will be liable to osmotic influences: it cannot therefore be in the form of simple sugars or even oligosaccharides, because of the osmotic problem this would cause to the cells. This is overcome by the synthesis of the macromolecule glycogen, so that the osmotic effect is reduced by a factor of many thousand compared with monosaccharides. The synthesis of such a polymer from glucose, and its breakdown, are brought about by enzyme systems which are themselves regulated, thus giving the opportunity for precise control of the availability of glucose.

(4) Glycogen in an aqueous environment (as in cells) is highly hydrated; in fact, it is always associated with about three times its own weight of water. Thus, storage of energy in the form of glycogen carries a large weight penalty (discussed further in Chapter 8).

1.2.2.2 Fats

Just as there are many different sugars and carbohydrates built from them, so there are a variety of types of fat. The term *fat* comes from Anglo-Saxon and is related to the filling of a container or vat. The term *lipid*, from Greek, is more useful in chemical discussions since 'fat' can have so many shades of meaning. Lipid materials are those substances which can be extracted from tissues in organic solvents such as petroleum or chloroform. This immediately distinguishes them from the largely water-soluble carbohydrates.

Amongst lipids there are a number of groups (Fig. 1.4). The most prevalent, in terms of amount, are the *triacylglycerols* or *triglycerides*, referred to in older literature as '*neutral fat*' since they have no acidic or basic properties. These compounds consist of three individual fatty acids, each linked by an ester bond to a molecule of glycerol. As discussed above, the triacylglycerols are very non-polar, hydrophobic compounds. The *phospholipids* are another important group of lipids – constituents of membranes and also of the lipoprotein particles which will be discussed in Chapter 9. *Steroids* – compounds with the same nucleus as cholesterol (see Fig. 1.6) – form yet another important group and will be considered in later chapters, steroid hormones in Chapter 5 and cholesterol metabolism in Chapter 9.

Fatty acids are the building blocks of lipids, analogous to the monosaccharides. The fatty acids important in metabolism are mostly unbranched, long-chain (12 carbon atoms or more) carboxylic acids with an even number of carbon atoms. They may contain no double bonds, in which case they are referred to as *saturated fatty acids*, one double bond (*mono-unsaturated fatty acids*), or several double bonds – the *polyunsaturated fatty acids*. Many individual fatty acids are named, like monosaccharides, according to the source from which they were first isolated. Thus, *lauric acid* (C12, saturated) comes from the laurel tree, *myristic acid* (C14, saturated) from the *Myristica* or nutmeg genus, *palmitic acid* (C16, saturated) from palm oil, and *stearic acid* (C18, saturated) from suet (Greek *steatos*). *Oleic acid* (C18, mono-unsaturated) comes from the olive (from Latin: *olea*, olive, or *oleum*, oil). *Linoleic acid*, C18 with two double bonds, is a polyunsaturated acid common in certain vegetable oils; it is obtained from linseed (from the Latin *linum* for flax and *oleum* for oil).

The fatty acids mostly found in the diet have some common characteristics. They are composed of even numbers of carbon atoms, and the most abundant have 16 or 18 carbon atoms. There are three major series or families of fatty acids, grouped according to the distribution of their double bonds (Box 1.2).

Differences in the metabolism of the different fatty acids are not very important from the point of view of their roles as fuels for energy metabolism. When considering the release, transport and uptake of fatty acids the term *non-esterified fatty acids* will therefore be used without reference to particular molecular species. In a later section (Box 9.5) some differences in their effects on the serum cholesterol concentration and propensity to heart disease will be discussed.

It will be seen from Figs 1.4 and 1.9 that saturated fatty acids, such as palmitic (16:0), have a natural tendency to fit together in nice orderly arrays. The unsaturated fatty acids, on the other hand, have less regular shapes (Fig. 1.9). This is reflected in the melting points of the corresponding triacylglycerols – saturated fats, such as beef suet with a high content of stearic acid, 18:0, are relatively solid at room temperature, whereas unsaturated fats such as olive oil are liquid. This feature may have an important role in metabolic regulation, although its exact significance is not yet clear. We know that cell membranes with a high content of unsaturated fatty acids in their phospholipids are more 'fluid' than those with more saturated fatty acids. This may make them better able to regulate metabolic processes – for instance, muscle cells with a higher content of unsaturated fatty acids in their membranes respond better to the hormone, insulin, probably because the response involves the movement of proteins (insulin receptors, glucose transporters) within the plane of the membrane (discussed in Box 2.4), and this occurs faster if the membrane is more fluid.

An important feature of the fatty acids is that, as their name implies, they have within one molecule both a hydrophobic tail and a polar carboxylic acid group. Long-chain fatty acids (12 carbons and more) are almost insoluble in water. They are carried in the plasma loosely bound to the plasma protein albumin. Nevertheless, they are more water-miscible than triacylglycerols, which are carried in plasma in the complex structures known as lipoproteins. The simpler transport of non-esterified fatty acids is perhaps why they serve within

---

Box 1.2   The structures and interrelationships of fatty acids

In the orthodox nomenclature, the position of double bonds is counted from the carboxyl end. Thus, α-linolenic acid (18 carbons, three double bonds) may be represented as cis-9,12,15-18:3, and its structure is:

$$CH_3 - CH_2 - CH = C^{15}H - CH_2 - CH = C^{12}H - CH_2 - CH$$
$$= C^9H - (CH_2)_7 - C^1OOH$$

(where the superscripts denote the numbering of carbon atoms from the carboxyl end). However, this is also known as an n-3 (or sometimes as an ω-3) fatty acid, since its first double bond counting from the non-carboxyl (ω) end is after the third carbon atom. On the latter basis, unsaturated fatty acids can be split into three main families, n-3, n-6 and n-9.

The saturated fatty acids can be synthesised within the body. In addition, many tissues possess the desaturase enzymes to form cis-6 or cis-9 double bonds, and to elongate the fatty acid chain (elongases) by addition of 2-carbon units at the carboxyl end. But these processes do not alter the position of the double bonds relative to the ω end, so fatty acids cannot be converted from one family to another: an n-3 fatty acid (for instance) remains an n-3 fatty acid. Oleic acid (cis-9-18:1, n-9 family) can be synthesised in the human body, but we cannot form n-6 or n-3 fatty acids. Since the body has a need for fatty acids of these families, they must be supplied in the diet (in small quantities). The parent members of these families, that need to be supplied in the diet, are linoleic acid for the n-6 family and α-linolenic acid for the n-3 family. These are known as essential fatty acids. They can be converted into other members of the same family although there seem to be health benefits of consumption of other members of the n-3 family, particularly 20:5 n-3 (eicosapentaenoic acid) and 22:6 n-3 (docosahexaenoic acid), found in high concentrations in fish oils. This is discussed further in Box 9.5. Some patients receiving all their nutrition intravenously have become deficient in essential fatty acids. The problem may be cured by rubbing sunflower oil into the skin!

Table 1.2.1

Family	Source	Typical member	Simplified structure
Saturated	Diet or synthesis	Myristic	14:0
		Palmitic	16:0
		Stearic	18:0
n-9	Diet or synthesis	Oleic	9-18:1
n-6	Diet	Linoleic	9,12-18:2
n-3	Diet	α-linolenic	9,12,15-18:3

Based on Gurr et al. (2002).

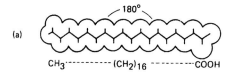

(a)

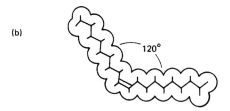

$CH_3\text{----------}(CH_2)_{16}\text{--------}COOH$

(b)

Fig. 1.9 Pictures of the molecular shapes of different fatty acids: (a) a saturated fatty acid, stearic acid (18:0), (b) a monounsaturated fatty acid, oleic acid (18:1n-9). From Gurr *et al.* (2002).

the body as the immediate carriers of lipid energy from the stores to the sites of utilisation and oxidation; they can be released very rapidly from stores when required and their delivery to tissues is regulated on a minute-to-minute basis.

But non-esterified fatty acids would not be a good form in which to store lipid fuels in any quantity. Their amphipathic nature means that they aggregate in micelles (small groups of molecules, formed with their tails together and their heads facing the aqueous environment); they would not easily aggregate in a very condensed form for storage. Triacylglycerols, on the other hand, do so readily; these hydrophobic molecules form uniform lipid droplets from which water is completely excluded, and which are an extremely efficient form in which to store energy (in terms of kJ stored per g weight). This is illustrated in Fig. 1.10. Thus, in brief, triacylglycerols are the form in which fat is mostly stored in the human body, and in the bodies of other organisms; hence they are the major form of fat in food. Non-esterified fatty acids, on the other hand, are the form in which lipid energy is transported in a highly regulated manner from storage depots to sites of utilisation and oxidation.

1.2.2.3 Proteins

Proteins are chains of amino acids linked through peptide bonds. Individual proteins are distinguished by the number and order of amino acids in the chain – the sequence, or primary structure. Within its normal environment, the chain of amino acids will assume a folded, three-dimensional shape, representing the secondary structure (local folding into α-helix and β-sheet) and tertiary structure (folding of the complete chain on itself). Two or more such folded peptide chains may then aggregate (quaternary structure) to form a complete enzyme or other functional protein.

In terms of energy metabolism, the first aspect we shall consider is not how this beautiful and complex arrangement is brought about; we shall consider how it is destroyed. Protein in food is usually *denatured* (its higher-order structures disrupted) by cooking or other treatment, and then within the intestinal tract the disrupted chains are broken down to short lengths of amino acids before absorption into the bloodstream. Within the bloodstream and within

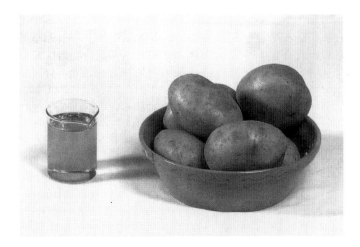

Fig. 1.10 The comparison of fat and carbohydrate as fuel sources. Raw potatoes (right) are hydrated to almost exactly the same extent as glycogen in mammalian cells. Olive oil (left) is similar to the fat stored in droplets in mature human adipocytes. The potatoes (1.05 kg) and olive oil (90 g) here each provide 3.3 MJ on oxidation. This emphasises the advantage of storing most of our energy in the body as triacylglycerol rather than as glycogen.

tissues we shall be concerned with the transport and distribution of individual amino acids. These are mostly sufficiently water-soluble to circulate freely in the aqueous environment of the plasma. Only tryptophan is sufficiently hydrophobic to require a transporter; it is bound loosely (like the non-esterified fatty acids) to albumin. Amino acids, not surprisingly, do not cross cell membranes by simple diffusion; there are specific transporters, carrying particular groups of amino acids (see Chapter 2, Table 2.3).

Protein is often considered as the structural material of the body, although it should not be thought of as the *only* structural material; it can only assume this function because of the complex arrangements of other cellular constituents, especially phospholipids forming cell membranes. Nevertheless, apart from water, protein is the largest single component in terms of mass of most tissues.[1] Within the body, the majority of protein is present in the skeletal muscles, mainly because of their sheer weight (around 40% of the body weight) but also because each muscle cell is well packed with the proteins (actin and myosin) which constitute the contractile apparatus. But it is important to remember that most proteins act in an aqueous environment and are therefore associated with water. This is relevant if we consider the body's protein reserves as a form of stored chemical energy. Since protein is associated with water, it suffers the same drawback as a form of energy storage as does glycogen; with every gram of protein are associated about 3 grams of water. It is not an energy-dense storage medium. Further, although protein undoubtedly represents a large source of energy that is drawn upon during starvation, it should be remembered that there is, in animals, no specific storage form of protein; all proteins have some function other than storage of energy. Thus, utilisation of protein as an energy source involves loss of the substance of the body. In evolutionary terms we might expect that this will be minimised (i.e. the use of the specific storage compounds glycogen and triacylglycerol will be favoured) and, as we shall see in later chapters, this is exactly the case.

1.3   Some physiological concepts

The emphasis of this book on the integration of metabolism in different tissues and organs is more closely related to physiology than to molecular biology. This short section is intended to fill in some physiological concepts for those from more biochemical backgrounds.

1.3.1   Circulation, capillaries, interstitial fluid

Blood is pumped around the body by the heart (Fig. 1.11). Strictly, it is pumped by the left ventricle, out into the *aorta* – the main artery – and its various

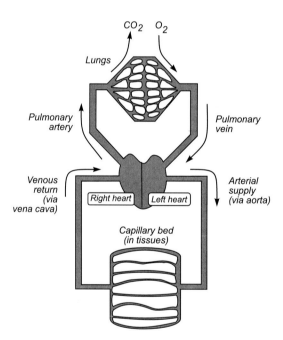

Fig. 1.11 The circulatory system. Oxygenated blood from the lungs returns in the pulmonary veins to the left heart, from where it is pumped through the aorta and its various branches (arteries) to the tissues and organs. It returns from the tissues and is pumped to the lungs for reoxygenation and expiration of CO_2. The key feature from the point of view of integration of metabolism is that blood returning from all tissues (and from endocrine glands) is mixed within the heart and lungs, and then redistributed to tissues. Thus, the bloodstream ('the circulation') acts as an efficient means for interchange of nutrients, metabolites and hormones between tissues.

branches, which supply blood to all tissues. Within tissues, the arterial vessels supplying blood divide into smaller and smaller vessels, and eventually into the *capillaries* – small vessels whose interior lumen is approximately 0.01 mm diameter, just large enough for red blood cells to pass through in single file.

The density of capillaries (numbers of capillaries per unit area when the tissue is examined in cross-section under the microscope) varies between different tissues, but in most tissues at least one capillary is in close proximity to each cell. The inner walls of the capillaries are lined with flat endothelial cells, but in most tissues there are gaps between the endothelial cells, and/or 'fenestrations' (passages) through the endothelial cells – not large enough to let red blood cells through, but large enough for proteins and other molecules such as metabolites and hormones to pass. Outside the capillaries, surrounding the cells of the tissue, is an aqueous medium known as the interstitial fluid. For the most part, it is believed that substances diffuse from cells through the interstitial fluid into the capillaries, and from the capillaries through the interstitial fluid to cells, following concentration gradients (Fig. 1.12). Thus oxygen, at its highest concentration in the blood supply at the arterial end of the capillary, will diffuse towards cells which are using it and thus depleting its local concentration in interstitial

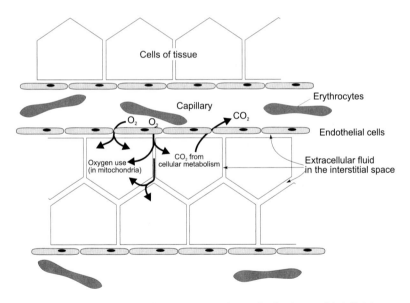

Fig. 1.12 Diffusion of chemical substances through the interstitial fluid. A typical tissue is shown (schematically) in cross-section. The diffusion of oxygen from erythrocytes to cells in the tissue is shown as an example. Oxygen diffuses down a concentration gradient, from the erythrocytes, via the plasma and the interstitial fluid, into the cells where its concentration is depleted as it is used in mitochondrial oxidation. CO_2 diffuses back to the plasma in the same way. The interstitial fluid occupies the space between cells known as the *extracellular space*; this is not a true empty space, but in reality is occupied by glycoproteins and other molecules joining the cells. Nevertheless, it offers a path for diffusion of substances.

fluid; carbon dioxide will diffuse from cells which are generating it, and thus creating a high local concentration, into the capillaries where the concentration is lower because it is continuously being removed by the flow of blood. There are some substances for which this cannot be entirely true, especially the non-esterified fatty acids; this will be discussed in more detail later.

There are different types of capillaries: those with abundant fenestrations in the endothelial cells occur in tissues where there are high rates of exchange with the cells, for instance the mucosa (absorptive lining) of the small intestine, where substances are absorbed, and in endocrine tissues where there is rapid secretion of hormones. In the brain the endothelial cells are tightly joined to one another, and this is believed to be the structural basis of the 'blood–brain barrier'; a number of substances, including non-esterified fatty acids and many drugs, are thus denied access to the cells of the brain.

The capillaries in turn lead to larger and larger vessels, merging to form the major veins, through which blood returns to the heart. The returning blood enters the right ventricle, from where it is pumped through the lungs, collecting O_2 and losing CO_2; it then returns to the left heart and starts its journey anew.

The bloodstream is the major means of carrying substances from one tissue to another – for instance, it carries non-esterified fatty acids liberated from adipose tissue to other tissues where they will be oxidised, and it carries hormones from endocrine organs to their target tissues. The term *the circulation* is often used to mean 'the bloodstream'; we speak of a substance being carried in the circulation, or even of *circulating glucose* (for instance), meaning glucose in the bloodstream. In the metabolic diagrams used extensively later in this book, the clear area in which different organs and tissues sit is meant to represent the bloodstream, and it may be assumed that substances will be efficiently carried across these blank spaces from one tissue to another.

1.3.2   Blood, blood plasma and serum

The blood itself is an aqueous environment, consisting of the liquid *plasma* – a solution of salts, small organic molecules such as glucose and amino acids, and a variety of peptides and proteins – and the blood cells, mostly red blood cells (*erythrocytes*). The erythrocyte membrane is permeable to, or has carriers for, some molecules but not others. Glucose, for instance, partially equilibrates across the erythrocyte membrane. Its concentration is somewhat lower inside the cell than outside, since the erythrocyte uses some for glycolysis and transport across the cell membrane must be somewhat limiting for this process. But nevertheless, glucose and some amino acids are carried around both in blood cells and in the plasma. On the other hand, lipid molecules are excluded from red blood cells and carried in the plasma. On the whole, the term 'in the plasma' will be used for those substances confined to that compartment, and 'in the blood' or 'in the bloodstream' for those which are carried in both compartments.

If blood is allowed to clot and then centrifuged, a yellow fluid can be removed: this is *serum*. It is like plasma but lacks the protein *fibrinogen*, which is used in the clotting process. Serum is often collected from patients for measurement of the concentration of cholesterol or triacylglycerol, mainly because it is convenient to let the blood clot. The term 'serum cholesterol', for instance, then simply refers to the concentration of cholesterol in the serum; it would be almost exactly the same as the plasma cholesterol concentration.

1.3.3   Lymph and lymphatics
The interstitial fluid is formed by filtration of the blood plasma through the endothelium (vessel lining), as described earlier. Some of the fluid which leaves the bloodstream in this way will naturally find its way back to the blood vessels, but some is drained away from tissues in another series of vessels, the lymphatics. These are for the most part smaller than blood vessels. The fluid within them, the lymph, resembles an ultrafiltrate of plasma – i.e. it is like plasma but without red blood cells and without some of the larger proteins of plasma. The lymphatic vessels merge and form larger vessels and eventually discharge their contents into the bloodstream. We shall be concerned with one particular branch of the lymphatic system – that which drains the walls of the small intestine. The products of fat digestion enter these lymphatic vessels, which collect together and form a duct running up the back of the chest, known as the *thoracic duct*. The thoracic duct discharges its contents into the bloodstream in the upper chest. The lymphatic system also plays an important role in defence against infection, but this immunological role is beyond the scope of this book.

1.4   Further reading

General metabolic biochemistry and nutrition: other useful textbooks
Fell, D. (1997) *Understanding the Control of Metabolism.* London: Portland Press.
Salway, J.G. (1999) *Metabolism at a Glance,* 2nd edn. Oxford: Blackwell Scientific Publications.
Murray, R.K., Granner D.K., Mayes, P.A. & Rodwell, V.W. (2000) *Harper's Biochemistry,* 25th edn. Stamford, CT: Appleton & Lange.
Bender, D.A. (2002) *Introduction to Nutrition and Metabolism,* 3rd edn. London: Taylor & Francis.

You may also need one of the 'classical' biochemistry textbooks to give more detail of pathways and structures, for example:

Nelson, D.L. & Cox, M.M. (2000) *Lehninger Principles of Biochemistry,* 3rd edn. New York: Worth Publishers.
Stryer, L. (1995) *Biochemistry,* 4th edn. New York: W.H. Freeman.

Harper's Biochemistry (Murray *et al.* 2000, above) may be a good compromise as it takes a 'physiological' approach to metabolism.

Note

1   Two important exceptions are mature white adipose tissue, in which triacylglycerol is the major constituent by weight, and the brain, of which 50–60% of dry weight is lipid (mostly phospholipid).

2

Some Mechanisms Involved in Metabolic Regulation

2.1 How is metabolic regulation achieved?

Metabolic regulation, as we have discussed it in Chapter 1, is achieved by controlling the flow of metabolites along metabolic pathways according to the body's needs.[1] There are various aspects to this. One is the partitioning of nutrients or metabolic substrates between tissues and organs in different nutritional states. This may be achieved by the expression of particular enzymes or proteins that impart specific metabolic properties to that tissue. For instance, some tissues do not express particular enzymes, others do. An example is *glucose-6-phosphatase*, the enzyme for making glucose from glucose 6-phosphate (produced either from glycogen breakdown or from gluconeogenesis). The liver expresses this enzyme: skeletal muscle does not. Therefore liver glycogen breakdown can contribute directly to blood glucose: skeletal muscle glycogen breakdown cannot. In addition, many key enzymes in metabolism have more than one isoform (often called *isoenzymes* or *isozymes*), related in structure and function, but produced from different genes, and with different regulatory properties. Both glycogen synthase and glycogen phosphorylase have different isoforms expressed in liver and muscle, and coded for by distinct genes. They catalyse identical reactions but their regulatory properties are subtly different. The family of glucose transporters, to be described below, is another example: tissue-specific expression gives different characteristics to tissues in terms of glucose uptake.

But there is also a dynamic aspect. Metabolic fluxes may need to change, gradually or sometimes very rapidly. Rapid changes occur in many situations. A sprinter starting from the blocks, or a high-jumper at take-off, has a very sudden need to supply energy for muscular contraction, and metabolic flux through the relevant pathways must change greatly within a fraction of a second. Even after eating a meal there are rapid changes in metabolic flux through certain pathways (as we shall see in later chapters). Glucose uptake into skeletal muscles increases, and the release of fatty acids stored in adipose tissue decreases, within about 60 minutes of eating a normal meal. (Even this period reflects the relatively slow entry of glucose from the small intestine into the bloodstream: if glucose is injected directly into a vein, then these changes happen correspondingly more rapidly.) Rapid changes in metabolic flux such as these usually reflect changes in the activity of key enzymes or other proteins brought about by a number of mechanisms. Some of these are listed in Table 2.1.

Other changes need to take place more gradually, perhaps over a period of hours, days or longer, for instance in response to a change in diet or activity pattern. Such gradual changes often involve changes in the amount of enzyme (or other proteins) present, and reflect changes in the rate of protein synthesis, or, less often, in the rate of protein degradation. An increase in the rate of protein synthesis can in turn reflect either an increased rate of transcription of messenger-RNA (mRNA) from DNA – often called *gene expression* – or (less often) a lower rate of mRNA degradation. It can also reflect an increase in the rate at which proteins are synthesised from the mRNA template by increasing the rate at which new protein chains are started (the process called *initiation*). This mechanism is known as *translational control*. The control of gene expression is a very general mechanism pervading much of metabolic regulation, and will be referred to many times in this book. Different stages at which the amount of any particular protein may be controlled are summarised in Fig. 2.1. Beyond the amount of protein present, the activity of an enzyme or transcription factor may then be altered by *post-translational control*, using mechanisms such as phosphorylation (see Table 2.1) or proteolytic cleavage (as for the sterol regulatory element binding proteins, discussed in Section 2.4.2.3 below).

There is no absolute division between 'rapid' and 'longer-term' changes. Often enzymes that are regulated in a certain way in the short term – for instance, activated by phosphorylation – are also increased in amount by increased gene transcription if the situation persists for longer. Nevertheless, the mechanisms are distinct. These various mechanisms for achieving changes in substrate flux are illustrated in Fig. 2.2.

Another form of control that will be discussed in many places in this book is achieved through alteration of the flow of substrates through the circulation. To give just one example, fatty acids are usually a preferred fuel (over glucose) for skeletal muscle. When glucose is present in increased concentrations in the circulation after a carbohydrate-rich meal, how do muscles reduce their fatty acid utilisation so that glucose can be utilised instead? The answer lies in adipose tissue, responsible for releasing fatty acids into the circulation. Fatty acid release is very effectively switched off by insulin, so muscles no longer have the option of using fatty acids. This apparent cooperation between tissues is typical of metabolic regulation when viewed on a whole-body basis.

Some the aspects just discussed can be illustrated by a puzzle (Fig. 2.3). We

Table 2.1 Common mechanisms for rapid alteration of cellular metabolic flux.

	Examples	Comments
Covalent modification: phosphorylation or dephosphorylation of serine, threonine or tyrosine residues	Glycogen phosphorylase (activated by phosphorylation) (see Box 2.4 and Box 4.1) Glycogen synthase (activated by dephosphorylation) (see Box 4.1) Hormone-sensitive lipase (activated by phosphorylation) (see Box 2.4 and Section 4.5.3.2)	Brought about by specific enzymes (kinases, phosphatases) that may themselves be controlled in the same way
Allosteric	Activation of phosphofructokinase-1 by fructose 2,6-bisphophate (see Box 4.2) Inhibition of fructose-1,6-bisphosphatase by fructose 2,6-bisphophate (see Box 4.2) Inhibition of carnitine-palmitoyl transferase-1 by malonyl-CoA (see Section 4.1.2.2)	Binding of a small molecule at a site distinct from the catalytic site alters protein conformation and changes activity
Competitive or uncompetitive inhibition	There are possible examples in serine biosynthesis [phosphoserine phosphatase is uncompetitively inhibited by its product, serine (Fell 1997, page 189)]; and in ketone body synthesis [acetyl-CoA acetyl transferase is competitively inhibited by its product, acetoacetyl-CoA].	Inhibitor competes with normal substrate for binding to enzyme active site. Common for xenobiotics (drugs, etc.) but apparently less so as a natural means of controlling flux
Interaction with another protein	Glucokinase regulatory protein (see Box 4.2)	Also a common mechanism in 'signal chains' for hormone action (see Box 2.4)
Translocation	GLUT4 moves from intracellular store to cell membrane in response to insulin (see Section 2.2.1.1) Hormone-sensitive lipase translocates to lipid droplet in adipocyte on phosphorylation (see Section 4.5.3.2)	

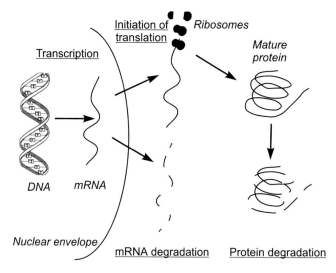

Fig. 2.1 Different stages at which the amount of a protein present in a cell may be controlled (underlined). For many proteins the major control is at the level of transcription (mRNA synthesis from the DNA template). Not shown in this figure is a further layer of complexity added by *alternative splicing* of the mRNA after transcription. The initial, nuclear full-length mRNA molecule is a faithful reproduction of all the DNA sequence of the gene. This includes introns (junk DNA) and exons (DNA that codes for mRNA that will be exported from the nucleus). The introns are removed in the nucleus and the ends of the remaining mRNA 'spliced' together before export from the nucleus. The resulting mRNA may start with alternative exons, giving a range of possible transcripts from one gene.

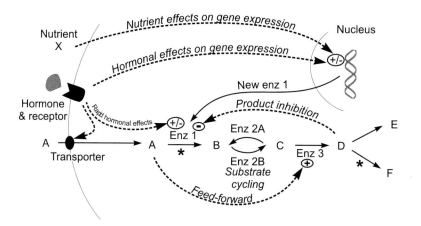

Fig. 2.2 Different methods for achieving changes in metabolic flux within a cell. A hypothetical metabolic pathway is shown. Enz 1, Enz 2, etc. are the enzymes converting substrate A to substrate B, B to C, etc. For many pathways, important control points are often the first step, and also the first step after a branch point (marked *).

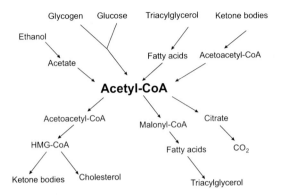

Fig. 2.3 A metabolic regulation puzzle. Illustrated are some of the pathways by which acetyl-CoA may be generated, and some of the pathways by which it is utilised. Think about this: what determines its fate in any particular cell at any particular time? And what prevents 'futile' metabolic cycling: e.g. fatty acids make acetyl-CoA, acetyl-CoA makes fatty acids; or ketone bodies make acetyl-CoA, acetyl-CoA makes ketone bodies? How can the control of ketone body synthesis (a pathway active in 'catabolic' conditions) be achieved when the initial steps in the pathway seem similar to those for cholesterol synthesis (active in 'anabolic' conditions)? The answers will be touched upon in passing and by the end of the book all should be clear.

will return to this puzzle in later chapters (see Section 6.4.1.1 and other sections in Chapters 4 and 6).

2.2   Metabolic regulation brought about by the characteristics of tissues

The characteristics of individual cells or tissues 'set the scene' for metabolic regulation. For instance, the metabolic characteristics of the liver mean that it will inevitably be able to take up excess glucose from plasma, whereas other tissues cannot adjust their rates of utilisation so readily. Therefore the liver is likely to play an important role in glucose metabolism whenever plasma glucose levels are high. The brain, in contrast, has a pathway for utilising glucose at a rate that is relatively constant whatever the plasma glucose concentration, a very reasonable adaptation, since we would not want to be super-intelligent only after eating carbohydrate, and intellectually challenged between meals.

Individual tissues and organs will be discussed in more detail in the next chapter, but here we will look at some general features, especially the means by which nutrients cross cell membranes, which differ from tissue to tissue.

2.2.1   Movement of substances across membranes

Cell membranes, as we saw in Chapter 1, are composed of bilayers of phospholipid molecules (Fig. 1.5). Molecules crossing this membrane must pass through both the hydrophilic, polar faces and the hydrophobic interior. In general, this presents less of a problem for non-polar hydrophobic molecules, and many hydrophobic drugs are able to enter cells readily. It has long been assumed that all hydrophobic molecules can enter cells by simple diffusion, but this is now increasingly under question as more and more specific transporter proteins are described. One example which will be common in this book is that of long-chain fatty acids entering cells: this process was for many years thought to occur by diffusion, but within the past few years specific *fatty-acid transporters* have been described. This should not surprise us, because the movement of molecules in and out of cells by simple diffusion is, by its very nature, not a process over which any control can be exerted. On the other hand, if the movement occurs by a carrier-mediated process, then immediately there are possibilities for regulation: some cells may have more carriers than others, or the number or activity of the carriers may be altered by hormones. General characteristics of the movement of substances across membranes are discussed in Box 2.1.

Box 2.1   Movement of molecules across membranes

The cell membrane, and membranes within cells, are formed from a phospholipid bilayer (see Fig. 1.5). Most biological molecules, especially polar molecules and ions, will not diffuse freely across such a membrane. Instead, there are specific proteins embedded in the membranes, which 'transport' molecules and ions from one side to the other. This box describes some general properties of the movement of molecules across membranes.

A substance will cross a membrane to move from one solution to another if (1) the membrane is permeable to the substance, and (2) there is a *concentration gradient* in the appropriate direction: i.e. a substance will move from a region of high concentration to a region of lower concentration. (In reality, there will be movement in both directions because of random molecular movements, but the *net* movement will be down the concentration gradient.)

There are two major means by which such movement may occur: *free diffusion*, i.e. unassisted movement by diffusion, brought about simply by the overall effect of random molecular motions, and *facilitated diffusion (carrier-mediated diffusion)*, i.e. movement assisted by a specific transporter protein. In addition, there is a third means of movement: *active transport*, in which substances may move *up* a concentration gradient – i.e. from a lower concentration to a higher one. This can only be brought about by the supply of energy, either electrical (charge on the membrane) or chemical; for instance, the *Na^+-K^+-ATPase* is a membrane protein that hydrolyses ATP and pumps sodium ions out of cells against a strong concentration gradient, and potassium ions in – also against a strong concentration gradient.

The two forms of movement down concentration gradients – free diffusion and facilitated diffusion – can be distinguished by their kinetic characteristics.

Since the movement of substances by a transporter protein is similar in many ways to enzyme catalysis, it has similar characteristics: there is a characteristic *affinity* of the transporter protein for the molecule, and a maximum rate of transfer of the molecule which will depend, in turn, on the intrinsic 'rate of action' of the protein, and the number of transporters available in the membrane. Thus, if we measure the rate of transport at differing concentrations of the substrate to be transported, we will find a hyperbolic curve similar to a Michaelis–Menten plot of enzyme action. On the other hand, if transport occurs by free diffusion, there is no limitation to the rate, and it will be simply proportional to the concentration gradient of the substrate across the membrane. These are illustrated in Fig. 2.2.1.

The presence of *active transport* will usually be identified by its need for energy. Blocking of ATP synthesis (for instance, by inhibition of oxidative phosphorylation) will usually reduce or abolish such transport.

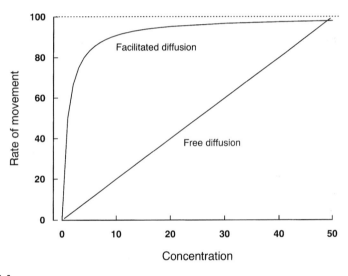

Fig. 2.1.1

2.2.1.1   Glucose transport

A particularly important mechanism from the point of view of energy metabolism is the way that glucose crosses cell membranes. There are two families of glucose transporters, each family comprising a number of homologous proteins synthesised from different genes and having different kinetic properties. These are summarised in Box 2.2. The 'GLUT' family are all facilitative (passive) transporters, whereas the sodium-glucose cotransporter (SGLT) family are active glucose transporters. SGLT-1, expressed in the small intestine, needs to be able to move glucose from a low to high concentration, in order to ensure virtually complete absorption from the intestinal lumen. This is achieved by

Box 2.2 Transport of glucose across cell membranes

It has long been known that glucose enters cells by carrier-mediated diffusion (facilitated diffusion) rather than by free diffusion across the cell membrane (see Box 2.1 for definitions). In recent years the genes for the specific glucose transporter molecules have been cloned and sequenced; the transporters have been expressed in cell lines and their characteristics studied. There are two families of glucose transporters. The more widespread family consists of *passive* transporters, allowing the movement of glucose across cell membranes *only* down a concentration gradient. They are called GLUTn, where *n* is a number distinguishing different members. There are 12 known members of this family but only five (shown in the table below) have well-characterised function. The other family consists of active transporters in which glucose may move up a concentration gradient (i.e. it may be concentrated by the transporter) because sodium ions, co-transported with the glucose, are moving down a concentration gradient (see Fig. 2.4). These are known as the sodium-glucose cotransporter family, SGLT-n. The expression of all these transporters is tissue-specific, and their properties are an integral part of the regulation of glucose metabolism in the particular tissue.

The effect which the characteristics of the glucose transporter may have on the rate of glucose entry into cells is illustrated in Fig. 2.2.1. (This refers to facilitated diffusion, i.e. passive transport, only.)

With a glucose transporter whose K_m for glucose entry is 1.6 mmol/l (e.g. GLUT3), the rate of glucose uptake is relatively independent of the extracellular glucose concentration over the normal, physiological range of plasma

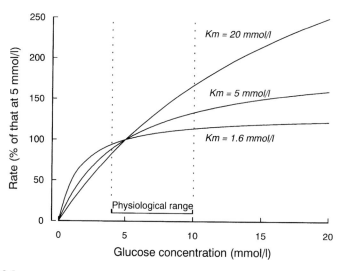

Fig 2.2.1

Table 2.2.1

Name	Tissue distribution	Approximate K_m (for inward transport of glucose or a glucose analogue)	Size (no. of amino acids)	Important features
GLUT1	Erythrocytes, fetal tissue, placenta, brain blood vessels	5–7 mmol/l	492	
GLUT2	Liver, kidney, intestine, pancreatic β-cell	High (7–20 mmol/l)	524	High K_m allows glucose to 'equilibrate' across the membrane
GLUT3	Brain (neuronal cells)	Low (1.6 mmol/l)	496	Low K_m allows relatively constant rate of glucose uptake independent of extracellular concentration over the normal range
GLUT4	Muscle, adipose tissue	5 mmol/l	509	The 'insulin-regulatable' glucose transporter: see Fig. 2.5
GLUT5	Jejunum	5 mmol/l for fructose	501	Probably responsible for fructose uptake from intestine
SGLT-1	Duodenum, jejunum, renal tubules		664	The sodium-glucose cotransporter of the small intestine (not part of the same family as GLUT1–5). Co-transports 1 mol sugar with 2 mol Na$^+$
SGLT-2, 3	Renal tubules			Homologous to SGLT-1; SGLT-2 in particular has high capacity and low affinity (high K_m for glucose). SGLT-2 co-transports 1 mol sugar with 1 mol Na$^+$; SGLT-3 co-transports 1 mol sugar with 2 mol Na$^+$

Based on Gould & Holman 1993; Joost et al. 2002; Thorens 1996; Wallner et al. 2001; Wright 1993.

glucose concentrations. This would be appropriate in, for instance, the brain, where the rate of glucose uptake needs to be constant despite cycles of feeding and fasting. With a K_m for glucose entry of 20 mmol/l (e.g. GLUT2), the rate of glucose entry is almost proportional to the extracellular glucose concentration (the higher the external concentration, the greater the rate of entry). The lines are plotted assuming Michaelis–Menten kinetics. This is oversimplified because it assumes that glucose *within* the cells is removed as fast as it enters. Therefore, the enzyme responsible for phosphorylation of glucose (hexokinase or glucokinase) must have similar characteristics to (or a greater capacity than) the glucose transporter in order for these kinetics to be expressed. The removal of glucose 6-phosphate must also occur at approximately the same rate as glucose enters the cell; the pathways of glucose metabolism are regulated hormonally so as to coordinate all these events (see Fig. 4.2).

The terminology is that GLUT refers to the proteins. These are related and all have 12 membrane-spanning regions. The genes encoding them are called SLC2A1 (the gene for GLUT1), SLC2A2 (for GLUT2), etc.

linking glucose transport to that of sodium: i.e. sodium moves down a strong concentration gradient, carrying glucose with it up a concentration gradient. This process is illustrated in Fig. 2.4. SGLT-1 to -3 are expressed in the renal tubule and are involved in kidney function; this will be described further in Section 4.6.2.

GLUT4 has special characteristics relevant for metabolic regulation. Many years ago it was recognised that when insulin stimulates glucose uptake by muscle preparations, it appears to do so by increasing the maximal rate of uptake (the V_{max}) rather than by changing the K_m. There is a large cellular store of the

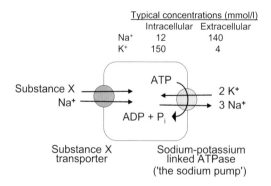

Fig. 2.4 Sodium-linked active transport. By co-transport with Na^+ ions, substance X may move up a concentration gradient. The Na^+ ions move down a gradient maintained by the activity of the Na^+-K^+-linked ATPase or 'sodium pump', which uses energy derived from ATP to pump Na^+ ions out of, and K^+ ions into the cell, both against concentration gradients. Substance X may be glucose (if the transporter belongs to the SGLT family) or an amino acid.

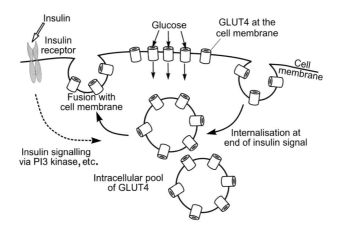

Fig. 2.5 GLUT4 recruitment to the cell membrane. There is an intracellular pool of GLUT4 in membranous vesicles that can translocate to the cell membrane when insulin binds to its receptor. When the insulin signal is withdrawn, the GLUT4 proteins return to their intracellular pool. Based loosely on Shepherd & Kahn (1999).

transporter GLUT4, sequestered in membrane vesicles within the cell. When insulin binds to its receptor, these vesicles move to, and become incorporated in, the cell membrane and therefore the amount of GLUT4 available for glucose transport into the cell is increased. When insulin action ceases, these transporters recycle into intracellular vesicles (Fig. 2.5).

2.2.1.2   Amino acids

The concentration of most amino acids is considerably higher inside cells than outside: this is illustrated in Table 2.2 for some amino acids in skeletal muscle. This implies the existence of active transporters to move amino acids into the cells up a concentration gradient. In fact, like glucose in the small intestine, amino acids are mostly actively transported by sodium-linked carriers. Again, therefore, energy is required to pump the sodium ions out and maintain their concentration gradient. There are a number of amino acid transporters, common to the intestinal cells and to many other tissues. Each has a fairly broad specificity and transports a number of amino acids. They are described further in Table 2.3.

2.2.1.3   Fatty acids

Fatty acids arrive at cells in two ways. They may come in the form of non-esterified fatty acids that have been carried through the plasma bound to albumin. Alternatively they may be liberated from triacylglycerol in the plasma (carried in lipoprotein particles, to be discussed further in Chapter 9) by the enzyme *lipoprotein lipase* attached to the endothelial cells that line the capillaries. They cross the endothelial cell lining and enter cells (e.g. liver, skeletal muscle, cardiac muscle, adipose tissue) down a concentration gradient, which is generated by

Table 2.2 Free amino acids in skeletal muscle.

Amino acids are found free (i.e. not as constituents of proteins) both in plasma and in the intracellular water of tissues. They may be present at considerably higher concentrations inside cells than out, reflecting the presence of active transport mechanisms for their entry into cells. The best data are available for skeletal muscle since small samples can be taken from human subjects with a special needle with a cutting edge. The sample (*biopsy*) is then frozen rapidly in liquid nitrogen to prevent further metabolism, and the amino acids are analysed. A correction is made for the amount of amino acid present in extracellular fluid (using the measurement of Cl^- ions, which are present mainly in the extracellular fluid). Some typical results are given below:

Amino acid	Plasma concentration (mmol/l)	Intracellular concentration (mmol/l)	Ratio intra-/extracellular concentrations
Glutamine	0.57	19.5	34 : 1
Glutamic acid	0.06	4.4	73 : 1
Alanine	0.33	2.3	7 : 1
Serine	0.12	0.98	7 : 1
Asparagine	0.05	0.47	10 : 1

1 kg of skeletal muscle contains about 650 g of intracellular water. Skeletal muscle represents about 40% of the body weight. In the whole body, the intracellular pool of free amino acids in muscle will be about 80 g, of which glutamine, glutamic acid and alanine contribute almost 80%.

Based on Bergström *et al.* (1974).

Table 2.3 Some amino acid transporters.

Transporter/family	Na$^+$-dependence	Tissues	Amino acids
A	Yes	Widespread	Ala, Ser, Gln
ASC	Yes	Widespread	Ala, Ser, Cys
L	No	Widespread	BCAA, aromatics
N$^{(m)}$	Yes	Liver; m in muscle	Gln, Asn, His

At least nine distinct transporters are known (McGivan & Pastor-Anglada 1994; Palacín et al. 1998). The amino acid transporters are often referred to as systems (e.g. system A transporters), partly because until recently few had been cloned and those shown may represent families. Now progress is being made in cloning and identifying individual transport proteins.

BCAA, branched-chain amino acids.

avid binding to specific fatty acid binding proteins within the cells. The gradient is maintained because the fatty acids are utilised for further metabolism within the cells. The first step in this process is always esterification to coenzyme A to form acyl-CoA thioesters. This step is sometimes called activation (it requires ATP and releases AMP and pyrophosphate, PP_i). It has been estimated that in muscle the gradient is from (around) 500 nmol/ml in plasma to (around) 100 nmol/ml (cardiac muscle) or 30 nmol/ml (skeletal muscle) within the tissue (van der Vusse & Reneman 1996).

There is still debate about how fatty acids cross cell membranes. They may do so by passive diffusion using a movement usually called 'flip-flop' in which the polar carboxyl group enters the polar face of the membrane, the hydrophobic fatty tail flips into the lipid bilayer, and then a reversal takes it out of the other side. The rate at which this could happen (based on physico-chemical calculations and measurements in artificial membranes) seems just about sufficient to account for rates of fatty acid utilisation observed. However, as mentioned above, there is increasing evidence for specific fatty acid transport proteins in the cell membrane. It is probable that fatty acids enter cells by a combination of routes, partially facilitated and partly passive diffusion. Some researchers, however, believe that intracellular sequestration of fatty acids by fatty acid binding proteins, and further metabolism of fatty acids (e.g. by acyl-CoA synthase) can give the appearance of carrier-mediated transport. Some of the putative fatty acid transporters are listed in Table 2.4.

In adipose tissue, fatty acids also need to leave the cell (during fat mobilisation). In this case the concentration gradient is reversed because hormone-sensitive lipase within the adipocyte liberates fatty acids at a high rate from stored triacylglycerol. It is not clear whether the same transporters are involved.

There is now growing evidence that fatty acid transport across cell membranes is regulated. This is an active field of research and new data are constantly emerging. Recent evidence suggests that CD36/FAT (see Table 2.4) in skeletal muscle may be recruited to the cell membrane from an intracellular pool when fatty acid utilisation is high during exercise, in a similar manner to GLUT4 (Fig. 2.5), and that insulin can also bring about a similar translocation.

2.2.1.4   Cholesterol

Like fatty acids, it has long been assumed that cholesterol can cross membranes by a flip-flop mechanism. Recent discoveries show this to be an oversimplification. The diet contains many plant- and fish-derived substances that are chemically very similar to cholesterol, some of which are termed sitosterols. It has long been recognised that, whereas absorption of cholesterol from the small intestine is relatively efficient (around 50%), the amount of the chemically similar sitosterols that enters the plasma is very small. Thus, absorption must in some way be very selective and that immediately suggests a carrier mechanism. However, there is an inherited condition known as sitosterolaemia in which

Table 2.4 Some putative cell membrane fatty acid transporters.

	Tissue distribution	Relative molecular mass	Comments
Fatty acid translocase (FAT)	White adipose tissue, myocardium, skeletal muscle, small intestine	88 kDa	Also known as CD36 and a member of the family of 'scavenger receptors'. Some people are deficient in CD36 and appear to have abnormalities of fat metabolism, especially in the heart.
Fatty acid transport protein (FATP)	FATP1 (the best characterised) mainly skeletal muscle, adipose tissue, small intestine, brain; other members (especially FATP5) in liver	63 kDa	There is a family of at least six related proteins in humans, known as FATP1 to FATP6; some members have since been shown to have acyl-CoA synthase activity (see below).
Fatty acid binding protein (plasma membrane) (FABPpm)	Widespread	43 kDa	Related to the family of fatty acid binding proteins but restricted to the plasma membrane; may cooperate with other proteins in fatty acid uptake.
Acyl-CoA synthase	Widespread	70–80 kDa (different family members)	It has been suggested that acyl-CoA synthase (which esterifies fatty acids with CoA) is intimately involved in the transport of fatty acids into cells. It is associated with membranes. Some members of FATP family (see above) may have this enzymatic activity

Information from (amongst others) Dutta-Roy (2000); Abumrad et al. (1999); Hirsch et al. (1998).

high levels of sitosterols are found in the plasma and this results in atherosclerosis just as when cholesterol levels are high. Tracing the gene responsible led to the identification of two transporters known as ABC-G5 and ABC-G8, where ABC refers to the presence in the protein of a motif called an ATP-Binding Cassette. In addition, a related transporter, ABC-A1, was identified through a genetic disorder of lipid metabolism (to be discussed later, in Section 9.2.3.1 and Fig. 9.5). All these proteins, ABC-A1, ABC-G5 and ABC-G8, are expressed in enterocytes (small intestinal absorptive cells). (ABC-A1 is also expressed in other tissues where it plays a crucial role in facilitating the movement of excess cholesterol from cells onto high-density lipoprotein (HDL) particles: see Fig. 9.5.) Current understanding is that cholesterol and other dietary sterols enter the enterocytes relatively non-specifically. ABC-A1 then re-exports a proportion of cholesterol back into the intestinal lumen; ABC-G5 and -G8 do the same (and very efficiently) for other sterols. When ABC-G5 or -G8 are mutated, this re-export does not happen and the plant sterols enter the plasma.

2.3   Hormones and short-term control of enzyme activity

Many metabolic pathways are subject to control by metabolites related to that pathway. The precursor metabolite may activate steps in the pathway (sometimes called feed-forward); intermediates in the pathway may regulate flux through the pathway; or the product(s) of the pathway may suppress metabolic flux (usually called product inhibition) (see Fig. 2.2). We will deal with some specific examples as we meet them in this book.

Many pathways are also controlled by factors external to the pathway, and here we will look at some general mechanisms involved in such control. In this section we will look particularly at how some pathways are rapidly controlled by hormones, and in a later section at how nutrients and hormones can affect gene expression.

Pathways may be controlled by hormones, secreted from *endocrine glands* (see Chapter 5), carried through the plasma and acting on the cell where the pathway takes place (the *target cell*). The nervous system also relays signals from distant organs (often the brain) that can alter metabolic flux and there are many parallels between nervous system activity and hormone action.

Hormones act on target cells by binding to specific *receptor proteins*. There are two major types of hormone–receptor interaction: on the cell surface (peptide hormones, catecholamines) and within the cell (thyroid hormones, steroid hormones). All the hormones that act through intracellular receptors exert their effects on gene expression. At present we will just consider hormones acting through cell-surface receptors.

Most metabolic pathways occur within cells (although some involve transport of substances through the cell membrane: e.g. glycogen synthesis requires transport of glucose into the cell). Therefore the binding of the hormone to its receptor embedded in the cell membrane must cause events to take place within the cell that alter metabolic flux. These links between hormone binding and metabolic effects are known as *signal chains* or *signal transduction*. The molecules that participate in those signal chains are sometimes called 'second messengers'. Many signal chains are complex and at the time of writing (2001–02) relatively few have been described in full detail. Boxes 2.3 and 2.4 describe some of the components common to many signal chains, and illustrate

Box 2.3   Components of signal transduction chains

Receptors

Each hormone or neurotransmitter has its own receptor protein. (There are some exceptions: insulin-like growth factors can bind to and act through the insulin receptor; the catecholamines adrenaline and noradrenaline share a family of receptors.) Here we are considering only those receptors that are expressed on the cell surface.

The insulin receptor: This is synthesised as one polypeptide chain but then cleaved to make two identical α-subunits and two β-subunits, which co-operate as shown schematically in Fig. 2.4.1, Box 2.4. When insulin binds, the β-subunits develop tyrosine kinase activity and phosphorylate themselves; this leads to interaction with other membrane-associated proteins, and the beginning of the insulin signal chain (see Box 2.4 for more details).

Adrenoceptors: The catecholamines – adrenaline (a hormone) and noradrenaline (a neurotransmitter) – share receptors called adrenergic receptors or adrenoceptors: there is a family of these described in Chapter 5 (see Table 5.1). Adrenergic receptors belong to a large family of receptors that share a similar structure, with seven hydrophobic regions that are considered to snake in and out of the cell membrane – hence alternative terms, serpentine receptors or, more prosaically, '7TMs' (i.e. with seven *trans*-membrane domains). These receptors are also known as G-protein coupled receptors (or GPCRs) for reasons described below. The glucagon receptor is also a GPCR.

G-proteins

G-proteins are so called because they bind and hydrolyse GTP. Those that interact with serpentine receptors are composed of three subunits, α, β and γ, that bind GTP when the receptor is occupied. Upon binding of GTP, these subunits dissociate and the α-subunit moves within the membrane and interacts with an enzyme. There are three different types of G-proteins involved in energy metabolism: stimulatory G-proteins, G_s, that activate adenylyl cyclase; inhibitory G-proteins, G_i, that inhibit adenylyl cyclase; and G_q, G-proteins that activate phospholipase C. In diagrams this system will only be shown very schematically (e.g. see Fig. 2.4.2, Box 2.4).

Small molecules

A variety of small molecules play a role as 'second messengers'.

Cyclic adenosine 3′,5′-monophosphate (cyclic AMP or cAMP). cAMP was the first second messenger to be characterised. It is involved in a very large number of cellular responses that include gene expression: many genes have cAMP response elements or CREs. cAMP is formed from ATP by the enzyme *adenylyl cyclase* (see below).

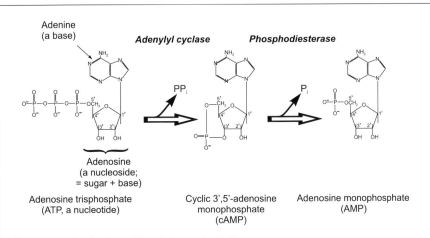

Fig. 2.3.1 Synthesis and breakdown of cAMP.

Cyclic GMP (cGMP): cGMP is analogous to cAMP. It is formed by guanylyl cyclase from GTP: its roles include regulation of ion transport in the kidney and relaxation of smooth muscle.

Calcium ions (Ca^{2+}): These regulate many enzymatic processes including aspects of glycogen metabolism, skeletal muscle contraction and secretion of hormones including insulin. There are large cellular stores of Ca^{2+} within the endoplasmic reticulum (or the sarcoplasmic reticulum in muscle). Ca^{2+} can be liberated into the cytosol from these stores very rapidly in response to opening of specific ion channels. After the stimulus is removed, Ca^{2+} are pumped back into the stores. Many responses to elevation of cytosolic Ca^{2+} are mediated by their binding to a 17 kDa protein called *calmodulin*. Calmodulin has four high-affinity Ca^{2+}-binding sites. It is related to the protein troponin that triggers skeletal muscle contraction (see Box 8.3).

Phosphatidylinositol and related compounds: Phosphatidylinositol is a phospholipid that is associated with the inner leaflet of the cell membrane. The hydroxyl groups of the inositol ring may be phosphorylated. One particular form, phosphatidylinositol (4′,5′)-bisphate (PIP_2), is the starting point for a number of important events. It may be cleaved by *phospholipase C* (see below) to release inositol (1′,4′,5′)-trisphosphate (IP_3) and diacylgylcerol (Fig. 2.3.2). IP_3 is water-soluble and diffuses to the endoplasmic reticulum where it interacts with specific receptors to release Ca^{2+} into the cytoplasm. Diacylglycerol, which remains associated with the membrane, acts in concert with Ca^{2+} to activate *protein kinase C* (see below). Alternatively, the enzyme *phosphatidylinositol-3-kinase* (see below) may phosphorylate the 3′-position on the inositol ring of PIP_2, forming phosphatidylinositol (3′,4′,5′)-trisphosphate (PIP_3). Note that PIP_3 is still a phospholipid, unlike IP_3 with which it should not be confused! PIP_3 plays a key role in insulin signalling (see Box 2.4).

☞

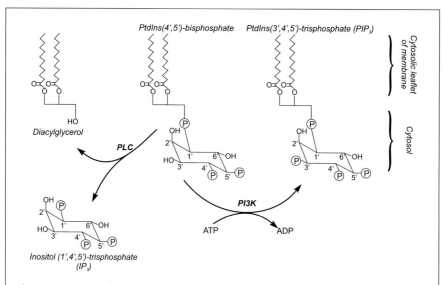

Fig. 2.3.2   PI3K, phosphatidylinositol-3-kinase; PLC, phospholipase C. Ⓟ represents a phosphate group (-PO$_4^{2-}$).

Enzymes

This box briefly describes some of the enzymes common to many of the control processes discussed in this book.

   Adenylyl cyclase (or **adenylate cyclase**): This is an integral protein of the plasma membrane. It is activated or inhibited by interaction with membrane-associated G-proteins. Adenylyl cyclase catalyses the production of cAMP from ATP (see Fig. 2.3.1).

   Phospholipase C: This is also a cell membrane-bound enzyme, activated by another class of G-proteins, G$_q$. It catalyses the cleavage of PIP$_2$ to release IP$_3$ and diacylglycerol (see Fig. 2.3.2).

   Phosphatidylinositol-3-kinase (PI3K, see Fig. 2.3.2) is activated by docking with protein targets of insulin receptor phosphorylation known as insulin receptor substrates (IRSs). It phosphorylates the 3′-position on the inositol ring of PIP$_2$, forming phosphatidyl-inositol (3′,4′,5′) trisphosphate (PIP$_3$).

Protein kinases

There is a family of protein kinases, of which the following are particularly relevant to this discussion. The following are serine or threonine kinases, involved in regulation of enzyme activity.

   cAMP-dependent protein kinase (protein kinase A, or PKA) was the first protein kinase to be identified. It is involved in rapid regulation of many pathways of energy metabolism. In its inactive state it is composed of four subunits, two regulatory (R) subunits and two catalytic (C). When cAMP binds to the R subunits, they dissociate, leaving the catalytic subunits active against protein targets.

Protein kinase B (PKB, also known as Akt) was first cloned as a homologue of PKA; because its properties were somewhere between those of PKA and PKC (see below) it was termed PKB!

Protein kinase C (PKC): There is a large family of PKCs, divided into four subgroups. One subgroup, the 'classical' PKCs, are activated by calcium ions (hence the name PKC). Other subgroups, the 'atypical PKCs', are activated by various lipid mediators that are generated in the cell membrane in response to other enzyme activities. These activators include diacylglycerol and PIP_3.

AMP-activated protein kinase (AMP-PK): This member of the protein kinase family is activated by AMP; this activation is antagonised by ATP. There-fore AMP-PK 'senses' the cell's energy status: when there is a drain on ATP, the AMP/ATP ratio rises and AMP-PK is activated, leading in turn to inhibition of ATP-utilising pathways (particularly biosynthetic pathways) and increased ATP generation. This enzyme has therefore been described as a 'cellular fuel gauge'.

Glycogen synthase kinase 3 (GS3K): As its name suggests, GS3K was first identified as a kinase responsible for phosphorylation, and inactivation, of glycogen synthase. It is now recognised to play a role in several signal chains relevant to energy metabolism although it has retained its original name (see Box 2.4, Fig. 2.4.1).

Mitogen-activated protein kinase (MAPK) is part of a signal chain that links cell-surface receptors, especially those for growth factors includ-ing insulin-like growth factors 1 and 2 (IGF-1 and IGF-2), with altered gene transcription in the nucleus, altered post-translational processing of proteins and control of the cell cycle. At one time the MAPK pathway was thought to be involved in insulin regulation of glycogen synthase, but it is now known that this is not so: it may be involved, however, in the regulation of gene expression by insulin. The pathway is complex, with a MAP-kinase-kinase and also a MAP-kinase-kinase-kinase!

3′-Phosphoinositide dependent kinase-1 (PDK1) is a serine/threonine kinase expressed in many tissues. It binds phosphatidylinositides that are phos-phorylated in the 3′ position, particularly phosphatidylinositol (3′,4′,5′)- tris-phosphate (PIP_3 on Fig. 2.4.1, Box 2.4). This activates it, and it phosphorylates and activates (amongst other proteins) PKB.

Protein phosphatases
There is a large family of protein phosphatases involved in dephosphorylation of serine, threonine and tyrosine residues and hence regulation of enzyme activity.

Protein phosphatase-1 (PP-1) is a serine phosphatase that plays a particular role in energy metabolism. PP-1 may have a subunit that associates it with glycogen, the *glycogen targeting subunit*. PP-1 that is associated with glycogen is known as *PP-1G*. There are glycogen targeting subunits that are specific to liver and muscle. The activity of PP-1 is itself regulated: for instance, it is activated by insulin, leading to dephosphorylation and hence inactivation of glycogen synthase. (For many dephosphorylation reactions, however, it seems that the phosphatase activity is constitutively expressed (i.e. always present) and not regulated. An example is the suppression of hormone-sensitive lipase (HSL) activity in the adipocyte by insulin. Insulin reduces phosphorylation of HSL by reducing cAMP concentration and hence PKA activity; the enzyme is dephosphorylated (and inactivated) by protein phosphatases that are always active.)

Protein-tyrosine phosphatases are also important in metabolic regulation. One particular isoform, PTP1B, is responsible for dephosphorylation of tyrosine residues in the insulin receptor, and therefore turning off insulin action. PTP1B is itself regulated by phosphorylation. Insulin, via the insulin receptor tyrosine kinase, phosphorylates tyrosine residues in PTP1B and reduces its activity. cAMP leads, presumably via PKA, to serine phosphorylation of PTP1B and an increase in activity. Signalling from catecholamines can then be seen to reduce insulin signalling. PTP1B has been described as a 'critical point for insulin and catecholamine counter-regulation'.

the events involved by looking at some well-established signal chains. The signal chains drawn out as examples in Box 2.4 make an important point. One molecule of enzyme can bring about the transformation of many molecules of its substrate. Therefore signal chains such as these open up the possibility of 'amplification' of a hormonal signal within a cell, with each successive step involving larger and larger numbers of molecules. This is also often described as a *'cascade'* of events following hormone-receptor binding.

Many events in signal transduction are mediated by phosphorylation, in which serine, threonine or tyrosine residues in proteins are phosphorylated (using ATP) or dephosphorylated by specific enzymes (*kinases* and *phosphatases* respectively). In general, tyrosine phosphorylation is involved in receptor function and early in signal chains. When enzymes are regulated by phosphorylation, it mostly involves serine residues. Sometimes the enzymatic activity is intrinsic to a protein with another function: for instance, the insulin receptor has tyrosine kinase activity which is activated when insulin binds. Phosphorylation or dephosphorylation of a protein leads to a conformational change, which may alter the protein's catalytic activity, or may lead to interaction with other proteins (sometimes called 'docking'). Both the kinases and the

---

Box 2.4   Signal transduction chains: some examples

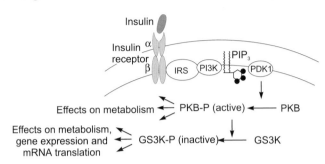

Fig. 2.4.1   Signal chain for regulation of many metabolic processes by insulin. Insulin binds to its receptor in the cell membrane leading to auto-phosphorylation of tyrosine residues in the receptor protein. This leads to interaction with a family of proteins known as insulin receptor substrates (IRS), which themselves become phosphorylated and then interact with the enzyme phosphatidylinositol-3-kinase (PI3K on figure). PI3K generates phosphatidylinositol (3′,4′,5′)-trisphosphate (PIP₃ on figure; see Box 2.3, Fig. 2.3.2 for structure) in the inner surface of the membrane, which acts through the enzyme 3′-phosphoinositide dependent kinase-1 (PDK1) to phosphorylate (and activate) protein kinase B (PKB). Activated PKB leads to several cellular responses to insulin including inhibition of lipolysis (see Fig. 2.4.3), increased glucose transport (see Fig. 2.5), effects on DNA transcription, and also phosphorylation and inactivation of glycogen synthase kinase 3 (GSK3). Inactivation of GSK3 also leads to multiple cellular effects including stimulation of glycogen synthesis (discussed later; see Box 4.1) and, again, effects on gene expression and also effects on protein chain initiation (i.e. mRNA translation). Although it seems odd to speak of *inactivation* of an enzyme leading to downstream events, these are brought about by specific phosphatases that are then free to dephosphorylate the proteins involved.   ☞

---

phosphatases may themselves be regulated, in some cases also by phosphorylation and dephosphorylation.

2.4   Longer-term control of enzyme activity

2.4.1   Hormones and longer-term control of enzyme activity
The events shown in Box 2.4 involve mainly reversible phosphorylation of enzymes, changing their activity rapidly. These are mechanisms for producing rapid changes in flux. But binding of hormones to cell-surface receptors can also regulate pathways over a longer time-scale by altering the expression of genes coding for enzymes of the pathway.

2.4.1.1   Insulin and control of gene expression
Insulin controls the expression of a large number of genes; some are suppressed, some are up-regulated (expression increased). Some of the genes whose expression is altered by insulin and which produce proteins involved in energy

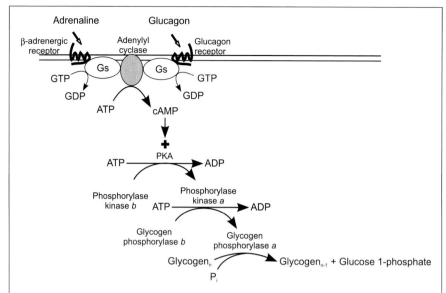

Fig. 2.4.2 Signal chain for stimulation of glycogen breakdown by adrenaline (or no-radrenaline) and glucagon. Adrenaline or glucagon bind to 7-transmembrane domain G-protein-coupled receptors in the cell membrane. These interact with stimulatory G-proteins (G$_s$) that bind GTP, and which in turn interact with and stimulate adeny-lyl cyclase. This forms cyclic adenosine 3′,5′-monophosphate (cAMP) from ATP (see Fig. 2.3.1, Box 2.3, for structure). cAMP binds to, and activates, the cAMP-dependent protein kinase, PKA. This in turn phosphorylates and activates phosphorylase kinase (in its inactive, dephosphorylated form known as phosphorylase kinase *b*; in its ac-tive, phosphorylated form known as phosphorylase kinase *a*). Phosphorylase kinase *a* in turn phosphorylates and activates glycogen phosphorylase (again, in its inactive, dephosphorylated form known as phosphorylase *b*; in its active, phosphorylated form known as phosphorylase *a*). Glycogen phosphorylase hydrolyses the α-1,4 bonds in glycogen (or strictly *phosphorylyses* them, using inorganic phosphate, P$_i$), forming glu-cose 1-phosphate. Phosphorylase kinase is a complex of four types of subunit, one of which (the δ-subunit) is calmodulin, a widespread regulatory protein that binds Ca^{2+}. This means that a rise in cytoplasmic Ca^{2+} concentration will, through activation of phosphorylase kinase, activate glycogen breakdown.   ☞

metabolism are listed in Table 2.5. The signal chains that lead from binding of insulin to alteration of gene expression are complex and will not be described here although some at least involve GSK3 (see Fig. 2.4.2 in Box 2.4). Others involve increased expression of the sterol-regulatory element binding protein (SREBP), SREBP-1c. (The SREBP system is described further below.) SREBP-1c is involved in regulation of lipogenic genes by insulin (leading to fat synthesis rather than fat oxidation).

These mechanisms are involved in adaptation to reduced or increased food intake, or a change in dietary composition, over a period of one or more days, but may play little role in the (major) changes in metabolic flux that occur after meals or during exercise.

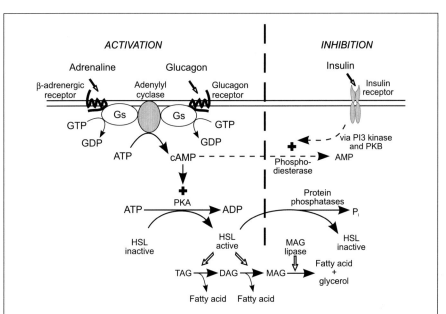

Fig. 2.4.3 Signal chain for control of hormone-sensitive lipase in adipocytes. Hormone-sensitive lipase (HSL) is the enzyme responsible for regulation of breakdown of triacylglycerol (TAG) stored in adipocytes, to deliver fatty acids to the plasma. HSL is activated by phosphorylation by PKA (see Fig. 2.4.2 for description of the early part of this signal chain). In its active state it catalyses the hydrolysis of TAG to diacylglycerol (DAG), and of DAG to monoacylglycerol (MAG), with release of two fatty acids. A constitutively active MAG lipase removes the final fatty acid. HSL is dephosphorylated and inactivated by constitutively active protein phosphatases. Insulin acts through the signal chain shown in Fig. 2.4.1 to phosphorylate and activate a phosphodiesterase that breaks down cAMP, so reducing the cellular cAMP concentration and allowing inactivation of HSL.

For more details on the components of these signal chains, see Box 2.3.

2.4.1.2   Steroid and thyroid hormones

Steroid and thyroid hormones enter cells and bind to intracellular receptors, which then migrate to the nucleus and bind directly to DNA. The hormone-receptor complexes bind to particular sequences ('response elements') in the promoter regions of the genes whose expression they regulate. Therefore these are 'longer-term' rather than rapid effects. Recently it has been recognised that some steroid hormones also have rapid effects, not mediated by alteration of gene transcription.

2.4.2   Nutrients and control of gene expression

In terms of adaptation to changes of diet, it makes sense that some nutrients themselves (or metabolic products of these nutrients) can alter gene expression. Several systems by which this occurs have been identified.

Table 2.5 Some genes involved in energy metabolism whose expression is controlled by insulin.

Increased	Comments	Suppressed	Comments
Glucose metabolism		*Glucose metabolism*	
GLUT1, 2, 3, 4	Glucose entry into the cell and glycolysis (Box 4.2)	Glucose-6-phosphatase	Gluconeogenesis‡ (Box 4.2)
Hexokinase II		Fructose-1,6 bisphosphatase	
Glucokinase (hexokinase IV) Glyceraldehyde-3-phosphate dehydrogenase		Phosphoenolpyruvate carboxykinase	
Pyruvate kinase BFE*		*Amino acid metabolism*	
		Aspartate aminotransferase	Amino acid catabolism and urea synthesis (Section 4.1.2.3 and Fig. 4.7)
		Carbamoyl phosphate synthetase I§	
De novo lipogenesis			
ATP:citrate lyase	Export of acetyl-CoA from mitochondrion (Fig. 4.6)		
Malic enzyme†			
Acetyl-CoA carboxylase	Synthesis of fatty acids from acetyl-CoA (Fig. 4.6)		
Fatty acid synthase			
Lipid metabolism			
Lipoprotein lipase	Gets fatty acids into cells		
Acyl-CoA synthase	'Activates' fatty acids		
Glycerol-3-phosphate acyltransferase	Triacylglycerol synthesis		
Transcriptional regulation SREBP-1c			

*BFE: the bifunctional enzyme 6-phosphofructo-2-kinase/fructose-2,6-bisphosphatase (see Box 4.2).

†Malic enzyme is strictly malate dehydrogenase (decarboxylating) (converts malate to pyruvate in cytoplasm: see Fig. 4.6).

‡GSK-3 is part of the signal chain (see text).

§Carbamoyl phosphate synthetase I is a key enzyme of the urea cycle (Fig. 4.7). The alternative isoform, carbamoyl phosphate synthetase II, is a cytosolic enzyme involved in purine and pyrimidine synthesis.

This list is rather selective: over 100 genes are known to be regulated by insulin.

Based on O'Brien & Granner (1991; 1996).

2.4.2.1   Carbohydrate responsive genes

The expression of some genes is increased in response to increases in carbohydrate availability. Some examples are given Table 2.6. Of course, increased carbohydrate availability also leads to higher insulin concentrations (discussed further in Chapter 5), but it has been shown with cellular preparations that the expression of some genes is increased by glucose without the need for additional insulin. It is now accepted that there are independent pathways for regulation of gene expression by insulin and glucose (Fig. 2.6). The molecular mechanism by which glucose regulates gene expression is not yet completely clear. Clearly glucose itself cannot bind to DNA. Recently a protein has been identified, known as the *carbohydrate responsive element binding protein* (ChREBP, Fig. 2.6) (other names have been used, for instance ChoRF for carbohydrate response factor). ChREBP is regulated in opposite ways by glucose and by cAMP. Phosphorylation of ChREBP by PKA (see Box 2.3 for definition) leads to inactivation. Dephosphorylation, stimulated by glucose availability, leads to activation, DNA binding and increased expression of the genes whose promoter regions contains the carbohydrate responsive element (ChRE). Glucose has to be metabolised in order to bring about these effects, and there are suggestions that the active metabolite is not glucose itself, but perhaps glucose 6-phosphate or fructose 2,6-bisphosphate. In the pancreatic β-cell, expression of the insulin gene is regulated by glucose (discussed later, Section 5.2.2). Here the immediate transcription factor is known as PDX1, and is different from ChREBP or ChRE identified in liver and other tissues. PDX1 is phosphorylated

Table 2.6 Some genes whose expression is increased by glucose (at a cellular level) or by carbohydrate availability.

Gene	Comments
Liver isoform of pyruvate kinase	Glycolysis
Acetyl-CoA carboxylase	Synthesis of fatty acids from cytosolic acetyl-CoA (see later, Box 4.3)
Fatty acid synthase	
S_{14} (or Spot 14)	Lipogenesis*
SREBP-1c	Transcriptional regulation
Insulin	(In the pancreatic β-cell)
SGLT-1	Increased by presence of glucose in the intestinal lumen
PDX1	Transcription factor in pancreatic β-cell increasing insulin gene expression

*S_{14} is believed to be involved in lipogenesis in liver and adipose tissue.

Note that the expression of several genes is increased by insulin and glucose acting in concert, and the definition of a 'glucose-regulated' gene is not always clear.

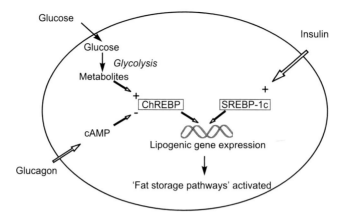

Fig. 2.6 Insulin and glucose control expression of lipogenic genes by independent routes. Insulin probably signals via increased SREBP-1c expression, glucose via a carbohydrate responsiveness element binding protein (ChREBP) (or, in the pancreatic β-cell, by a transcription factor known as PDX1). Glucagon (in the liver) may antagonise the glucose effect via cyclic AMP. There is considerable 'cross-talk' between the pathways: SREBP-1c expression is also increased by glucose; and SREBP-1c induces enzymes of glucose metabolism such as glucokinase. Based loosely on Koo *et al.* (2001) with additional information from Kawaguchi *et al.* (2001).

when glucose levels rise and moves from its location on the nuclear membrane, into the nucleus to interact with DNA. PDX1 expression is also up-regulated by glucose, giving longer-term control.

The sodium-linked glucose transporter SGLT-1 increases in activity in the small intestine when dietary carbohydrate is abundant. The mechanism seems to involve both increased gene expression and increased translation of mRNA into protein. SGLT-1 is induced by glucose within the intestinal lumen but not by a rise in blood glucose concentration.

2.4.2.2 Fatty acids and gene expression

A particular type of nuclear receptor (or transcription factor, since it regulates gene transcription) is activated by fatty acids. It was recognised as early as the 1960s that an apparently diverse group of xenobiotics (pesticides, etc.) cause the proliferation of the small, oxidative organelles called peroxisomes in rat liver. More recently these compounds have been shown to bind to a nuclear receptor, known for obvious reasons as a *peroxisome proliferator-activated receptor* (PPAR). We now know that the normal, endogenous ligands for PPARs (i.e. the substances that normally bind to and activate these receptors) are fatty acids, or compounds derived from fatty acids such as certain prostaglandins. These PPARs seem to be a way of regulating gene expression according to the availability of fatty acids. There are three major isoforms of PPAR, described in more detail in Table 2.7. The overall effect of increased fatty acid availability is that fatty acid oxidation is up-regulated in the liver through PPARα, while fatty acid storage as triacylglycerol in adipose tissue is also increased through PPARγ.

Table 2.7 Peroxisome proliferator-activated receptors (PPARs): tissue distribution and effects of activation.

Receptor	Other names	Main tissue distribution	Genes whose expression is increased by PPAR activation	Genes whose expression is suppressed by PPAR activation
PPAR-α		Liver (main site) Also kidney, heart, muscle, brown adipose tissue	Apolipoprotein AI* Apolipoprotein AII Enzymes of peroxisomal fatty acid oxidation Liver FABP CPT-1 Enzymes of mitochondrial fatty acid oxidation	Apolipoprotein CIII
PPAR-δ	PPAR-β, NUC 1, FAAR (fatty-acid activated receptor)	Widespread	Not known although HDL concentrations increase with activation	Not known
PPAR-γ1†		Widespread at low levels		
PPAR-γ2		Adipose tissue	Factors involved in adipocyte differentiation Adipose tissue FABP (also known as aP2) Lipoprotein lipase Fatty acid transport protein Acyl-CoA synthase GLUT4 Phosphoenolpyruvate carboxykinase	Leptin

CPT-1, carnitine palmitoyltransferase-1 (see Fig. 4.3); FABP, fatty acid binding protein.

*The apolipoproteins and their functions are described in Chapter 9.

†The isoforms PPARγ1 and PPAR-γ2 are produced from the same gene by use of different promoters.

Based on Gurr et al. (2002).

Not all fatty acids are equally active in activating the PPARs. Polyunsaturated fatty acids are more potent than saturated fatty acids, and amongst the former, the *n*-3 series are more potent than the *n*-6 series. This probably relates also to the marked effect of *n*-3 polyunsaturated fatty acids in lowering plasma triacylglycerol concentrations, discussed in a later chapter (see Box 9.5). Fatty acids also interact with the sterol regulatory element binding protein system described in the next section.

The PPAR system has aroused intense interest because of the potential for pharmacological manipulation. Again, in the 1960s it was observed by chance that a new pesticide was causing illness amongst farmers, and on investigation they were found to have low serum cholesterol concentrations. This led to the discovery of *clofibrate*, the first drug reliably able to lower serum cholesterol levels. Clofibrate is a peroxisome proliferator: it is a ligand for PPARα. Clofibrate turned out to have some undesirable side effects, but a group of drugs was developed from it: the *fibrates* or fibric acid derivatives. These drugs play an important role in lowering elevated serum lipid concentrations. In fact they are more potent in lowering elevated triacylglycerol concentrations than elevated cholesterol, as we might predict knowing the effects of PPARα activation. They also have beneficial effects on some proteins involved in lipid metabolism; this will be discussed in Chapter 9 (Section 9.4.3).

During the search for new agents acting like the fibrates, a group of drugs was discovered that has the effect of lowering blood glucose concentrations, apparently by improving the sensitivity of tissues to the actions of insulin. These drugs are now called the *thiazolidinediones* or '*glitazones*' and they are already in use for the treatment of diabetes. After their discovery, it was found that they are ligands for PPARγ. One possibility is that they act by increasing the ability of adipose tissue to store excess fatty acids as triacylglycerol: thus, circulating fatty acid concentrations are reduced, and tissues such as skeletal muscle are able to utilise more glucose because of reduced substrate competition.

2.4.2.3 Cholesterol and gene expression

One of the first systems to be fully understood by which nutrients or cellular constituents regulate gene expression was that for cholesterol. This will be discussed again in more detail in Chapter 9, but is covered here because the system is now recognised to have more general importance. All cells with nuclei can synthesise cholesterol from cytosolic acetyl-CoA, and can also acquire it from the plasma through a specific cell-surface receptor (the *LDL receptor*, described in detail in Chapter 9). Cells regulate their own cholesterol content by adjusting expression of the key enzymes of cholesterol synthesis, particularly the first committed step in cholesterol synthesis from cytosolic acetyl-CoA, *3-hydroxy-3-methyl-glutaryl-CoA reductase* (HMG-CoA reductase; described later, Box 4.3). Expression of the LDL receptor is also regulated in parallel. These genes were considered to have a regulatory element responsive to sterols (i.e. to cholesterol or related compounds), i.e. a *sterol regulatory element*. The sterols

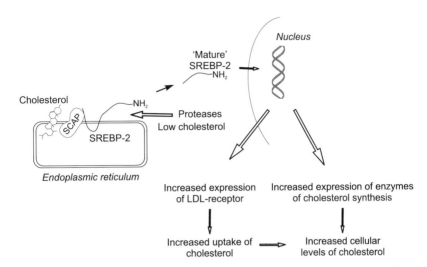

Fig. 2.7 The SREBP system. The full-length SREBP protein is located in the endoplasmic reticulum (a system of membranous cavities within the cytoplasm). It is associated with the SREBP cleavage activating protein (SCAP), which 'senses' the level of cholesterol, or related sterols, within the cell. When the cellular cholesterol content is low, specific proteases cleave SREBP to release the N-terminal portion, known as 'mature' SREBP. (Note that cholesterol does not float around in the cytosol: in fact it is associated with membranes in the cell.) Mature SREBP moves to the nucleus where it binds to sterol response elements in the promoter regions of many genes. If SREBP-2 is concerned (as shown in the figure), these are mainly genes concerned with cholesterol metabolism (LDL receptor, enzymes of cholesterol synthesis). SREBP-1 appears to be regulated more by expression of the full-length protein (which is increased by insulin in the case of SREBP-1c); proteolytic cleavage then seems to be constitutive, so the more SREBP-1 protein that is produced, the more the relevant genes are activated. These are mainly genes concerned with fat storage (including acetyl-CoA carboxylase and fatty acid synthase).

themselves do not bind to DNA, so the protein doing this was called the *sterol regulatory element binding protein* (SREBP). SREBP is synthesised initially as a protein associated with the membrane of the endoplasmic reticulum, but after proteolytic cleavage, the N-terminal portion can move to the nucleus and regulate gene expression. The system is illustrated and explained in Fig. 2.7.

There are two SREBP genes, producing SREBP-1 and SREBP-2. SREBP-2 regulates cholesterol homeostasis in the manner described above. This system has also been exploited pharmacologically, as described in Chapter 9 (Section 9.4.2.1). There are, in turn, two isoforms of SREBP-1, produced by alternative splicing of the mRNA. One in particular, SREBP-1c, seems to be intimately involved with insulin regulation of gene expression (see above), especially for genes involved in fatty acid metabolism. SREBP-1c is the main isoform expressed in liver and adipose tissue, in which fat storage (at the expense of oxidation) is likely to be an important pathway.

It is now recognised that fatty acids can also affect the SREBP system. Polyunsaturated fatty acids (but not apparently saturated fatty acids) markedly down-regulate expression of SREBP-1c. This makes sense, because increased fat availability then down-regulates the expression of lipogenic enzymes.

2.4.2.4 Amino acids and gene expression

If carbohydrates and lipids can regulate gene expression, it should not surprise us that amino acids can do the same. This is a newly emerging area of research and not much can be said definitely. Molecular mechanisms have not been elucidated. Amino acid availability can increase expression of, amongst other proteins, amino acid transporters (especially the System A transporters, see Table 2.3), and an enzyme involved in amino acid catabolism in skeletal muscle, 2-oxoacid dehydrogenase kinase (described further in Section 6.3.2.2).

2.4.2.5 Oxygen and gene expression

Oxygen is just as important for the body as are the fuels it will oxidise. It is therefore not surprising that the availability of O_2 can alter gene expression. Chronic reduction in O_2 availability (as would occur at high altitude, for example) leads to up-regulation of the expression of many genes relating to O_2 transport and energy metabolism. These include the glycoprotein hormone *erythropoietin* produced in the kidney, which stimulates erythrocyte (red blood cell) production. The glucose transporters GLUT1 and GLUT3 and enzymes of glycolysis are also up-regulated (phosphofructokinase, aldolase and lactate dehydrogenase; particular isoforms are involved in each case). The process of angiogenesis, formation of new blood vessels, is also stimulated, so that regions of tissue that are not receiving enough O_2 become better perfused. The molecular mechanisms by which this is achieved are outside the scope of this book, but there is an important transcription factor complex that is activated when O_2 availability is low, known as *hypoxia-inducible factor-1* or HIF-1.

2.5   Further reading

Membrane transporters

Palacín, M., Estévez, R., Bertran, J. & Zorzano, A. (1998) Molecular biology of mammalian plasma membrane amino acid transporters. *Physiol Rev* 78: 969–1054.

Shepherd, P.R. & Kahn, B.B. (1999) Glucose transporters and insulin action. Implications for insulin resistance and diabetes mellitus. *N Engl J Med* 341: 248–257.

Abumrad, N., Coburn, C. & Ibrahimi, A. (1999) Membrane proteins implicated in long-chain fatty acid uptake by mammalian cells: CD36, FATP and FABPm. *Biochim Biophys Acta* 1441: 4–13.

Zorzano, A., Fandos, C. & Palacín, M. (2000) Role of plasma membrane transporters in muscle metabolism. *Biochem J* 349: 667–688.

Watson, R.T. & Pessin, J.E. (2001) Intracellular organization of insulin signaling and GLUT4 translocation. *Recent Prog Horm Res* 56: 175–193.

Schmitz, G., Langmann, T. & Heimerl, S. (2001) Role of ABCG1 and other ABCG family members in lipid metabolism. *J Lipid Res* 42: 1513–1520.

(See also Further Reading in Chapter 9 for additional reviews on ABC family transporters)

Signal transduction

Cohen, P. (1999) The Croonian Lecture 1998. Identification of a protein kinase cascade of major importance in insulin signal transduction. *Philos Trans R Soc Lond B Biol Sci* 354: 485–495.

Newgard, C.B., Brady, M.J., O'Doherty, R.M. & Saltiel, A.R. (2000) Organizing glucose disposal: emerging roles of the glycogen targeting subunits of protein phosphatase-1. *Diabetes* 49: 1967–1977.

Vanhaesebroeck, B. & Alessi, D.R. (2000) The PI3K-PDK1 connection: more than just a road to PKB. *Biochem J* 346: 561–576.

Downward, J. (2001) The ins and outs of signalling. *Nature* 411: 759–762

Frame, S. & Cohen, P. (2001) GSK3 takes centre stage more than 20 years after its discovery. *Biochem J* 359: 1–16.

Vanhaesebroeck, B., Leevers, S.J., Ahmadi, K. *et al.* (2001) Synthesis and function of 3-phosphorylated inositol lipids. *Annu Rev Biochem* 70: 535–602.

Winder, W.W. (2001) Energy-sensing and signaling by AMP-activated protein kinase in skeletal muscle. *J Appl Physiol* 91: 1017–1028.

Bickel, P.E. (2002) Lipid rafts and insulin signaling. *Am J Physiol Endocrinol Metab* 282: E1–E10.

PPARs and SREBPs

Kersten, S., Desverg Kersten, S., Desvergne, B. & Wahli, W. (2000) Roles of PPARs in health and disease. *Nature* 405: 421–424.

Osborne, T.F. (2000) Sterol regulatory element-binding proteins (SREBPs): key regulators of nutritional homeostasis and insulin action. *J Biol Chem* 275: 32379–32382.

Shimano, H. (2001) Sterol regulatory element-binding proteins (SREBPs): transcriptional regulators of lipid synthetic genes. *Prog Lipid Res* 40: 439–452.

Torra, I.P., Chinetti, G., Duval, C., Fruchart, J.C. & Staels, B. (2001) Peroxisome proliferator-activated receptors: from transcriptional control to clinical practice. *Curr Opin Lipidol* 12: 245–254.

Horton, J.D., Goldstein, J.L. & Brown, M.S. (2002) SREBPs: activators of the complete program of cholesterol and fatty acid synthesis in the liver. *J Clin Invest* 109: 1125–1131.

Walczak, R. & Tontonoz, P. (2002) PPARadigms and PPARadoxes: expanding roles for PPARγ in the control of lipid metabolism. *J Lipid Res* 43: 177–186.

Nutrient and hormone control of gene expression

O'Brien, R.M. & Granner, D.K. (1996) Regulation of gene expression by insulin. *Physiol Rev* 76: 1109–1161.

Duplus, E., Glorian, M. & Forest, C. (2000) Fatty acid regulation of gene transcription. *J Biol Chem* 275: 30749–30752.

Rutter, G.A., Tavaré, J.M. & Palmer, D.G. (2000) Regulation of mammalian gene expression by glucose. *News Physiol Sci* 15: 149–154.

Sanderson, I.R. & Naik, S. (2000) Dietary regulation of intestinal gene expression. *Annu Rev Nutr* 20: 311–338.

Bruhat, A. & Fafournoux, P. (2001) Recent advances on molecular mechanisms involved in amino acid control of gene expression. *Curr Opin Clin Nutr Metab Care* 4: 439–443.

Christie, G.R., Hyde, R. & Hundal, H.S. (2001) Regulation of amino acid transporters by amino acid availability. *Curr Opin Clin Nutr Metab Care* 4: 425–431.

Ferraris, R.P. (2001) Dietary and developmental regulation of intestinal sugar transport. *Biochem J* 360: 265–276.

Semenza, G.L. (2001) Hypoxia-inducible factor 1: oxygen homeostasis and disease pathophysiology. *Trends Mol Med* 7: 345–350.

Towle, H.C. (2001) Glucose and cAMP: adversaries in the regulation of hepatic gene expression. *Proc Natl Acad Sci USA* 98: 13476–13478.

Note

1   Some biochemists distinguish carefully between metabolic *regulation*, which concerns maintaining homeostasis, and metabolic *control*, which implies altering rates of metabolic flux. The distinction is often difficult when applied to real-life situations. This book deals with many mechanisms for metabolic control, in that terminology, but their aim is almost always to bring about matching of energy supply and demand (or homeostasis, therefore regulation). I apologise here to anyone who feels I use the term 'regulation' when 'control' would be more strictly appropriate. For discussion of this, see Chapter 1 in Fell (1997).

3

Digestion and Intestinal Absorption

In a book that describes the events connecting the eating of food and the utilisation of nutrients within the body, it is necessary to look at the processes that come between food entering the mouth, and its components appearing in the bloodstream. These are the processes of digestion and intestinal absorption. The aim of this chapter is to show the relationships between food and the substrates whose metabolism will be considered in later chapters. In addition, the process of digestion illustrates some interesting examples of integration by hormones and by the nervous system. The general layout of the digestive tract is shown in Fig. 3.1, and typical amounts of the major nutrients eaten each day on a Western diet are given in Table 3.1. We shall deal here only with the macronutrients. Vitamins and minerals are also taken in with the diet, of course, but their handling is outside the scope of this book.

3.1 The strategy of digestion

3.1.1 Carbohydrate

Dietary carbohydrate may take a number of forms. In most real meals (as opposed to the pure glucose loads studied in many experimental situations) there is a mixture of simple sugars, oligosaccharides and complex carbohydrates. Of the complex carbohydrates, some will be readily digestible *starch*, composed of the straight-chain *amylose* and the branching *amylopectin*, together with very small amounts of glycogen in animal tissues. Amylose consists of long chains of glucosyl units joined by α-1,4 links; amylopectin consists of chains of α-1,4-linked glucosyl units, with α-1,6-linked branches very like glycogen (see Fig. 1.8). There are other types of starch which are resistant to digestion in the small intestine, but fully digested in the large intestine; they are referred to as

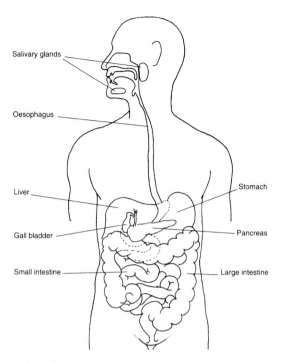

Fig. 3.1 Anatomy of the digestive tract and associated organs. Typical measurements are given in the text.

resistant starch. Their chemical structure is identical to more easily digestible starch, but the polysaccharide chains are in a semicrystalline state that makes the bonds inaccessible to the usual enzymes of starch digestion. The remaining, less digestible, carbohydrate is referred to as *non-starch polysaccharide* or more generally as *dietary fibre.* Cellulose, one of the main components of the non-starch polysaccharide fraction, consists of long β-1,4 linked chains of glucosyl units.

The digestible carbohydrates are for the most part absorbed from the small intestine in the form of monosaccharides. The strategy of the digestive process, then, is to have them in that form as they reach the small intestine. Digestion of dietary carbohydrate to monosaccharide units takes place in two stages: *luminal digestion* – digestion occurring in the intestinal lumen – and *membrane digestion*, the hydrolysis of certain small oligosaccharides by enzymes forming part of the microvillus membrane, the absorptive surface of the cells lining the small intestine.

3.1.2   Fats
The majority of dietary fat is in the form of triacylglycerol, together with some cholesterol and small amounts of other lipids such as phospholipids (Table 3.1). Fat-soluble vitamins are ingested with other foods. Some are taken in as relatively water-soluble precursors, or *provitamins*, such as carotene in carrots and

Table 3.1 Average daily intake of the macronutrients.

Nutrient	Amount per day (g)	Constituents	Percentage
Carbohydrate	300	Polysaccharides:	
		Starch	65
		Glycogen	0.5
		Disaccharides:	
		Sucrose	25
		Lactose	6
		Monosaccharides:	
		Fructose and glucose	3
Fats	100	Triacylglycerols	94
		Phospholipids	5
		Cholesterol	1
Protein	100		100

The figures apply to a typical Western diet. The figure for fat intake was correct in around 1990 but some data suggest average fat intake has declined since then. Not shown is a very variable amount of non-digestible carbohydrate (fibre), typically 10–20 g per day.

other vegetables. Others, such as vitamin D, are taken in with fatty foods and absorbed with the fat.

The digestion and absorption of fat necessitates that the fat is made accessible to the enzymes which break it down for digestion. This is achieved by emulsification – formation of microscopic droplets in which the ratio of surface area, where enzymes can act, to mass is very large. Thus, in considering the digestion and absorption of fat, we are concerned both with physico-chemical changes and with enzymatic processes.

3.1.3   Protein and amino acids

Protein in the diet may take many forms. For the most part, this makes little difference to its handling in the digestive process; proteins are hydrolysed to free amino acids and dipeptides for absorption.

3.2   Stages of digestion

3.2.1   The mouth

The process of digestion and preparation for the absorption of food may begin even before food enters the mouth. The *cephalic phase* represents the brain's anticipation of food, through the sight or smell or even thought of food; it is reinforced by the taste of food in the mouth. Cephalic stimulation of the flow of saliva occurs through activation of the parasympathetic nervous supply to the salivary glands. (The parasympathetic nervous system will be discussed in detail in Section 7.2.2.2.) Stimulation of gastric juice secretion also occurs, and there is cephalic-phase secretion of insulin, showing the control of insulin secretion by the nervous system (to be discussed in more detail later; see Section 7.4). The presence of food in the mouth stimulates nerve receptors both mechanically and chemically through taste receptors to reinforce the stimulus to saliva production.

Saliva is produced in pairs of glands which are located along the line of the jaw: the parotid, submandibular and sublingual. It is slightly buffered by its content of bicarbonate and phosphate ions, and contains a number of enzymes as well as the glycoprotein *mucin* which gives it its lubricating properties. The major enzyme in saliva is an α-*amylase* which hydrolyses α-1,4 links to begin the process of carbohydrate digestion. This is probably not extensive unless the food is chewed for an abnormal length of time before swallowing. The most important process occurring in the mouth is mechanical breakdown of the food and its hydration with saliva.

3.2.2   The stomach

3.2.2.1   General description

After swallowing, the chewed food is propelled rapidly, in a matter of seconds, through the oesophagus to enter the stomach. The stomach is a distensible muscular sac, about 25 cm long, with a volume of around 50 ml when empty, but which can expand to hold up to 1.5 litres or more. Its muscular walls are made of three layers of smooth muscle running in different directions, giving the stomach the ability to churn food around and physically break it up further and mix it with the stomach's own digestive juices.

The cells of the *epithelium* (inner lining) of the stomach produce both mucus and an alkaline, bicarbonate-containing fluid, which protect them from attack by the stomach's own acidic digestive juices. Interspersed with these cells are many millions of small holes, visible microscopically; these are the openings of the *gastric pits* or *gastric glands*. The gastric pits are lined with further epithelial, mucus-secreting cells but also contain specialised cells secreting different substances: the *parietal* or *oxyntic cells* secreting HCl (hydrochloric acid), and the *chief cells*, also known as *zymogenic* or *peptic cells*, which secrete proteins, particularly the pro-enzyme *pepsinogen*. The oxyntic cells also secrete the glycoprotein known as *intrinsic factor*, which is necessary for absorption of vitamin B12.

3.2.2.2   Regulation of digestive processes in the stomach

The theme of this book is the coordination of processes within the body, and it will not be surprising that the secretion of these various substances is not continuous in time; it is coordinated with the ingestion of food and its arrival in the stomach.

The control of acid secretion is summarised in Fig. 3.2. Secretion of HCl is stimulated by three factors acting at specific receptors on the oxyntic

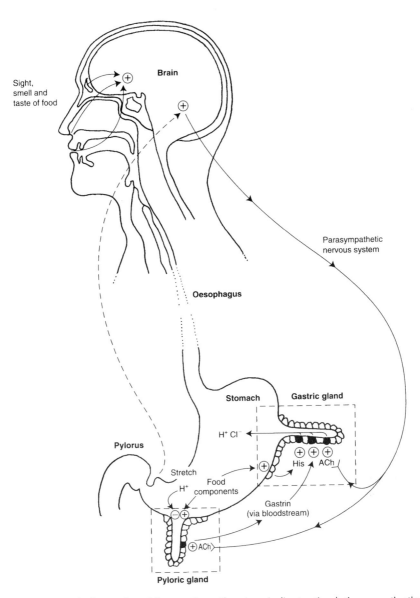

Fig. 3.2 Control of gastric acid secretion. Plus signs indicate stimulation or activation; a negative sign indicates inhibition. The gastric and pyloric glands within the dotted boxes are greatly enlarged relative to the rest of the drawing.

cells: *acetylcholine*, the parasympathetic neurotransmitter (discussed in Section 7.2.2.2); *histamine*; and the peptide hormone *gastrin*. Maximal acid production is only achieved when all three signals are present; any one of the three will only give weak stimulation of acid production.

Histamine is released from cells in the stomach wall in response to food in the stomach. It acts locally, on nearby cells; it is thus not a true hormone, but acts in a *paracrine* manner. It acts at specific receptors, known as H_2-receptors, on the oxyntic cells; drugs which block binding at these receptors, the H_2-antagonists (e.g. cimetidine, ranitidine), have found widespread use as anti-ulcer agents, since they reduce acid secretion. The parasympathetic nervous system is activated during digestion, as noted earlier, by the taste, smell and sight of food; when food enters the stomach, distension of its walls activates *stretch receptors* which send signals to the brain, which in turn causes further activation of the parasympathetic nervous system (the *vagus nerve*), and enhances acid secretion. A traditional surgical treatment for gastric ulcers (now out of fashion) was to sever the vagus nerve, thus removing one stimulus for acid secretion. When we consider later other effects of the vagus nerve (e.g. the modulation of insulin secretion) we shall see that this could have widespread, unwanted effects. In more recent years, *highly selective vagotomy* was introduced, in which only those branches innervating the stomach were cut, but even this treatment has now been superseded by the use of H_2-antagonists. Nowadays there is an even more direct treatment: drugs that bind to and inhibit the pump that extrudes H^+ ions from the oxyntic cells (proton pump inhibitors).

Gastrin, the third regulator of acid secretion, is a 17-amino acid peptide produced by *enteroendocrine* cells, which are found in gastric pits in the region of the *pylorus* – the exit from the stomach, leading to the first part of the small intestine (the *duodenum*). Gastrin is a true hormone; it is released from these cells into the bloodstream and circulates in the bloodstream. There is no apparent short cut for it, although the cells it affects are near to the cells secreting it. The release of gastrin is stimulated by a number of factors arising from the food in the stomach: some amino acids and peptides released from partially digested protein in the stomach, caffeine, calcium and alcohol. In addition, stimulation of gastrin secretion is reinforced by the parasympathetic nervous system, activated during the digestive process. Gastrin acts directly on the oxyntic cells to stimulate acid secretion. It also has other actions in the small intestine, which will be considered below.

The secretion of gastrin is inhibited by too high an acidity in the stomach; when the pH falls below about 2 (the optimum for the action of pepsin) gastrin secretion declines. This seems to be brought about by release from adjacent cells of the 14-amino acid peptide *somatostatin*. Somatostatin is a widespread inhibitor of peptide hormone secretion: it is found throughout the intestine, in the brain and in the pancreas, and, when given intravenously, will inhibit the secretion of many peptide hormones including growth hormone, gastrin, insulin and glucagon. (Its name comes from the inhibition of growth hormone, or somatotropin, secretion.) Clearly, it could have very non-specific effects if released in sufficient quantities into the circulation, and somatostatin appears, like histamine, to act locally on adjacent or nearby cells; it is a paracrine regulator of hormone secretion. Excess acidity appears to act directly to stimulate somatostatin secretion and thus inhibit gastrin release.

The inhibition of gastrin release by excess acidity is a good example of feedback inhibition brought about by a hormonal regulator. Large amounts of protein in the stomach act as a buffer, 'soaking up' excess acid, so the pH will rise and more gastrin will be released; as the pH falls below the optimum for pepsin action, gastrin release, and thus acid production, is diminished. The system maintains a relatively constant, and optimum, hydrogen ion concentration for digestion.

3.2.2.3 Digestive processes in the stomach

It is quite possible to live without a stomach (except for the need for injections of vitamin B12, which cannot be absorbed because of the lack of intrinsic factor), and yet the stomach normally plays an important role in digestion of food.

The mechanical activity of the stomach results in disruption and liquefaction of food particles. The acidity of the stomach also has an antibacterial action. But specific digestive activity also takes place here.

The acidic environment in the stomach stops the action of the salivary amylase. Nevertheless, the contractile activity of the stomach is greatest near the pylorus, and after a large meal, boluses of food which arrive from the oesophagus may remain relatively undisturbed, and salivary amylase continue to act, for up to an hour in the upper part of the stomach. It has been estimated that up to 50% of dietary starch (but usually less) may be digested by the time food leaves the stomach.

A triacylglycerol lipase is secreted from glands in the stomach (*gastric lipase*). This is an acid lipase, with a pH optimum of around 4–6, although it is still active even at a pH of 1. In other mammals a homologous lipase may be secreted higher up the gastrointestinal tract, e.g. from the serous glands of the tongue in rodents (lingual lipase). (The realisation that humans secrete a gastric lipase is relatively recent, and there are still references to human lingual lipase in the literature.) Gastric lipase may be responsible for 25% of the partial triacylglycerol hydrolysis necessary for fat absorption. In addition, its action seems to 'prepare' fat droplets for the action of pancreatic lipase in the small intestine.

Most proteins are denatured (that is, their quaternary, tertiary and secondary structures are lost) in an acidic environment. (Adding lemon juice to milk or egg white will 'curdle' it.) This makes the peptide chains more accessible to proteolytic enzymes, which break the peptide bonds linking the amino acids. The proteolytic enzyme produced by the chief or zymogenic cells is *pepsin*. This is released, as with all extracellular proteolytic enzymes, as an inactive precursor, *pepsinogen*. It is activated by hydrolysis, catalysed by hydrogen ions, of a single peptide bond, releasing a 42-amino acid peptide and the active enzyme. Pepsin has a very acidic pH optimum, around 2. It acts preferentially on peptide bonds in the middle of peptide chains (i.e. it is an *endopeptidase*), to the C-terminal side of aromatic amino acids. Thus, proteins are broken down into shorter chains.

Little absorption into the bloodstream occurs from the stomach: ethanol and some lipid-soluble drugs are absorbed, but not the normal dietary constituents. The stomach is primarily an organ of mechanical digestion, comparable to a food liquidiser. By the rhythmic contractions of the lower part of the stomach, the food is pounded into a creamy mixture known as *chyme*. Entry to the duodenum is regulated by a circular muscle, the *pyloric sphincter.* It opens at regular intervals (about twice each minute) and about 3 ml of chyme is squirted into the duodenum. The pyloric sphincter only opens partially, so that large particles are retained for further pummelling. Thus, a creamy acidic mixture of lightly digested starch, partially digested protein and coarsely emulsified fat enters the duodenum.

3.2.3   The small intestine

3.2.3.1   General description

The small intestine is often said to be about 6 m (20 feet) long and about 2.5 cm (one inch) in diameter. This is a generalisation and its length actually differs in life and after death; in life, it is somewhat contracted by virtue of the 'tone' of its muscular walls. Measurements made by passing tubes through the small intestine in adult, living humans show the length to vary between about 3 and 4.5 m. Of this, the first 25 cm (or so) is the *duodenum*, curving downwards after leaving the stomach and running roughly horizontally across the middle of the abdomen. (It gets its name from the Latin *duodecim* for 12, because it is about 12 inches or 12 finger-breadths long.) The *jejunum* begins after a sharp downward bend; it accounts for around another 2 m, and is the site of much of the absorption of the macronutrients. Finally, the *ileum*, about 2.5–3 m in length, leads to the large intestine at the ileo-caecal valve.

Two important glands discharge into the small intestine. The *gall bladder,* the storage reservoir for bile salts produced in the liver, discharges its contents via the *common bile duct*, and the exocrine part of the pancreas releases its secretions through the *pancreatic duct*; the common bile duct joins this, and they both discharge into the duodenum. The regulation, and the content, of their secretions will be covered in detail below.

The small intestine, like all parts of the intestine, has layers of smooth muscle running lengthways and around its circumference. The inner surface, or mucosal layer, is folded into finger-like projections (*villi*), each villus being about 1 mm long. There are 20–40 villi per mm². This enormously increases the surface area, to a total of about 300 m²; this surface area is where absorption takes place. The surface area is increased still further by the presence of the *brush border.* Each cell making up the surface of a villus has its own microscopic finger-like projections, the *microvilli*, giving under the electron microscope a brush-like appearance. There are around 2000–4000 microvilli per cell. The presence of the microvilli increases the surface area about a further thirty-fold.

Each villus has a characteristic structure (Fig. 3.3). Within its core there is a dense network of capillaries surrounding a channel (the *lacteal*), which is a branch of the lymphatic system. (The name, from the latin *lactis*, means related to milk, because the products of fat absorption give these vessels a milky appearance.) The venous blood vessels leaving the intestinal mucosa merge and eventually form the hepatic portal vein. The lymphatic vessels also merge and

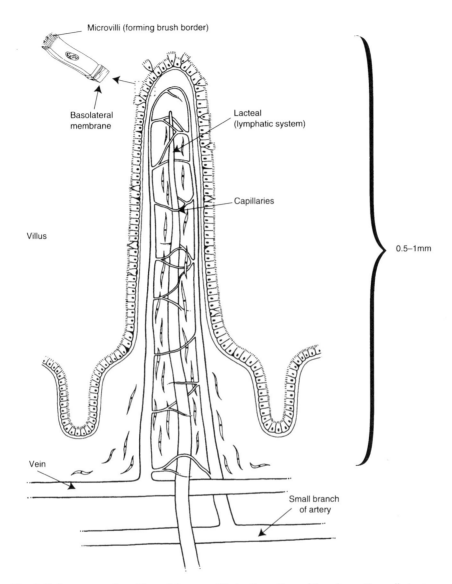

Microvilli (forming brush border)

Basolateral
membrane

Villus

Lacteal
(lymphatic system)

Capillaries

0.5–1mm

Vein

Small branch
of artery

Fig. 3.3 Structure of a villus of the small intestine. One of the absorptive cells (entero-cytes) on the surface is enlarged to illustrate the *microvilli* of the brush-border membrane.

form one single vessel, the *thoracic duct* (see Section 1.3.3), so called because it leads upwards through the thorax (chest), and finally discharges its contents into the great veins in the neck, near where they return to the heart (Fig. 3.4).

There are four important sources of digestive agents in the small intestine: the gall bladder, which provides the bile salts necessary for emulsification of fat; the exocrine pancreas, which provides bicarbonate to neutralise the acidic chyme entering through the pylorus, and a mixture of digestive enzymes; secretory cells in glands located throughout the small intestinal wall which produce an isotonic, neutral, mucus-containing juice; and the brush border membrane,

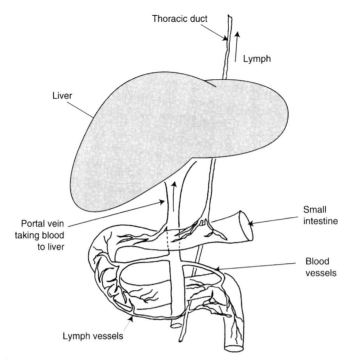

Fig. 3.4 Vessels carrying the products of digestion away from the small intestine.
Substances entering the bloodstream reach the hepatic portal vein, and are thus carried to
the liver. The products of fat digestion are carried in the vessels of the lymphatic system.

in which are incorporated several digestive enzymes. These, and the other digestive juices, are summarised in Table 3.2.

3.2.3.2 Regulation of digestive processes in the small intestine

The efficiency of digestion and absorption is very high. Usually the energy we
excrete in faeces represents only about 5% of the energy we ingest, and even
then much of the weight of faeces consists of bacteria from the colon together
with material that we are unable to digest. Maintaining this efficiency requires
control mechanisms. For instance, if the contents of a meal were to pass too
rapidly through the gastrointestinal tract, there would not be sufficient time for
digestive enzymes to act and for absorption to take place. These control mechanisms, in general, respond to the presence of food (or its components) at various
points in the gastrointestinal tract and regulate movement of further food along
the tract; they also control the production of digestive juices.

The presence of chyme in the duodenum activates receptors in its walls via
both stretch and chemical effects. These receptors trigger the *enterogastric
reflex*, in which the brain reduces parasympathetic activity (one of the main
stimulants of gastric secretion and gastric contraction) and increases sympathetic nervous stimulation of the pyloric sphincter, which causes it to contract;
these effects combine to retain food in the stomach and reduce the loading

Table 3.2 Digestive enzymes and juices.

Source	Enzyme/juice	Function
Mouth		
– Salivary glands	α-Amylase	Initial digestion of starch
Stomach		
– Gastric glands	HCl	Denaturation/swelling of proteins; acidification for pepsin action; antibacterial; activation of pepsinogen
	Pepsin (secreted as pepsinogen)	Initial digestion of proteins
	Gastric lipase	Lipid hydrolysis in stomach
Small intestine and associated organs		
– Small intestinal wall	*Succus entericus* (intestinal juice)	Dilution, lubrication
– Gall bladder	Bile	Neutralisation of acidic chyme
	Bile salts	Emulsification of fats
– Exocrine pancreas	Pancreatic juice	Neutralisation of acidic chyme
	Proteases: trypsin (secreted as trypsinogen); chymotrypsin (secreted as chymotrypsinogen); carboxypeptidases A,B (secreted as procarboxypeptidase)	Digestion of protein to oligopeptides and free amino acids
	Pancreatic lipase	Triacylglycerol hydrolysis
– Brush border membrane	Disaccharidases (more detail in Table 3.3)	Disaccharide hydrolysis
	Peptidases	Hydrolysis of peptides to di- and tripeptides

of the small intestine until it is ready for more. Acidity in the duodenum also causes the secretion of *secretin*, a 27-amino acid peptide, into the bloodstream from cells in the duodenal and jejunal mucosa. Secretin was the first hormone to be discovered, by the English physiologist W.M. Bayliss and the physician E.H. Starling in 1902. (Gastrin was the second, in 1905, by J.S. Edkins in London.) Secretin gets its name from its effects on pancreatic secretion (see below), but it has an additional effect in inhibiting gastric contractions and secretion; these effects are reinforced by other hormones, *cholecystokinin* and *gastric inhibitory peptide*, both also secreted in response to distension of the duodenum and the presence of acidic chyme. This is another example of negative feedback: the entry of chyme into the duodenum is inhibited as it accumulates there.

Two of these hormones, secretin and cholecystokinin, also have important effects on digestive enzyme secretion. Secretin stimulates the exocrine pancreas to produce a fluid which is high in bicarbonate (and is thus alkaline, to neutralise the acidic chyme) but relatively low in enzyme content. Cholecystokinin stimulates the exocrine pancreas to produce a digestive juice which is relatively lower in bicarbonate but higher in enzyme content. The name cholecystokinin, however, relates to its effect on the gall bladder: it causes the gall bladder to contract, releasing its contents via the common bile duct into the duodenum. (At one time there were thought to be two separate hormones, known as *pancreozymin*, responsible for stimulation of pancreatic juice secretion, and *cholecystokinin*, acting on the gall bladder. Now they are known to be one and the same.) Thus, the arrival of chyme in the duodenum causes the secretion of digestive juices via the release of these two hormones: this is a further example of the role of hormones in integrating events within the body. The role of hormones in integration of digestion is illustrated in Fig. 3.5.

In addition, gastrointestinal hormones modulate the secretion of other hormones, particularly of insulin secretion from the pancreas. This means that

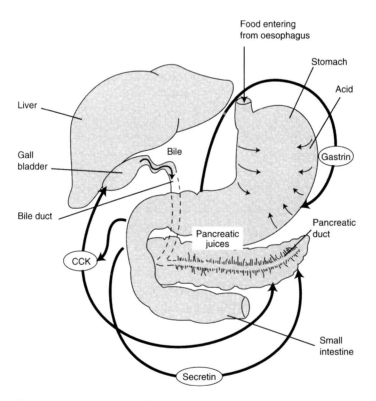

Fig. 3.5 Hormonal regulation of the secretion of digestive juices. Gastrin stimulates hydrochloric acid secretion by the oxyntic cells in the gastric glands. Secretin and cholecystokinin (CCK) promote the secretion of pancreatic juices. CCK also causes the gall bladder to contract, releasing bile into the duodenum.

the arrival of food in the gastrointestinal tract will amplify the secretion of insulin that is otherwise stimulated by a rise in the blood glucose concentration. This aspect of gastrointestinal hormone action will be considered more fully in Chapter 5 (Section 5.7).

And yet further, cholecystokinin, in particular, may have a role in regulation of food intake. The suggestion has been made that cholecystokinin, released in response to food in the intestine, can signal to the brain to induce satiety, the feeling that leads to termination of a meal. The same effect has also been attributed to apolipoprotein-AIV, a protein produced by small-intestinal enterocytes and secreted with chylomicron particles. The role of apolipoprotein-AIV in lipid metabolism is not clear, and it may be that its real role is to signal to the brain that fat is being processed in the small intestine and it's time to stop eating. There is also a recently discovered peptide secreted from the stomach, ghrelin, that may play the opposite role: ghrelin secretion falls after meals and rises during fasting and it seems to stimulate appetite. These and other mechanisms for induction of hunger and satiety will be discussed in Chapter 11 (see Box 11.1).

Although most lipid absorption occurs in the jejunum (see below), some lipids may reach the later part of the small intestine, the ileum. Here a further mechanism is activated. Lipids in the ileum slow the transit of material through the earlier parts of the small intestine. This is referred to as the 'ileal brake'. The mechanism may involve a peptide known as peptide-YY (Y here is the single letter code for the amino acid tyrosine) which can act as both neurotransmitter and hormone.

3.2.3.3   Digestive processes occurring in the small intestine
The pancreatic juice contains amylases (for hydrolysis of starch), proteases and a lipase; thus, it plays a major role in luminal digestion of each of the macronutrients.

Starch digestion
The pancreatic juice contains two *α-amylases* – i.e. enzymes which hydrolyse the α-1,4 glycosidic bonds in starch. Their pH optimum is around 7.0, which is the pH of the small intestinal contents after the bicarbonate-containing pancreatic juice has neutralised its acidity. These enzymes will not hydrolyse the α-1,6 branch-point in the amylopectin molecule, nor α-1,4 links within two glucosyl units after a branch, so that α-*limit dextrins*, small oligosaccharides containing the α-1,6 link, are produced, along with tri- and disaccharides such as maltotriose and maltose (three and two α-1,4 linked glucosyl units respectively). These products, along with other disaccharides ingested in the food (such as sucrose and lactose), are then hydrolysed by the enzymes associated with the microvillus membrane of the absorptive cells. There are four different enzymes, which hydrolyse the various remaining bonds (including the α-1,2 linkage in sucrose), to liberate free monosaccharides (Table 3.3).

Table 3.3 Small intestinal brush-border disaccharidases.

Enzyme	Hydrolyses	Absorption of product
Sucrase/isomaltase	Glucose α1-β2 fructose bond in sucrose (see Fig. 1.7); α1,6 bonds in α-limit dextrins	Glucose: SGLT-1 Fructose: GLUT5
Maltase/glucoamylase	α1-4 bonds in maltose and isomaltose	Glucose: SGLT-1
Lactase	β1-4 bonds in lactose	Glucose: SGLT-1 Galactose: SGLT-1
Trehalase	α1-1α bonds in trehalose	Glucose: SGLT-1

For more on disaccharides see Section 1.2.2.1 and text around this table.

Trehalose is D-glucose α1-1α-D-glucose and is a disaccharide found in mushrooms and in insects (in insects, it replaces glucose as the main blood sugar).

Protein digestion

The pancreatic juice contains a number of enzymes with proteolytic activity. The most important of these are secreted as *pro-enzymes* or *zymogens* which are activated by proteolysis in the intestinal lumen, presumably to protect the pancreas from digesting itself. These proteases are *trypsin* (secreted as trypsinogen), *chymotrypsin* (secreted as chymotrypsinogen) and *carboxypeptidases* (the precursor procarboxypeptidase is activated to produce carboxypeptidases A and B). The enzyme trypsin is derived from trypsinogen by the action of an 'enterokinase' associated with the brush border membrane; trypsin then catalyses the activation of the other zymogens. Each of these enzymes has its own characteristic specificity for peptide bonds, but the net result of their combined action is the liberation of some free amino acids and a mixture of oligopeptides. These may be further hydrolysed by membrane-bound enzymes to tri- and dipeptides and amino acids for absorption.

Fat digestion

This is the most complex process because, as mentioned earlier, it involves both physico-chemical and enzymatic processes. Fat digestion and absorption depend upon emulsification of triacylglycerol, and finally formation of particles even smaller than those typical of emulsions, known as micelles. The main emulsifying agents are the *bile salts*, amphipathic molecules secreted in the bile (Box 3.1). As fat digestion proceeds, so further amphipathic molecules are formed which may help in emulsification; these include monoacylglycerols and phospholipids, particularly lysolecithin. Emulsification is brought about by the non-polar tails of the amphipathic molecules stabilising small groups of non-polar molecules, predominantly triacylglycerol and a smaller amount of cholesterol; their polar aspects face outwards to the aqueous intestinal contents. A net repulsive action of the outward facing polar groups also tends to further split the lipid droplets, resulting in a finer and finer emulsion. These emulsified particles are typically 1 μm in diameter. It is in this form that most of the hydrolysis of triacylglycerols proceeds.

Pancreatic lipase is a member of a family of lipases which includes lipo-protein lipase, an important enzyme in fat metabolism to be discussed in later chapters. These enzymes act on the ester links in the terminal (1,3) positions in an acylglycerol, but not the central fatty acid (2-position). Thus, fatty acids are liberated and 2-monoacylglycerols remain. Both fatty acids and mono-acylglycerols have amphipathic properties. Monoacylglycerols are effective emulsifying agents and aid the action of the bile salts, as noted above. Gradu-ally, much smaller groups of molecules are formed, the *mixed micelles* – mixed because they contain both bile salts (which can themselves form micelles) and other molecules, particularly fatty acids and monoacylglycerols. These micelles have a diameter of 4–6 nm, so small that they do not scatter light and produce an almost clear solution. They are able to move readily through the aqueous intestinal contents, and thus bring the products of triacylglycerol hydrolysis, fatty acids and monoacylglycerols, to the surface of the absorptive cells. Lipid digestion in the small intestine is summarised in Fig. 3.6.

The action of pancreatic lipase can be potently inhibited by a bacterial product called tetrahydrolipstatin (generic drug name orlistat). Orlistat is now available as a treatment for obesity: by preventing up to 30% of dietary fat digestion, nutrient (hence energy) absorption is decreased (discussed again in Section 11.5.2).

Other forms of lipid in the diet – phospholipids and cholesterol esters – are also hydrolysed by pancreatic and other lipases, and the products (fatty acids, monoacylglycerols and free cholesterol) are also incorporated into the mixed micelles.

3.3   Absorption from the small intestine

3.3.1   Monosaccharides

The hydrolysis of the digestible carbohydrates proceeds to the stage of mon-osaccharides, some of which are liberated by the enzymes of the brush border membrane. These must then enter the *enterocytes*, the absorptive cells of the intestinal mucosa. Mechanisms by which sugars cross cell membranes were summarised in Box 2.2. The role of the various monosaccharide transporters in carbohydrate absorption is summarised in Fig. 3.7. Glucose and galactose enter by active transport mediated by the sodium-glucose cotransporter SGLT-1; i.e. these sugar molecules may be absorbed against a concentration gradient (see Box 2.1). During the active phase of digestion, it is likely that the local concentration of free glucose or galactose on the luminal surface of the brush border membrane is so high that this is unnecessary, but during the early and late phases of digestion active transport ensures complete capture of almost all the intestinal sugar molecules. Energy is provided by a concentration gradient

Box 3.1   The bile acids and salts

These are derivatives of cholesterol (see Fig. 1.6), synthesised in the liver. A typical bile acid is shown. This is *cholic acid. Chenodeoxycholic acid* lacks the hydroxyl group at carbon 12. They are secreted in the bile in the form of covalent conjugates, formed with a base: either glycine as shown here, or taurine ($^+H_3NCH_2CH_2SO_3^-$). The conjugate shown is sometimes known as *glycocholate*. They are amphipathic molecules, with a predominantly non-polar ring structure but a highly polar acidic group (especially in the conjugated form).

The first committed step in bile acid synthesis from cholesterol is hydroxylation of carbon 7 (marked on figure). This is brought about by an enzyme formerly known as cholesterol 7-α hydroxylase. This enzyme, like many involved in hydroxylation reactions, is a member of a large family of haem proteins that has the characteristic (when it has bound CO) of absorbing light at a wavelength of 450 nm, known generally as cytochrome P-450. Because of this, it now has the 'family name' CYP7A1. CYP7A1 expression is controlled primarily at the transcriptional level by the relative levels of cholesterol and bile acids in the hepatocyte, through a nuclear receptor/transcription factor known as LXR (liver X-receptor).

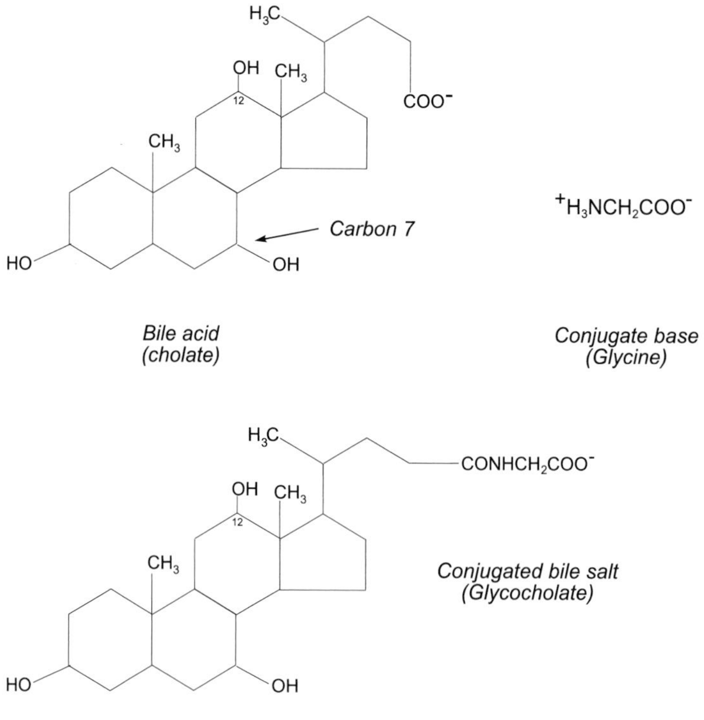

Bile acid
(cholate)

Carbon 7

$^+H_3NCH_2COO^-$

Conjugate base
(Glycine)

Conjugated bile salt
(Glycocholate)

—CONHCH$_2$COO$^-$

Fig. 3.1.1

The bile salts are not absorbed with the contents of the mixed micelles. Instead, they are absorbed from the terminal part of the ileum by an energy-requiring process. They then enter the portal vein and are re-utilised in the liver. This 'salvaging' of the bile acids is known as the *enterohepatic circulation*. Bile salts returning to the liver repress the conversion of further cholesterol to bile acids via LXR as described above.

If the reabsorption of bile salts is interrupted, they are excreted, after some bacterial modification, in the faeces. The consequence is that CYP7A1 expression is up-regulated and more cholesterol is converted to bile acids in the liver, depleting the body's cholesterol pool. The usefulness of this as a treatment for lowering of the serum cholesterol concentration will be discussed further in Chapter 9 (Box 9.4).

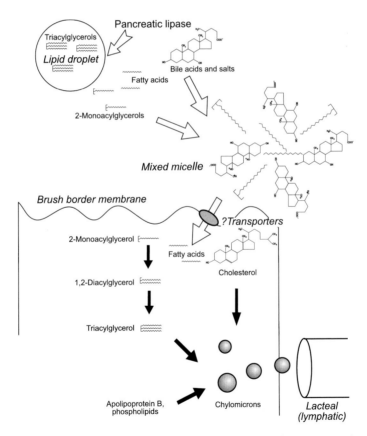

Fig. 3.6 Lipid digestion and absorption in the small intestine. Fatty acids probably enter the mucosal cells by facilitated diffusion (see Section 2.2.1.3). Within the mucosal cells, 2-monoacylglycerol and fatty acids are re-esterified largely by the monoacylglycerol pathway (see Fig. 3.8, later) and packaged into chylomicrons. Cholesterol absorption is not shown for simplicity; it is described in the text of this chapter and also in Section 2.2.1.4.

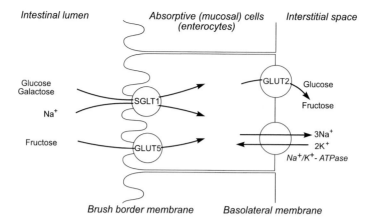

Fig. 3.7 Absorption of monosaccharides from the intestine. Monosaccharides enter the enterocytes across the brush border or *apical* membrane and leave the cell by the basolateral membrane using specific transporter proteins. Based on Thorens (1993); Wright (1993).

of sodium ions across the membrane, maintained in turn by the Na^+-K^+-ATPase (Fig. 3.7). Fructose, in contrast, is taken up into the mucosal cells by facilitated diffusion by the fructose transporter GLUT5.

The expression of these transporters is regulated by the availability of dietary carbohydrate. SGLT-1 expression is increased by glucose availability in the small intestinal lumen (see Table 2.6). Fructose availability is a specific signal increasing expression of GLUT5.

From within the mucosal cells, the sugars enter the capillaries that form a dense network within each villus (see Fig. 3.3). They must first cross the cell membrane at the 'back end' of the cell – the *basolateral membrane* (Fig. 3.7), to enter first the interstitial space and then the blood in the vessels draining the small intestine towards the portal vein. This basolateral transport is by facilitated diffusion mediated by GLUT2, which will transport both glucose and fructose. Active transport of sugar into the cell from the intestinal lumen must raise its intracellular concentration to the extent that it will move out, into the interstitial space, down a concentration gradient. Thus, carbohydrate from the diet appears ultimately in the form of monosaccharides in the blood in the hepatic portal vein.

However, not all of the sugars absorbed are liberated into the bloodstream in this way. Some are metabolised by the cells of the intestinal mucosa, which require a constant supply of ATP for maintenance of the sodium gradient. At least a proportion of the glucose used by these cells for ATP generation is metabolised to lactate, again released into the portal vein. The amount of absorbed carbohydrate which is converted to lactate in this way is presently unknown (and very difficult to estimate). The relevance of this pathway of lactate production will be considered again in Section 4.1.2.1.

3.3.2   Amino acids and peptides

The products of protein digestion are absorbed into the intestinal epithelial cells in two ways: absorption of free amino acids, by certain specific carriers, and absorption of di- and tripeptides.

Amino acids are mostly actively transported by sodium-linked carriers that were described in Table 2.3. Again, therefore, energy is required to pump the sodium ions out and maintain their concentration gradient. Amino acids thus enter the epithelial cells and eventually the capillaries of the intestinal mucosa. Like glucose, however, they may not escape some metabolism during their passage through the intestinal absorptive cells. Some amino acids are oxidised very effectively to provide energy for the intestinal cells, in particular glutamine, glutamate and aspartate. Glutamine is actually extracted from the blood flowing through the intestinal wall, and oxidised. Thus, as in the case of glucose, the energy required for active absorption of the amino acids is provided to some extent by oxidation of the molecules absorbed.

Some di- and tripeptides are absorbed intact by transporters known as PEPT1 and PEPT2, which are also expressed in renal tubules. It has been suggested that peptide uptake is more important quantitatively than uptake of free amino acids. Transport is hydrogen ion-linked, so is down a hydrogen ion gradient (or up a pH gradient). Cellular pH is maintained by a family of hydrogen ion transporters, in which hydrogen ion transport is coupled with movement of cations (e.g. the sodium-hydrogen cotransporter).

3.3.3   Lipid absorption

It is likely that fatty acid absorption is mediated to a major extent by facilitated transport by FAT and FATP (see Table 2.4). Monoacylglycerol uptake may occur by the same mechanism although it is easy to see that passive diffusion across the membrane would also be possible. Once inside the cell, the fatty acids are bound by a specific *fatty acid binding protein* which may aid or direct movement through the cytosol.

Within the enterocytes, fatty acids and monoacylglycerols are re-esterified to form new triacylglycerol molecules. This occurs mainly by the *monoacylglycerol esterification pathway* beginning with monoacylglycerol (Fig. 3.8), unlike most other tissues in which the formation of triacylglycerols occurs by the *phosphatidic acid pathway*, building upon glycerol 3-phosphate (Fig. 3.8).

The triacylglycerols are packaged with phospholipids and proteins, particularly the protein called *apolipoprotein B*, discussed more in Chapter 9 (Box 9.1). They form particles of around 100 nm to 1 μm diameter, the *chylomicrons*. The chylomicrons are the largest of the lipoprotein particles present in blood. They leave the absorptive cells and pass into the lacteals (Fig. 3.6). From there they flow slowly into more major branches of the lymphatic system, up the thoracic duct and thence into the circulation. Because the diameter of chylomicrons is of the same order as the wavelength of visible light, they scatter light, resulting in a turbid or milky appearance. Hence the name *lacteal*,

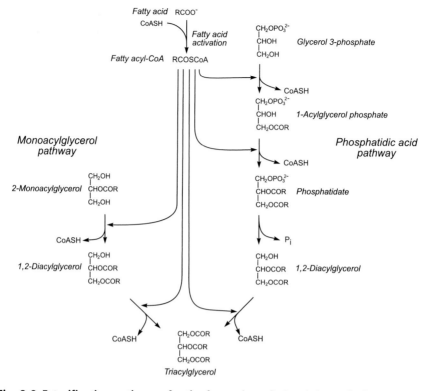

Fig. 3.8 Esterification pathways for the formation of triacylglycerol. The monoacyl-glycerol pathway is prevalent in enterocytes, the phosphatidic acid pathway in other tissues. Chemical structures are detailed in Fig. 1.4. CoASH, coenzyme-A; P_i inorganic phosphate; R represents the fatty acid hydrocarbon chain.

mentioned earlier. As chylomicrons enter the plasma they give it, too, a milky appearance; it is easy to see from visual inspection of the plasma whether someone has recently eaten a fatty meal.

Not all fatty acids are re-esterified to form triacylglycerol. Those with a shorter chain length, below 12–14 carbons, are not good substrates for esterification, because the specific medium-chain acyl-CoA synthase required for their activation is not present. They enter the capillary plasma directly in the form of non-esterified fatty acids. However, except when the diet contains a large amount of dairy produce, rich in short- and medium-chain fatty acids, most of the dietary fatty acids are long-chain (16 carbons upwards) and enter the bloodstream as chylomicron-triacylglycerol.

We also eat a certain amount of cholesterol (Table 3.1). This becomes incorporated into the mixed micelles (Fig. 3.6). About half ultimately enters the absorptive cells. It seems that cholesterol is actively re-exported from the enterocytes to maintain cholesterol homeostasis, by the transporter ABC-A1 (Section 2.2.1.4). This process also excludes plant- and fish-derived cholesterol-like substances in food (the transporters ABC-G5 and -G8 are involved, also discussed in Section 2.2.1.4). The remainder of cholesterol is lost in the faeces. The selectivity of cholesterol absorption is being exploited by the food industry. Some plant-derived cholesterol-like compounds such as phytosterols and phytostanols actually inhibit cholesterol absorption, presumably by competing for, and in some way blocking, the transporters. Margarines containing these compounds are therefore being promoted for their cholesterol-lowering properties.

Within the absorptive cells, some of the cholesterol is esterified with long-chain fatty acids by the action of the enzyme *acyl-CoA-cholesterol acyl transferase*, to form hydrophobic cholesteryl esters. Both cholesterol and cholesteryl esters are incorporated into the chylomicron particles and thus enter the bloodstream via the lymphatics.

3.3.4   Other processes occurring in the small intestine

Most of the absorption of sugars, amino acids and peptides, and fatty acids and monoacylglycerols is completed during passage through the duodenum and jejunum. In the ileum some further specific compounds are absorbed, particularly vitamin B12 and the bile salts (left behind when other components of the mixed micelles were taken up higher in the small intestine – Box 3.1). The reabsorption of bile salts has important implications for the whole-body store of cholesterol, and will be considered again in Chapter 9 (Box 9.4).

3.4   The large intestine

The large intestine is about 1.5 m in length, and extends from the end of the ileum, the *ileo-caecal valve*, to the anus. It contains, on average, over 200 g of material (water, bacteria, residual food particles, shed epithelial cells and mucus) at any one time. An important function of the large intestine is the absorption of water, but it is also the site of considerable bacterial activity on the carbohydrate that has escaped digestion in the small intestine. This process makes available some of the energy that would otherwise have been lost from the body. Bacterial breakdown, or *fermentation*, of dietary material also provides faecal bulk (most of the weight of faeces is bacteria from the colon) which assists intestinal transit, and has important effects on the colonic cells themselves. It has been estimated that this 'colonic salvage' (of energy-providing material that would otherwise be lost) may contribute 5% of basal energy requirements.

Carbohydrates such as cellulose, which are not susceptible to degradation by mammalian digestive enzymes, and resistant starch that was not accessible to these enzymes, are (at least partially) broken down by enzymes secreted by the resident bacteria of the colon. Amongst the products of this breakdown are short-chain fatty acids, also known as volatile fatty acids, such as acetate (two-carbon carboxylic acid), propionate (three carbons) and butyrate (four carbons). These short-chain fatty acids are absorbed by the epithelial cells of the large intestine. Acetate enters the bloodstream and can be converted to acetyl-CoA in the liver and other tissues, thus serving as a precursor for lipogenesis (fat synthesis) or as a substrate for oxidation. Propionate enters the portal vein and is almost entirely extracted by the liver for oxidation. Butyrate is mostly used as a fuel by the large-intestinal cells (often called *colonocytes*) themselves and little enters the bloodstream. The short-chain fatty acids are essential for the well-being of the large intestine. There is considerable evidence that the short-chain fatty acids, butyrate in particular, protect the colon against cancer development. This may be one reason for the strong protective effect of fruit and vegetable intake against colon cancer.

Because of these beneficial properties of colonic fermentation, products have been developed that will encourage this process. These are known as prebiotics and probiotics. Prebiotics are carbohydrates that will largely escape small-intestinal digestion, for instance polysaccharides composed of fructose units (called inulin or fructo-oligosaccharides). By reaching the large intestine they stimulate bacterial activity. Probiotics are the bacteria themselves, usually in the form of 'live yoghurts'. A proportion of these will escape death in the acidity of the stomach and will colonise the colon. These dietary supplements, or 'functional foods', may have beneficial effects on health for the reasons given above.

There is a further form of colonic salvage. Urea, produced in hepatic amino acid metabolism (discussed later, Section 4.1.2.3), can enter the colon from the bloodstream via a specific urea transporter. Within the colon, bacteria may split this urea to release ammonia, and that ammonia, together with some amino acids produced by the bacteria, may be reabsorbed. Ammonia can be used within tissues for amino acid formation (discussed later; see Section 6.3.2.3). It is believed that in some way this 'urea salvage' pathway is up-regulated when dietary protein is restricted, thus conserving nitrogen that would otherwise be excreted in urine.

3.5   Further reading

Digestion and absorption and their control

Lentze, M.J. (1995) Molecular and cellular aspects of hydrolysis and absorption. *Am J Clin Nutr* 61: 946S–951S.

Gudmand Høyer, E. & Skovbjerg, H. (1996) Disaccharide digestion and maldigestion. *Scand J Gastroenterol* 31 Suppl 216: 111–121.

Kunze, W.A. & Furness, J.B. (1999) The enteric nervous system and regulation of intestinal motility. *Annu Rev Physiol* 61: 117–142.

Nutting, D.F., Kumar, N.S., St Hilaire, R.J. & Mansbach, C.M. (1999) Nutrient absorption. *Curr Opin Clin Nutr Metab Care* 2: 413–419.

Chawla, A., Saez, E. & Evans, R.M. (2000) 'Don't know much bile-ology'. *Cell* 103: 1–4.

Edwards, P.A., Kast, H.R. & Anisfeld, A.M. (2002) BAREing it all: the adoption of LXR and FXR and their roles in lipid homeostasis. *J Lipid Res* 43: 2–12.

Intestinal endocrinology

Sachs, G., Zeng, N. & Prinz, C. (1997) Physiology of isolated gastric endocrine cells. *Annu Rev Physiol* 59: 243–256.

Rehfeld, J.F. (1998) The new biology of gastrointestinal hormones. *Physiol Rev* 78: 1087–1108.

Dockray, G.J., Varro, A., Dimaline, R. & Wang, T. (2001) The gastrins: their production and biological activities. *Annu Rev Physiol* 63: 119–139.

Drucker, D.J. (2001) Minireview: the glucagon-like peptides. *Endocrinology* 142: 521–527.

Colon

Topping, D.L. & Clifton, P.M. (2001) Short-chain fatty acids and human colonic function: roles of resistant starch and nonstarch polysaccharides. *Physiol Rev* 81: 1031–1064.

4

Organs and Tissues

The aim of this book is to show how the major metabolic pathways are regulated and how they interrelate in the whole body, rather than to provide a detailed description of each pathway. In this chapter we shall look at the specific features of metabolism in different tissues. This will enable us to integrate them more easily in later chapters.

The distinction between an organ and a tissue is not absolute. Either may be composed of more than one cell type. For instance, the kidney is composed of two distinctive tissue types, the *cortex* and *medulla*, and each of these in turn is composed of various types of cell. The most important tissues in metabolism, such as skeletal muscle and adipose tissue, are arranged in fairly discrete groups, and under many circumstances all of one type of tissue in the body behaves in a broadly similar manner: thus, adipose tissue throughout the body is sometimes referred to as the adipose organ. In this chapter some of the major organs and tissues involved in the utilisation and interconversion of substrates for cellular energy generation – energy metabolism – will be described. Some emphasis will be given to the way in which the various organs and tissues are interconnected by blood vessels, since this is essential to a full understanding of the way in which they interact metabolically.

4.1   The liver

4.1.1   General description of the liver and its anatomy

The word 'liver' seems to come from old Norse, *lifr*. The adjective 'hepatic', describing things to do with the liver, comes from the Greek *hepatos*. The adult human liver weighs 1–1.5 kg and lies immediately under the diaphragm. It is supplied with blood from below through two major vessels: the *hepatic artery* (which supplies about 20% of the blood) and the *hepatic portal vein*, often called simply the *portal vein*. The portal vein carries blood which has passed through the complex system of blood vessels around the intestinal tract (see Fig. 3.4). This unusual feature – that the liver receives its major blood supply via a vein – gives the liver a special role in metabolism.

The portal vein is short – about 7–8 cm long. It is formed by the joining of veins coming from different parts of the intestinal tract including the stomach, and also from the spleen. These veins carry the substances absorbed from the intestinal tract into the blood – particularly, from the point of view of energy metabolism, monosaccharides and amino acids. Thus, the water-soluble substrates arising from the diet are transported first to the liver, before entering the general circulation.

Another important, although small, group of veins joins the portal vein just before it enters the liver – the *pancreatic veins*. These veins carry blood from the endocrine part of the pancreas (described in more detail in Chapter 5), containing the pancreatic hormones insulin and glucagon. These hormones therefore exert their effects first on the liver, before being diluted in the general circulation.

Blood leaves the liver through a number of *hepatic veins*, which enter the *inferior vena cava*, the main blood vessel returning blood from the lower part of the body up towards the heart.

There is one other important system of vessels associated with the liver – those that carry *bile* to the gall bladder. Bile (see Section 3.2.3.3) contains the bile salts (Box 3.1), which are essential to the digestion and absorption of fats from the intestine. It is also a route for excretion of organic compounds detoxified in the liver, and having a molecular mass greater than 400 Da. The 500–1000 ml of bile produced each day travels through a system of *hepatic ducts* to the gall bladder, a pear-shaped organ (about 8 cm long by 2–3 cm in diameter) located immediately under the liver (see Fig. 3.5). Here it is stored between meals, and emptied during digestion through the *common bile duct* to the duodenum.

The major part of the liver (80% by volume) is composed of one cell type, the *hepatocyte*. Other cell types include the phagocytic Kupffer cells (macrophages, see Section 4.7.3) and endothelial cells. These other cell types are generally smaller than hepatocytes and so may make up a larger proportion of total cell number. Hepatocytes are arranged in a very characteristic manner (Fig. 4.1) which appears in cross-section as hexagonal units or *lobules*, each around 1 mm across. At each corner of the hexagon is a *triad* of three vessels: tiny branches of the portal vein, the hepatic artery and the bile duct. In the centre of the lobule is a branch of a hepatic vein, carrying blood away. The hepatocytes radiate out from the central vein. Blood flows from the triads towards the central vein in small passages between the hepatocytes, the *sinusoids*. The sinusoids are therefore the equivalent of the capillaries found in other tissues, and are lined by flat *endothelial cells*, as are all capillaries. The

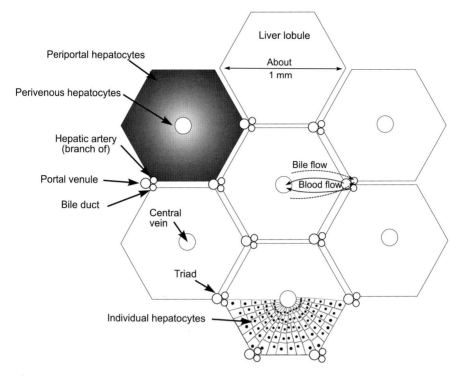

Fig. 4.1 Arrangement of hepatocytes. In a cross-section of the liver, the hepatocytes appear to radiate out from the central vein. (Individual hepatocytes are not to scale – they are much magnified.) The anatomical features are described in more detail in the text.

blood in the sinusoids is in intimate contact with the hepatocytes. Bile formed in the hepatocytes passes out to the bile duct branch in the triad along the lines of hepatocytes in fine tubes, the *bile canaliculi* (little canals).

The precise arrangement of hepatocytes within the liver is closely related to the function of the cells; this is known as *metabolic zonation* of hepatic metabolism. The hepatocytes on the 'outside' of each lobule (*periportal hepatocytes*) are exposed to blood which has recently arrived at the liver in the portal vein and hepatic artery. Thus, these cells are well oxygenated and supplied with substrates, and oxidative metabolism predominates. The synthesis of glucose (*gluconeogenesis*) occurs mainly in these cells, whereas the cells nearer the centre of each lobule (*perivenous hepatocytes*) are more involved in glycolysis and also ketone body production. It appears that this arrangement is quite flexible, and each individual cell can perform either function depending upon its location in the lobule and the prevailing physiological circumstances.

4.1.2 Liver metabolism

By understanding how the liver is placed within the circulatory system, we can understand the rationale behind many of its metabolic functions. It is the first organ to 'get its pick' of the nutrients which enter the body from the intestine after a meal, and we might therefore predict that it would have a major role in energy storage after a meal. This is indeed so, at least for carbohydrate; storage and later release of glucose are major functions of the liver. It also has an important role in amino acid metabolism. Although most dietary fat bypasses the liver as it enters the circulation (see Section 3.3.3), the liver does have important roles in fat metabolism. Also, short- and medium-chain fatty acids from the diet reach the liver directly in the portal vein.

4.1.2.1   Carbohydrate metabolism in the liver

The major pathways of glucose metabolism in the liver, and their hormonal regulation, are summarised in Fig. 4.2.

Fed conditions

Glucose is absorbed from the intestine into the portal vein, where its concentration may reach almost 10 mmol/l after a meal. (Arterial blood glucose concentration is normally around 5 mmol/l.) The hepatocytes, especially the periportal cells, are therefore exposed to high concentrations of glucose during the absorptive phase. Liver cells have predominantly the *GLUT-2* type of

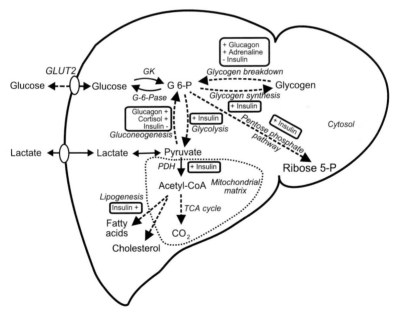

Fig. 4.2 Outline of glucose metabolism and its hormonal regulation in the liver. Dashed arrows in pathways indicate multiple enzymatic steps. The dotted shape is the mitochondrial membrane. GLUT2, hepatic glucose transporter (see Box 2.2); G 6-P, glucose 6-phosphate; GK, glucokinase; G-6-Pase, glucose-6-phosphatase; LDH, lactate dehydrogenase; PDH, pyruvate dehydrogenase; Ribose 5-P, ribose 5-phosphate; TCA cycle, tricarboxylic acid (Krebs) cycle. A 'plus' sign indicates stimulation, a 'minus' sign inhibition. Note that the pathway for gluconeogenesis is over-simplifed (see Box 4.2), and no detail of the pathways of fatty acid and cholesterol synthesis is shown (see Box 4.3).

glucose transporter (Box 2.2), which is not responsive to insulin, and has a relatively high K_m for glucose so that it normally operates well below saturation. In addition, because there are many transporters, there is a high maximal activity (V_{max}) for glucose transport. This means that the rate and direction of movement of glucose across the hepatocyte membrane are determined by the relative glucose concentrations inside and outside the cell.

Within the hepatocyte, glucose is phosphorylated to form glucose 6-phosphate – the initial step in its metabolism by any pathway – by the enzyme *glucokinase*. This enzyme belongs to the family of hexokinases (hexokinase Type IV), but differs from the other hexokinases found in muscle and other tissues in that it has a high K_m for glucose (12 mmol/l) and is not inhibited by its product, glucose 6-phosphate, at physiological concentrations.[1] Like the GLUT2 transporter it has a high capacity (high V_{max}) and is unaffected, in the short term, by insulin.

The overall result is that when the glucose concentration outside the hepatocyte rises, glucose will be rapidly taken into cells and phosphorylated; the liver is often described as acting like a 'sink' for glucose. Another way of expressing this is to say that it acts like a buffer, taking up glucose when the concentration outside is high (e.g. after ingestion of a carbohydrate-containing meal) and releasing it, by specific mechanisms discussed below, when it is required elsewhere in the body.

The presence of the high-K_m glucose transporter and the high-K_m glucokinase would not, alone, enable the hepatocyte to take up unlimited quantities of glucose, as glucose 6-phosphate would simply accumulate within the cell until glucose phosphorylation ceased. Instead, there are specific mechanisms for stimulating the disposal of glucose 6-phosphate.

Glucose 6-phosphate may enter the pathways of glycogen synthesis or glycolysis. Insulin and glucose both activate the storage of glucose as glycogen. They activate the main regulatory enzyme of glycogen synthesis (*glycogen synthase*) and inhibit glycogen breakdown (by *glycogen phosphorylase*). This control is brought about in both cases by changes in the phosphorylation of the enzyme (Box 4.1). The result is a rapid stimulation of glycogen synthesis and suppression of glycogen breakdown, so that net storage of glycogen occurs. Because insulin is secreted from the pancreas and reaches the liver directly, and because glucose from the small intestine also arrives in the hepatic portal vein, they can bring about precise coordination of this system.

Glucose 6-phosphate can also be metabolised via glycolysis to pyruvate in hepatocytes. This pathway is also activated in fed conditions. Details are given in Box 4.2. Some of the resulting pyruvate may be oxidised directly in the tricarboxylic acid cycle, some released after conversion to lactate. Most of the energy required by the liver for its multiple metabolic purposes is, however, derived from the oxidation of amino acids and fatty acids rather than glucose.

Note that expression of several of the enzymes of glycolysis is induced by insulin and glucose (Tables 2.5, 2.6). In a situation of prolonged high carbohydrate intake, this would reinforce the shorter-term mechanisms that have mainly been discussed above.

Overnight fasted conditions
Glycogen breakdown, controlled by reciprocal activation of glycogen phosphorylase and inhibition of glycogen synthase, is brought about by a change in the balance of hormones. The activation (by phosphorylation) of glycogen phosphorylase is regulated by a number of hormones including glucagon, and by the catecholamines, adrenaline and noradrenaline (Box 4.1). (The role of the catecholamines in metabolic regulation during normal daily life is probably small, although it becomes important in 'stress situations', considered in Chapters 7 and 8.) Activation of glycogen phosphorylase is opposed by insulin and glucose, as we have seen. As the absorption of a meal is completed, tissues such as brain and muscle are still using glucose, and its concentration in the blood will begin to fall, albeit slightly; the balance of the hormones insulin and glucagon secreted by the pancreas will then change in favour of glucagon. Again, the anatomical relationship of the liver to the endocrine pancreas means that hepatic metabolism is very directly regulated by this balance.

Glycogen will therefore be broken down when the concentration of glucose in the blood falls. The 'purpose' of this is to liberate the carbohydrate, stored in the liver after meals, into the bloodstream. The breakdown of glycogen leads to the production of glucose 1-phosphate, which is in equilibrium with glucose 6-phosphate (catalysed by the enzyme *phosphoglucomutase*). Glucose 6-phosphate cannot be converted to glucose by the enzyme glucokinase, which catalyses an essentially irreversible reaction, and the formation of glucose from glucose 6-phosphate is instead brought about by *glucose-6-phosphatase* (Fig. 4.2). Like glucokinase, the K_m of glucose-6-phosphatase is high relative to normal concentrations of its substrate, glucose 6-phosphate. Glucose-6-phosphatase is not free in the cytoplasm: it is a membrane-bound enzyme present in the membranes of the endoplasmic reticulum (a complex of membranes enclosing a compartment separate from the cell cytoplasm). Its catalytic site faces into the lumen of the endoplasmic reticulum and the enzyme is associated with subunits that act as specific transporters for the facilitated diffusion of glucose 6-phosphate (from the cytosol into the lumen), and glucose (from lumen to cytosol); the latter is a member of the GLUT family, possibly GLUT9.

Neither glucokinase nor glucose-6-phosphatase is directly regulated *in the short term* by hormonal signals (they are over a matter of some hours, by changes in the amount of enzyme protein present), and the net flux between glucose and glucose 6-phosphate is therefore determined by their relative concentrations. During glycogen breakdown, brought about because the plasma glucose concentration is falling, the net flux will be towards the formation and export from the cell of glucose.

The other important function of the liver in glucose metabolism is the synthesis of glucose from other precursors, *gluconeogenesis*. In terms of function,

Box 4.1   Hormonal regulation of glycogen breakdown (*glycogenolysis*) and synthesis (*glycogenesis*) in the liver

Glycogen breakdown

Adrenaline or noradrenaline, acting via β-adrenergic receptors, and glucagon act through the pathway shown in Fig. 2.4.2, Box 2.4, to activate protein kinase-A (PKA), which phosphorylates phosphorylase kinase (*phosph kinase* in Fig. 4.1.1), converting it from its dephosphorylated, inactive form (*b*) to its phosphorylated, active form (*a*). Phosphorylase kinase then phosphorylates and activates glycogen phosphorylase (*gly phosphorylase* in Fig. 4.1.1), converting it from its dephosphorylated, inactive form (*b*) to its phosphorylated, active form (*a*). Glycogen phosphorylase acts on glycogen, releasing (by phosphorolysis, which is similar to hydrolysis) one molecule at a time of glucose 1-phosphate; this may be converted to glucose and released into the circulation. Glycogenolysis is inhibited by insulin, which activates a protein phosphatase (protein phosphatase-1G, a form specifically found associated with glycogen); this dephosphorylates (and thus inactivates) phosphorylase kinase. [The regulation of protein phosphatase-1G by insulin is complex. It may involve reduction of cAMP by insulin and lowered activation of glycogen phosphorylase: phosphorylase *a* is an allosteric inhibitor of protein phosphatase-1G.]

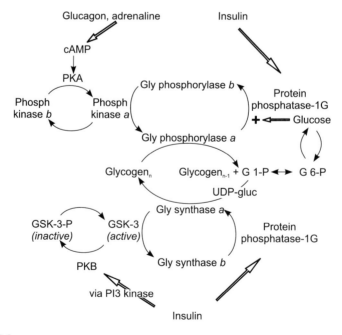

Fig. 4.1.1

Further regulation is brought about by glucose itself. Glucose binds to a specific site on phosphorylase a, causing a conformational change that makes the enzyme a better substrate for dephosphorylation by protein phosphatase-1G. Thus, in the liver, an increase in the intracellular glucose concentration will itself lead to inactivation of phosphorylase.

Glycogen synthesis
Insulin acts via PKB to phosphorylate and inactivate glycogen synthase kinase-3 (GSK-3: see Fig. 2.4.1, Box 2.4). It also activates protein phosphatase-1G, bringing about the dephosphorylation (and thus activation) of glycogen synthase, by conversion from its inactive, phosphorylated form (shown as *gly synthase b*) to its active, dephosphorylated form (*gly synthase a*). Insulin also inhibits glycogenolysis as described above. Thus, there is coordinated control of glycogen synthesis and breakdown: when one process is stimulated, the other is inhibited.

The pathways are similar in muscle although there are differences in regulation (see Fig. 8.8). For instance, in muscle glycogen breakdown is more susceptible to allosteric effects of AMP (activation) and glucose 6-phosphate (inhibition). Liver glycogen breakdown seems – very reasonably – to respond more to stimuli from outside the cell (i.e. hormones and the glucose concentration). Glycogen synthase in muscle is also phosphorylated by PKA, whereas liver glycogen synthase lacks the relevant phosphorylation sites. Therefore, in muscle adrenaline may also act via PKA to inhibit glycogen synthesis.

Information for this box taken from (amongst others) Cohen (1999); Bollen *et al.* (1998).

the pathway of gluconeogenesis is like glycolysis in reverse, but there are some essential differences in the enzymatic steps, and these are the points at which regulation occurs (Box 4.2). The substrates for gluconeogenesis are smaller molecules: usually, in order of importance, lactate, alanine, glycerol. Other amino acids can also serve as gluconeogenic precursors, although alanine is by far the most important, for reasons that will be discussed in Section 6.4.2.

The pathway of gluconeogenesis is controlled by two major factors: by the rate of supply of substrate, and by hormonal regulation of the enzymes concerned (discussed in detail in Box 4.2). As in the case of glycolysis, hormonal control involves both acute effects and effects on gene expression. As Table 2.5 shows, the expression of some enzymes of gluconeogenesis is down-regulated by insulin.

Overall, gluconeogenesis is stimulated by glucagon and inhibited by insulin whilst glycolysis is favoured under the opposite conditions. The stimulation of gluconeogenesis by glucagon also occurs in part because of direct stimulation of the transporters for uptake of substrates (particularly alanine) from the

Box 4.2   The pathways of glycolysis and gluconeogenesis and their hormonal regulation

Pathways and abbreviations

The pathways are shown as they occur in the liver. Fine-dashed arrows in pathways indicate multiple enzymatic steps. Dashed arrows indicate regulation. The dotted ellipse is the mitochondrial membrane. Co-substrates including ATP, ADP, P_i, GTP and CO_2 are not shown, for simplicity. Substrates: G 6-P, glucose 6-phosphate; F 6-P, fructose 6-phosphate; F 1,6-P_2, fructose 1,6 bisphosphate; F 2,6-P_2, fructose 2,6-bisphosphate; Glyc 3-P, glyceraldehyde 3-phosphate; DHAP, dihydroxyacetone phosphate; PEP, phosphoenolpyruvate. Enzymes: GK, glucokinase; G-6-Pase, glucose-6-phosphatase; PFK, phosphofructokinase; FBP, fructose-1,6 bisphosphatase; PK, pyruvate kinase; PC, pyruvate carboxylase; PEPCK, phosphoenolpyruvate carboxykinase; Glyc-K, glycerol kinase; LDH, lactate dehydrogenase; AAT, alanine aminotransferase. The enzyme marked *BFE* is a single, bifunctional enzyme known as *6-phosphofructo-2-kinase/fructose-2,6-bisphosphatase*, responsible for formation and breakdown of F 2,6-P_2, a compound with a crucial role in regulation of these pathways.

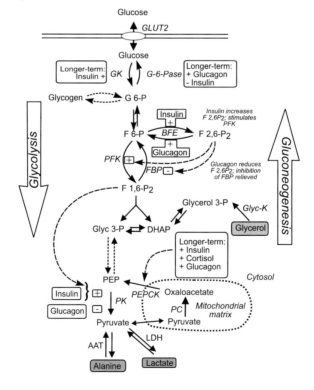

Fig. 4.2.1

Note that there are three places in which the pathways of glycolysis and gluconeogenesis are separate: glucokinase/glucose-6-phosphatase, phosphofructokinase/fructose-1,6 bisphosphatase; pyruvate kinase/(pyruvate carboxylase and phosphoenolpyruvate carboxykinase). Pyruvate carboxylase is present within the mitochondrion, but PEPCK in humans is equally distributed between cytosol and mitochondrion. [Since oxaloacetate cannot cross the mitochondiral membrane, it is converted to malate for transport to the cytosol; this is not shown.]

The three major substrates for gluconeogenesis are shown (dark boxes) together with the places at which they enter the pathway. They arise from tissues outside the liver.

Regulation

The pathways of glycolysis and gluconeogenesis catalyse opposite functions, and conditions that favour one tend to suppress the other. In general, glycolysis is favoured under 'fed' conditions, gluconeogenesis under 'starved' conditions. There are three major modes of regulation: allosteric, covalent (phosphorylation) and gene expression. The last of these is relatively long term (hours rather than minutes) and affects GK, G-6-Pase and PEPCK activities as shown. Allosteric and covalent regulation by hormones works mainly through adenylyl cyclase/cAMP (see Box 2.4 for more details). The principal features are as follows:

- Glucokinase is inhibited allosterically by a specific regulatory protein that is activated by fructose 6-phosphate (i.e. tending to limit glycolysis when flux is high), but fructose 1-phosphate, a product of fructose metabolism, relieves the inhibition of glucokinase.
- The bifunctional enzyme 6-phosphofructo-2-kinase/fructose-2,6-bisphosphatase is regulated by phosphorylation by PKA (glucagon high) and dephosphorylation by protein phosphatase 2A (insulin high). In the phosphorylated form it catalyses breakdown of F $2,6-P_2$; in the dephosphorylated form it catalyses formation of F $2,6-P_2$.
- F $2,6-P_2$ is a potent activator of PFK and inhibitor of FBPase; thus, when insulin is elevated glycolysis is favoured; when glucagon is high relative to insulin, the F $2,6-P_2$ concentration falls and gluconeogenesis is favoured.
- The enzyme PK (glycolysis pathway) is inhibited by phosphorylation by PKA (glucagon high); insulin inhibits this phosphorylation (i.e. maintains the enzyme active).
- In addition, PK is activated allosterically by F $1,6-P_2$ (thus, its activity is maintained when glycolytic flux is high).
- Other compounds within the cell also play a role in allosteric regulation. Of these, the most important are probably: (i) the adenine nucleotides (ATP,

ADP, AMP) regulate several steps such that when the cellular energy state is low (low ATP/ADP ratio) glycolysis is favoured; (ii) citrate inhibits PFK. The importance of these additional controls may lie in the fact that when cellular energy is plentiful, e.g. because the cell is oxidising fatty acids (and thus citrate concentrations are also high), gluconeogenesis will be favoured. There is much experimental evidence that an increased rate of fatty acid oxidation in the liver increases the rate of gluconeogenesis.

Glucagon is an example of a hormone counteracting insulin (a *counter-regulatory* hormone). In certain 'stress' conditions (see Section 7.3.1) adrenaline and noradrenaline may play the equivalent role, raising cyclic AMP concentrations through β-adrenergic receptors.

Based in part on Hue & Rider (1987), Pilkis & Granner (1992) and Nordlie *et al.* (1999).

blood into the liver cell. The net result is again that, in conditions where glucagon predominates over insulin, the liver will produce glucose 6-phosphate that is directed, by the mechanisms discussed earlier, into export as glucose into the circulation. It will be apparent that the processes of glycogenolysis and gluconeogenesis tend to be active at the same time in normal daily life. This is not so in more prolonged starvation, a condition in which gluconeogenesis becomes particularly important but there is little glycogen in the liver to mobilise; this will be discussed fully in Chapter 8.

Hepatic gluconeogenesis can also be stimulated by an increase in the supply of substrate from other tissues. One example is the period after physical exercise when there are elevated concentrations of lactate in the blood, some of which will be reconverted to glucose in the liver. During starvation, an increased concentration of blood glycerol arising from adipose tissue lipolysis (see Section 4.5.3.2) will have the same effect. However, there is one common situation in which hormonal factors will be tending to suppress gluconeogenesis whilst substrate supply increases it. This is the situation after a meal. It leads to a phenomenon known as the *glucose paradox*. It was noted some years ago that an isolated liver, perfused with an artificial 'blood' medium, will synthesise glycogen under appropriate conditions. However, the highest rates of glycogen synthesis are observed not when glucose alone is supplied at high concentration in the perfusate, but when it is supplied together with a precursor of gluconeogenesis such as lactate. Under these conditions lactate rather than glucose appears to be the true substrate for glycogen synthesis. (Lactate must first be converted to glucose 6-phosphate by the pathway of gluconeogenesis – see Box 4.2.) Findings in an isolated tissue like the perfused liver must be interpreted with caution for the reason discussed earlier, that in the body there are special relationships between different organs and tissues which are not reproduced in this laboratory situation. However, the result has since been confirmed in humans: hepatic glycogen synthesis after a meal comes about by a combination of the 'direct pathway' (glucose uptake, glucose 6-phosphate formation, glycogen synthesis) and the 'indirect pathway' (uptake of three-carbon gluconeogenic substrates, particularly lactate, formation of glucose 6-phosphate and glycogen synthesis). The origin of the lactate in this situation is not yet completely clear. One suggestion is that the small intestine itself, during the process of glucose absorption, metabolises a proportion of the glucose to lactate, which passes to the liver through the portal vein (see Section 3.3.1). Again, the anatomical relationship of liver to intestine is important. It is also possible that some hepatocytes produce lactate whilst others use it for gluconeogenesis. Other tissues may produce some lactate from glucose in the plasma: red blood cells, adipose tissue and muscle play some part in this, although it is not yet clear how important any particular tissue is in the postprandial period (the period after a meal). The essential point, however, is still that glycogen is synthesised by the liver after a meal, although the pathways involved are not quite so straightforward as we would have thought fifteen years ago.

The pentose phosphate pathway
Figure 4.2 shows an alternative fate for glucose 6-phosphate. It may be converted to five-carbon sugars (pentoses), particularly ribose 5-phosphate, which is required for synthesis of nucleic acids. This pathway is a relatively minor route for disposal of glucose 6-phosphate but is important because the partial oxidation that it brings about releases reducing power, in the form of NADPH (rather than NADH). NADPH is required for fatty acid synthesis. The first step in this pathway is catalysed by glucose-6-phosphate dehydrogenase, which forms 6-phosphogluconate. 6-Phosphogluconate dehydrogenase is the next step. Both these dehydrogenases produce NADPH. The activity of glucose-6-phosphate dehydrogenase is increased in conditions of carbohydrate excess, and it has been grouped with the 'lipogenic' enzymes because of its role in releasing the reducing power needed for lipogenesis. Activation of glucose-6-phosphate dehydrogenase by carbohydrate availability involves increased gene expression but also appears to involve increased stability of its mRNA. The pentose phosphate pathway is present in most tissues, but only in the liver and adipose tissue is the activity of glucose-6-phosphate dehydrogenase regulated by carbohydrate availability, stressing the link with fat synthesis.

4.1.2.2   Fat metabolism in the liver
The main pathways of fatty acid metabolism in the liver, and their hormonal regulation, are shown in Fig. 4.3. The liver can both oxidise and synthesise fatty acids. In humans the overall rate of fatty acid synthesis from other molecules (glucose in particular) is usually small in comparison with dietary fatty

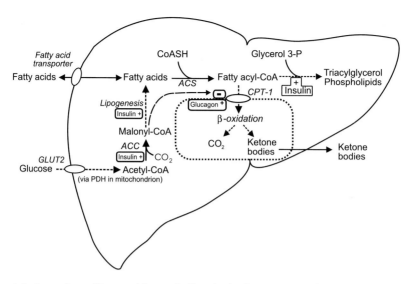

Fig. 4.3 Overview of fatty acid metabolism in the liver. Fatty acids cross the hepatocyte membrane mainly by a carrier-mediated process (see Table 2.4). Inside the liver cell they are transported through the cytosol by binding to specific *fatty acid binding proteins*, and *activated* by esterification to coenzyme-A (CoASH) by the enzyme *acyl-CoA synthase* (ACS). In order to enter the mitochondrion (dotted box) for oxidation in the tricarboxylic acid cycle (TCA cycle), fatty acyl-CoA esters are converted to acyl-carnitine derivatives by the action of carnitine-palmitoyl transferase-1 (CPT-1) (further details on Fig. 4.4). This enzyme is inhibited by malonyl-CoA, an intermediate in the pathway of *de novo lipogenesis.* Insulin inhibits fatty acid oxidation by (1) increasing the concentration of malonyl-CoA via activation of *acetyl-CoA carboxylase* (ACC) and (2) stimulating fatty acid esterification to form triacylglycerol. Glucagon increases fatty acid oxidation, possibly by a direct effect on CPT-1. Note that acetyl-CoA formation from glucose is over-simplified: see Fig. 4.5 for further details. PDH, pyruvate dehydrogenase.

acid intake, but this pathway has a special significance in coordinating glucose and fat metabolism as discussed below.

Like other tissues, the liver may take up non-esterified fatty acids from the plasma. These fatty acids have two major fates within the liver: oxidation or triacylglycerol formation.

Fatty acid oxidation

The liver may oxidise fatty acids by the mitochondrial β-oxidation pathway to produce energy for its many metabolic activities. An alternative β-oxidation pathway in peroxisomes operates mainly to shorten very-long-chain fatty acids. It uses different enzymes, but the same metabolic steps. It has been estimated to contribute from 5% to 30% of the total rate of hepatic fatty acid oxidation, and will not be considered here except to note that, in rodents although probably not in humans, it is up-regulated by ligands of the nuclear receptor PPARα (see Table 2.7). In humans, PPARα activation increases mitochondrial fatty acid oxidation. Given that the natural ligand for PPARα is thought to be a fatty acid derivative, this may be seen as a way of increasing the oxidation of fatty acids when fatty acid supply is high.

In particular, gluconeogenesis, a pathway that requires energy and reducing equivalents (NADH), appears to be 'fuelled' by oxidation of fatty acids. If fatty acid oxidation is prevented by using a specific inhibitor, then gluconeogenesis is suppressed: if fatty acid supply to the liver is increased experimentally, gluconeogenesis always increases.

The pathway of fatty acid oxidation diverges from that of glycerolipid synthesis when acyl-CoA enters the mitochondrion for oxidation. This step is closely regulated. The mitochondrial membrane is not permeable to acyl-CoA and the acyl group is transferred to the small molecule carnitine (Fig. 4.4). This transfer is catalysed by the enzyme *carnitine-palmitoyl transferase-1* (CPT-1). The activity of this enzyme is controlled by the cellular level of the compound *malonyl-CoA* (Fig. 4.3), which is a potent inhibitor. The significance of this will become clear soon. This role of malonyl-CoA provides a vital link between carbohydrate and fat metabolism. It was discovered in 1977 by the British-born biochemist, J. Denis McGarry, working at the University of Dallas, Texas with Daniel W. Foster (McGarry *et al.* 1977).

During the oxidation of fatty acids in the liver, the ketone bodies *aceto-acetate* and *3-hydroxybutyrate* are produced (Fig. 4.5) and exported into the circulation. The regulation of *ketogenesis* occurs at several steps (see Fig. 4.5) although it is clear that to a major extent ketone body production in the liver is determined by the rate of fatty acid oxidation (i.e. acetyl-CoA generation, determined in turn by the activity of CPT-1).

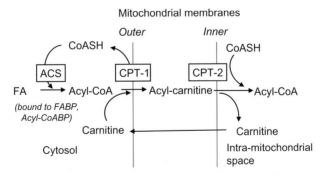

Fig. 4.4 Further detail of the transport of fatty acids into mitochondria. Carnitine is a highly charged molecule ($(CH_3)_3N^+CH_2CH(OH)CH_2COO^-$) and there is a specific translocase for it to move (with and without esterified acyl group) across the mitochondrial membranes. ACS, acyl-Co synthase (this is membrane-associated: it has been suggested that it may be linked with fatty acid transport into the cell so that the intracellular concentration of free fatty acids is very low); CPT, carnitine-palmitoyl transferase: CPT-1, so-called 'overt' CPT (outer mitochondrial membrane); CPT-2, inner mitochondrial membrane (not regulated); BP, binding proteins for fatty acids (FA) and acyl-CoA.

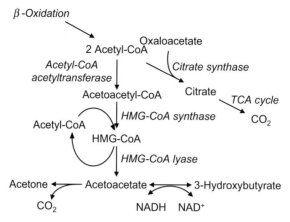

Fig. 4.5 The pathway of ketone body formation from acetyl-CoA (ketogenesis). This is all located within the mitochondrion. Acetyl-CoA is produced from β-oxidation of fatty acids. It may enter the tricarboxylic acid cycle (TCA cycle) or it may enter the ketogenesis pathway. For the latter, two molecules of acetyl-CoA condense to form acetoacetyl-CoA. A third is added to form 3-hydroxy-3-methylglutaryl-CoA (HMG-CoA) in a reaction catalysed by HMG-CoA synthase. This is split to release *acetoacetate* (a ketone body) and acetyl-CoA. The other major ketone body, *3-hydroxybutyrate*, is formed by reduction of acetoacetate. A minor one, *acetone*, is formed by non-enzymatic breakdown of acetoacetate. The ketone bodies cannot be re-utilised in the liver and are exported into the bloodstream. The major regulation appears to be the delivery of fatty acids to the mitochondrion for oxidation. Beyond that, the availability of oxaloacetate may limit entry of acetyl-CoA into the TCA cycle. HMG-CoA synthase is also regulated by covalent modification (succinylation) by succinyl-CoA, a TCA cycle intermediate. Succinyl-CoA competes with acetyl-CoA and can be displaced when acetyl-CoA concentration is high. Glucagon lowers succinyl-CoA concentration and so stimulates ketogenesis. See Further Reading for more details.

Lipid synthesis

The alternative fate for fatty acids taken up by the liver is esterification to form triacylglycerol, which is stored within hepatocytes. In addition, lipids – glycerolipids (phospholipids and triacylglycerol) and cholesterol – may be synthesised from non-lipid precursors such as glucose and amino acids, via acetyl-CoA (Box 4.3). In fact, much like the situation of the 'glucose paradox' described earlier (Section 4.1.2.1), in isolated hepatocytes the three-carbon compounds lactate and pyruvate are better substrates for this pathway than is glucose: it is not known which are the preferred substrates *in vivo*. These pathways are stimulated by insulin in the short term, and in the longer term by increased expression of key enzymes (see Box 4.3). Therefore, under conditions when glucose is in excess, it is converted to lipids (maybe via three-carbon intermediates), and in addition fatty acids taken up by the liver are used for glycerolipid synthesis rather than oxidation. Malonyl-CoA, the first committed intermediate in fatty acid synthesis, is a key coordinator of glucose and fat oxidation through its ability to inhibit fatty acid entry into the mitochondrion for oxidation.

It should be stressed again, however, that the rate of *de novo* fatty acid synthesis in humans is usually low (it will be considered again in Section 6.4.1.1), and the importance of this pathway under most circumstances relates to its link with fat oxidation via malonyl-CoA. But closely linked with this is a diversion of fatty acids from oxidation into glycerolipid, especially triacylglycerol, synthesis. In 'fed' conditions, when insulin is elevated, malonyl-CoA levels will be high and fatty acid oxidation will be inhibited. Fatty acids will be diverted into esterification with glycerol 3-phosphate, a process which is stimulated by insulin (although the exact locus of control is not clear). Thus, in the 'fed' state, the liver tends to store fatty acids as triacylglycerol rather than to oxidise them. Hepatic energy requirements under these circumstances will be met mainly by amino acid oxidation.

The hepatic triacylglycerol pool is not a major energy store for the rest of the body (that function is performed by the triacylglycerol stored in adipose tissue) but appears to be a local store for hepatic needs.[2] The stored triacylglycerol acts as the substrate for hepatic secretion of fat into the bloodstream, in the form of the lipoprotein particles known as *very-low-density lipoprotein* (VLDL). The bulk of the lipid in VLDL is in the form of triacylglycerol, derived from the hepatic store. The details and the regulation of lipoprotein metabolism will be discussed in detail in Chapter 9.

Longer-term control of hepatic fat metabolism
Most of the description above of the regulation of fat metabolism has related to short-term control. However, many of the enzymes involved are also subject to longer-term regulation of expression by insulin and carbohydrate availability, as well as via the SREBP and PPAR systems. We can therefore imagine the metabolic pattern of the liver as shifting rapidly, on an hour-to-hour basis, as meals are taken, digested and absorbed: but these rapid fluctuations may be overlaid on a longer-term trend to increases or decreases in particular pathways. Some of the genes involved have been mentioned in passing above, and were summarised in Tables 2.4 and 2.6. In general, fatty acid synthesis and diversion of fatty acids away from oxidation is favoured by high insulin (which would usually be associated with overfeeding), but activation of PPARα, perhaps brought about by increased fatty acid availability, tends to up-regulate fatty acid oxidation.

Other roles of the liver in fat metabolism
The liver has other specialised roles in fat metabolism. These include its production of bile salts, covered in Box 3.1, and its role in uptake of circulating cholesterol (Chapter 9).

4.1.2.3   Amino acid metabolism in the liver
Under normal circumstances in adult life, our bodies do not continuously accumulate or lose protein in a net sense. The rate of amino acid oxidation in the body must therefore balance the rate of entry of dietary protein (typically 70–100 g of protein per day on a Western diet). General features of amino acid metabolism in the body will be covered later (Section 6.3). The liver plays a

Box 4.3   Synthesis of fatty acids and cholesterol from glucose

De novo lipogenesis is the term used for synthesis of fatty acids from non-lipid precursors. It is in effect a pathway for disposing of excess carbohydrate, and it is stimulated by conditions of high carbohydrate availability.

Pathways and abbreviations

Acetyl-CoA cannot cross the inner mitochondrial membrane and so is converted to citrate, for which there is a transporter. Mitochondrial citrate is regenerated by the inward transport of pyruvate, as shown. The enzyme ATP : citrate lyase is the starting point for synthesis of both fatty acids and cholesterol and has been investigated by pharmaceutical companies as a potential target for both body weight regulation and cholesterol lowering. Note that the pathway of fatty acid synthesis from acetyl-CoA (in animals) involves just two enzymes. Fatty acid synthase (FAS) is a complex enzyme with seven different functional activities in a single polypeptide chain. Fatty acid synthesis proceeds by sequential addition of two-carbon units (from malonyl-CoA, a three-carbon intermediate: one carbon is then lost from each three-carbon unit added). The combination of fatty acids with glycerol 3-phosphate, derived from glycolysis, to form triacylglycerol and phospholipids (glycerolipids) is also shown.

   Cholesterol synthesis from acetyl-CoA is a more complex pathway with many enzymatic steps. 3-Hydroxy-3-methylglutaryl-CoA (HMG-CoA) is formed by reactions identical to those shown in Fig. 4.5 for ketone body synthesis, except that there are different isoforms of the enzymes expressed in the cytoplasm.

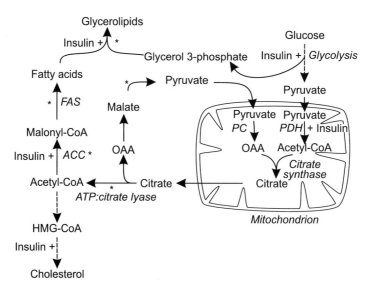

Fig. 4.3.1   Note: Small molecules such as CO_2, ATP, $NAD^+/NADH$ and $NADP^+/NADPH$ are not shown.

The first 'committed' step is the synthesis of cytosolic HMG-CoA, but an important regulatory step (and a target for drug action; see Section 9.4.2.1) is the reduction of HMG-CoA by HMG-CoA reductase.

   Other abbreviations: ACC, acetyl-CoA carboxylase; OAA, oxaloacetate; PC, pyruvate carboxylase; PDH, pyruvate dehydrogenase.

Regulation

The activity of several steps in the pathway of fatty acid synthesis is increased acutely by insulin (shown as insulin +) and in addition the expression of the enzymes marked * is increased by insulin (longer-term regulation). NADPH is required for fatty acid synthesis. This comes both from the pentose phosphate pathway (Section 4.1.2.1) and from the enzyme responsible for conversion of cytosolic malate to pyruvate (see Fig. 4.3.1), *malate dehydrogenase (oxalo-acetate-decarboxylating) (NADP+)*, commonly called *malic enzyme*. Expression of malic enzyme, like that of glucose-6-phosphate dehydrogenase (see Pentose phosphate pathway, Section 4.1.2.1), is increased by carbohydrate availability, and also by increased stability of its mRNA. In the pathway of cholesterol synthesis, HMG-CoA reductase is regulated by reversible phosphorylation and activated acutely by insulin. It is also subject to longer-term regulation by the SREBP system as described in Section 2.4.2.3 and later in Box 9.3.

special role in amino acid oxidation, not least because it is the organ that first receives the dietary amino acids, which enter the circulation via the portal vein. It is also the only organ capable of eliminating the nitrogen from amino acids, by synthesising urea. Therefore, with a few exceptions, amino acid catabolism occurs predominantly in the liver. (An important exception is that of the group of *branched chain amino acids*, whose catabolism is largely initiated in muscle; see Section 6.3.2.2.) Amino acid oxidation provides about half the liver's energy requirements. Figure 4.6 provides a general overview of hepatic amino acid metabolism.

   Amino acids are not merely substrates for energy production in the liver, however. They also provide a substrate for synthesis of glucose (particularly alanine – see Box 4.2), of fatty acids and of ketone bodies. Of course, amino acids also serve as precursors for hepatic protein synthesis: both proteins required within the liver, and proteins exported into the circulation such as albumin.

   An important general reaction in amino acid catabolism is the loss of the amino group by the process of *transamination* (Fig. 4.6), described in detail later (Box 6.2). The *2-oxoacid* (or *keto acid*) resulting may enter a catabolic or an anabolic pathway directly: for instance, the 2-oxoacid of alanine is pyruvate, the end-product of glycolysis; that of glutamic acid is 2-oxoglutarate,

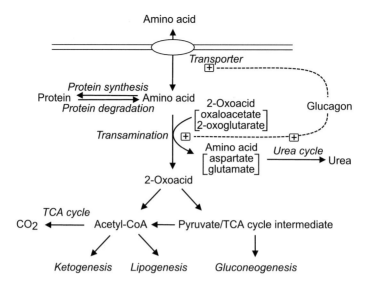

Fig. 4.6 Outline of amino acid metabolism in the liver. The intracellular effects of glucagon are relatively long-term, particularly increased expression of the enzymes for transamination and of the urea cycle. TCA cycle, tricarboxylic acid cycle.

and that of aspartic acid is oxaloacetate. The last two are intermediates of the tricarboxylic acid cycle. Each of these may lead to glucose synthesis by the pathway of gluconeogenesis (Box 4.2). Alternatively, the 2-oxoacid may undergo further metabolic transformations leading to a compound which can enter one of the catabolic pathways (acetyl-CoA for many amino acids, which can then be oxidised in the tricarboxylic acid cycle).

An important function of the liver is to synthesise urea, a relatively non-toxic compound, which is then excreted by the kidneys. Urea is the form in which we, as humans, excrete most of the amino nitrogen that is 'left over' after amino acid oxidation, although we also excrete some nitrogen in the form of ammonia, especially during starvation (see Section 8.3.2.4). The enzymes of the urea cycle are found at low levels also in the brain and adipose tissue, but the liver is the only organ contributing significant amounts of urea to the circulation.

We need to understand how amino acid nitrogen feeds into the urea cycle. This is illustrated in Fig. 4.7. The two nitrogen atoms of urea arise from ammonia and from the amino group of aspartate. Aspartate can arise, like any amino acid, from protein breakdown or from the diet, but is also readily formed by transamination of oxaloacetate (an intermediate of the tricarboxylic acid cycle), and hence many amino acids can feed their amino nitrogen in through this route. Ammonia arises essentially from two reactions: the catabolism of glutamine by glutaminase and the oxidative deamination of glutamate by glutamate dehydrogenase. The former will be covered again in Chapter 6 (Fig. 6.16). The latter is illustrated in Fig. 4.8. By linking transamination of

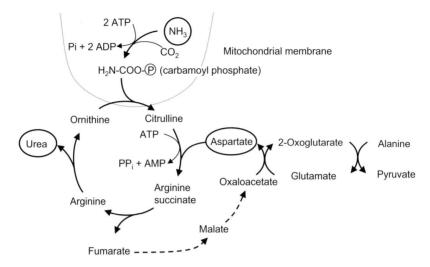

Fig. 4.7 Outline of the supply of nitrogen atoms to the urea cycle. The donors, ammonia and aspartate, are encircled, as is the end-product, urea. The source of ammonia is discussed in the text.

Amino acid + 2-Oxoglutarate $\longrightarrow$ Glutamate + 2-Oxoacid

Transamination

L-Glutamate + NAD(P)$^+$ + H$_2$O $\longrightarrow$ 2-Oxoglutarate + NAD(P)H + NH$_4^+$ + H$^+$

Glutamate dehydrogenase

Amino acid + NAD(P)$^+$ + H$_2$O $\longrightarrow$ 2-Oxoacid + NAD(P)H + NH$_4^+$ + H$^+$

Net: oxidative deamination of amino acid

Fig. 4.8 Importance of glutamate dehydrogenase. The reaction catalysed by glutamate dehydrogenase, when coupled with transamination of any amino acid, leads to production of the corresponding 2-oxoacid and ammonia. (Please note that, for simplicity, ionisation states are not always shown as they would be at physiological pH; ammonium ion shown here (NH$_4^+$) may be considered the same as ammonia shown in Fig. 4.7.)

any amino acid with the reaction catalysed by glutamate dehydrogenase, there is effectively an oxidative deamination of the amino acid with the production of ammonia that can enter the urea cycle.

Catabolism of amino acids by the liver is mainly regulated on a short-term basis by substrate supply. Substrate supply depends in the fed state on the arrival of dietary amino acids, and in the starved state on the net rate of body protein breakdown. The latter is itself under hormonal control (discussed later, Section 6.3.3). On a longer-term basis amino acid catabolism is regulated by the hormones glucagon and cortisol and again by the supply of amino acids. These hormones stimulate the synthesis of enzymes of amino acid catabolism and urea synthesis. Glucagon has a short-term effect by activating amino acid transporters, particularly that for alanine, to increase amino acid uptake. In addition, there is long-term control by the amount of dietary protein (Section 2.4.2.4); when the dietary protein content is low, the hepatic enzymes of amino acid catabolism are repressed; when dietary protein is more than adequate, their expression is stimulated. Thus, the liver regulates the body's overall store of amino acids.

4.2   The brain

The brain is a very heterogeneous structure, and different regions of the brain may have very different patterns of metabolism. Some generalisations may be made, however, which are relevant for understanding energy metabolism in the body as a whole. Some more specialised functions of the brain – coordination of the autonomic nervous system, and production of hormones, for instance – will be dealt with in Chapters 5 and 7.

The adult human brain weighs about 1.5 kg. It consists of a large number of cell types (Section 7.2.1), although the bulk of its mass consists of nerve cells: an outer layer of *grey matter*, largely nerve cell bodies, surrounding the *white matter*, largely myelinated fibres bundled into large tracts (like electrical cables). (These terms, and the structure of the brain, will be amplified in Chapter 7.) There are estimated to be around 100 billion (10^{11}) nerve cells and 900 billion glial cells (see Chapter 7 for a description of these cells) in an adult brain, so as you can imagine, it has a high rate of metabolism. The head is supplied with blood through the two *common carotid arteries* (one on either side of the neck). These each divide in the neck into an internal and an external carotid artery, the internal supplying blood to the brain, the external more to the face, neck and exterior of the head. Blood returns from the brain in the *internal jugular veins*, eventually reaching the heart via the superior vena cava. The rate of blood supply to the brain is high, about 750 ml/min (50ml blood per minute per 100 g of tissue). This can be compared with about 2–5 ml blood per minute per 100 g of tissue for *resting* skeletal muscle and for adipose tissue, or around 50 ml blood per minute per 100 g of tissue for skeletal muscle during vigorous exercise. This high rate of blood flow to the brain reflects its high metabolic rate.

The brain oxidises about 120 g of glucose per day, equivalent to about 2 MJ of energy, or 20% of the whole body energy expenditure in a typical day. This is known from studies in which samples of blood have been taken from jugular veins, and compared with arterial blood. It is not possible to detect any increase in this overall rate of metabolism during mental activities (such as mental arithmetic), presumably because the actual increase in metabolic rate in a small area adds very little to the overall rate of metabolism, although with specialised techniques for scanning metabolic activity (based on glucose utilisation and blood flow) it is possible to show local increases in metabolic activity when a subject performs certain tasks.

Many substances, such as metabolites and drugs, which gain ready access to other tissues from the blood, seem to be excluded from the brain. This gives rise to the concept of the *blood–brain barrier* which some substances cannot cross. This barrier is created by a closely-packed layer of endothelial cells without fenestrations (Section 1.3.1), which are surrounded by a layer of periendothelial cells or pericytes, forming another barrier. In general, the blood–brain barrier seems to prevent the access of lipid-soluble (hydrophobic) molecules to the brain, including the plasma non-esterified fatty acids. The brain as a whole does not appear to use fatty acids as a metabolic fuel. Instead it uses almost entirely glucose under normal circumstances, although in prolonged starvation (Section 8.3) it can use the ketone bodies. The glucose is for the most part completely oxidised (a small proportion is released as lactate), so the brain has a correspondingly high rate of oxygen consumption and carbon dioxide production. In general, the rate of utilisation of glucose by the brain is not affected by insulin, although there are particular insulin-sensitive areas where insulin receptors exist. Glucose is transported into nerve cells by the glucose transporter GLUT3, which has characteristics which make it particularly suitable for this role. It has a low K_m for glucose transport into the cell so that at normal plasma glucose concentrations it is saturated with substrate (Box 2.2): thus, quite wide variations in glucose concentration cause little change in the rate at which it is taken up by the brain. This is, of course, eminently sensible. If the rate of glucose uptake by the brain were to rise in response to increased plasma glucose concentrations after a meal, we might experience some strange effects. More importantly, the brain is protected against a fall in the plasma glucose concentration: not until the plasma glucose concentration falls below about 2 mmol/l does the rate of glucose uptake decrease so much that mental function is impaired. Again, therefore, the metabolic characteristics of the tissue seem ideally matched to its function.

The glucose transporter GLUT1 (Box 2.2) is also expressed in the brain. It appears to mediate glucose transport at the blood–brain barrier. Since its K_m for glucose is considerably higher than that of GLUT3, it might appear that it would pose a limitation to glucose entry to the interstitial fluid at low plasma glucose concentrations. However, it may be that its capacity is sufficiently high that this does not limit the rate of glucose utilisation by brain cells.

Although the brain does not use fatty acids as a metabolic fuel, during starvation the body has a need to preserve glucose. We will see how this conflict is reconciled in Chapter 8. Also, it should not be thought that the brain is not involved in lipid metabolism. Most of the wet weight of the brain is lipid, almost all phospholipid, since the structure of the brain is a large complex of cell membranes. These are interesting phospholipids and although they will not be discussed in detail here, one important point is a high content of the *n*-3 polyunsaturated fatty acids, especially docosahexaenoic acid (DHA, 22:6 *n*-3). As we saw in Chapter 1, the body has an absolute requirement for a small amount of n-3 polyunsaturated fatty acids, and this may be particularly important in early life when the brain is developing. How does the brain acquire its fatty acids if non-esterified fatty acids cannot be taken up? This is not absolutely clear. There may be a preferential transport mechanism for non-esterified polyunsaturated fatty acids into the brain. Alternatively, or in addition, there could be uptake of these fatty acids from lipoproprotein particles (lipoprotein metabolism will be covered in Chapter 9). Some experimental data suggest preferential uptake of lysophosphatidylcholine that contains DHA (lysophosphatidylcholine is phosphatidylcholine from which one fatty acid has been removed). This is all an active area of research, not least because of the importance of understanding the need of the developing brain for a supply of the *n*-3 polyunsaturated fatty acids.

4.3   Skeletal muscle

4.3.1   General description and structure of skeletal muscle

Skeletal or *striated muscle* is also known as voluntary muscle since we have conscious control over its use. Other muscles, such as those lining the wall of the intestine, are involuntary *smooth muscle*, which lacks striations.

The cells of skeletal muscle are also known as *muscle fibres* since they are long and fibril-like – they may be a few cm long. Individual cells are grouped together into bundles known as *fasciculi* (each one is a *fasciculus*), each surrounded by a sheath of connective tissue. A number of fasciculi are then grouped together and surrounded by a further covering of connecting tissue, the *epimysium* or *deep fascia*; this whole structure is what we call a muscle (Fig. 4.9).

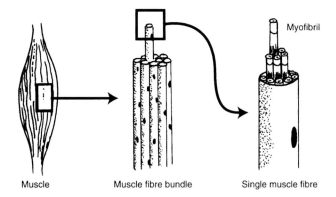

Fig. 4.9 Structural organisation of skeletal muscle. One cell is a *muscle fibre*. The whole muscle is made up of bundles of fibres, each filled with myofibrils. Reproduced from Jones, D.A. & Round, J.M. (1990) *Skeletal Muscle in Health and Disease. A Textbook of Muscle Physiology*, with permission of Manchester University Press.

Within each muscle fibre are many *myofibrils*, themselves highly organised bundles of long polymers of the proteins *myosin* and *actin*. These form, respectively, 'thick' and 'thin' filaments, that overlap in a characteristic pattern to form the striations that give skeletal muscle its alternative name. Muscle contraction is brought about through head-groups, that protrude from the myosin thick filaments, binding to the actin filaments. The head-groups can 'rock' to move the myosin relative to the actin, detach, and rebind further along the actin. This process requires energy in the form of ATP, which is hydrolysed to release ADP + P_i, and it is regulated by Ca^{2+} binding to a protein known as *troponin-C* that is associated with the thin (actin) filaments.

This is necessarily a brief description of the molecular basis of muscle contraction, and the reader is referred to Further Reading for more details of this process. The important point is that a supply of ATP is required at the point of action at the appropriate time. There is a 'buffer store' in the form of phosphocreatine, which is in equilibrium with ATP through the action of the enzyme creatine kinase (Fig. 4.10). Since this is an equilibrium reaction, any fall in the ATP concentration will lead to the formation of further ATP from ADP, using the energy of phosphocreatine. This section covers the major fuels used by skeletal muscle to form the ATP required for contraction, and for the many other functions involved in cellular metabolism.

4.3.2   Metabolism of skeletal muscle: general features

Muscle cells differ according to their relative capacity for oxidative metabolism as opposed to anaerobic, glycolytic metabolism. If a cross-section of muscle is stained for one of the enzymes associated with aerobic metabolism (for instance, succinate dehydrogenase) then it can be seen that individual fibres differ in the extent of their staining (Fig. 4.11).

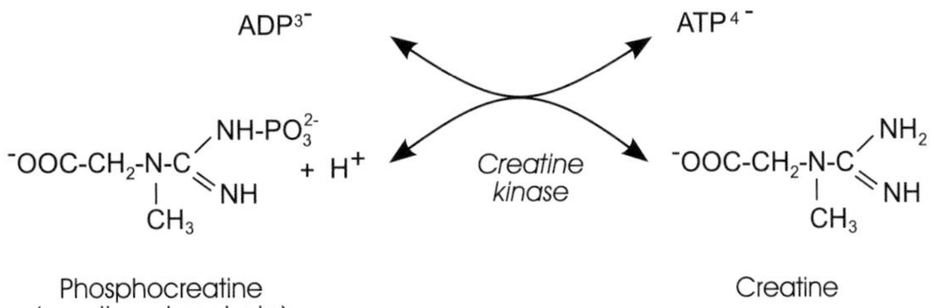

Fig. 4.10 The *creatine kinase* reaction in muscle. The reaction is referred to as the *Lohmann reaction* after the German biochemist who elucidated it. Creatine kinase operates near to equilibrium; therefore, as ATP is utilised rapidly at the beginning of contraction, the phosphocreatine pool is used to maintain the ATP concentration. In resting muscle, typical concentrations of ATP and phosphocreatine are 5 and 17 mmol per kg of muscle; therefore, the presence of phosphocreatine quadruples the ability to produce rapid contraction, before more ATP can be generated by other routes.

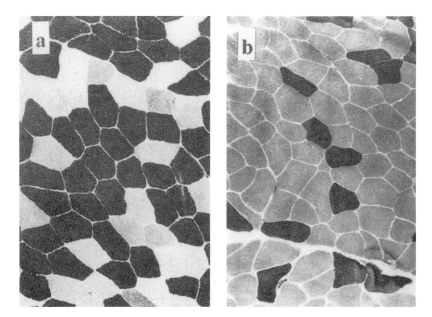

Fig. 4.11 Fibre-type composition of leg muscles in athletes. Different types of muscle fibre (muscle cell) are shown in a cross-section of muscle, by staining for the enzyme my-osin-ATPase (which reflects fast-twitch muscles): dark-stained fibres are Type II, lighter fibres are Type I. Left, quadriceps muscle from a high-jumper; right, from a marathon runner. Reproduced from Jones, D.A. & Round, J.M. (1990) *Skeletal Muscle in Health and Disease. A Textbook of Muscle Physiology,* with permission of Manchester University Press.

Broadly, there are two major types of muscle fibre (Table 4.1). Oxidative or *red* fibres are so-called because of their high content of *myoglobin*, a pigment related to haemoglobin, which assists the diffusion of oxygen into the muscle. They have a high density of capillaries perfusing them, and many mitochondria. These fibres use substrates, largely from the blood, and oxidise them to yield energy. Because the supply of substrate from the blood can be maintained for a long time – for instance, most of us have plenty of fat which can be supplied in this way – these muscle fibres are particularly important for sustained, but relatively low intensity, exercise such as walking or long-distance running. The oxidation of substrates from the blood requires time for diffusion of the substrate to the cell, diffusion of oxygen to the cell, and diffusion out of the cell of CO_2. Therefore, contraction of this type of fibre, when it is stimulated, is relatively slow. These fibres are called *red, slow-twitch* or *Type I* fibres.

At the other extreme are the *white* fibres, lacking myoglobin. These fibres have fewer mitochondria, and are more equipped for anaerobic glycolysis than oxidative metabolism. Their main substrate for glycolysis is glucose 6-phosphate produced by breakdown of glycogen stored within the same cells. The sequence of glycogen breakdown and generation of energy by glycolysis can be extremely rapid, since everything is 'on site'. Hence these are the *fast-twitch* fibres or *Type II* fibres (Table 4.1). Their role is to produce energy quickly, but

Table 4.1 Characteristics of fibre types in skeletal muscle.

Property	Type I (slow twitch) fibre	Type II (fast twitch) fibre
Speed of contraction	Slow	Fast
Myoglobin content	High	Low
Capillary density	High	Low
Myofibrillar ATPase activity	Low	High
Mitochondrial enzyme activity	High	Low
Glycogenolytic enzyme activity	Low	High
Glycogen content		May be somewhat higher
Triacylglycerol content	High	Low
Lipoprotein lipase activity	High	Low

The terms 'high' and 'low' are relative. Type II fibres are adapted to fast work using their endogenous stores (ATP, phosphocreatine and glycogen, using anaerobic glycolysis), but have limited endurance. Type I fibres are adapted to slower work using energy generated by the complete oxidation of fuels (their own glycogen and triacylglycerol, and also glucose and non-esterified fatty acids taken up from the plasma).

because they largely depend upon stored substrate, they cannot maintain this for long. They are therefore particularly important in the rapid generation of energy over short periods, such as sprinting. A third type of muscle fibre is described as fast-twitch oxidative glycolytic or *Type IIa*, as distinct from the very fast, anaerobic glycolytic *Type IIb* fibres.

In some animals, individual muscles are fairly uniform in their fibre type. In the rat, for example, there are some muscles which are composed almost entirely of red or white muscle fibres. For instance, the *soleus muscle* in the calf is used during movement such as running, and it is composed of consistently slow-twitch fibres. The *adductor longus* muscle in the thigh plays an intermittent role in maintaining posture and is a mainly fast-twitch muscle. In humans, most muscles are composed of a variety of fibre types. The composition of any particular muscle is not the same in everybody; some people have a preponderance of oxidative fibre types, some a preponderance of white, fast-twitch fibre types. This pattern is inherited to some extent. This is one reason why some people are naturally better than others at certain types of athletic events; for instance, someone with a preponderance of oxidative fibres will be better at endurance exercise than someone with more white, glycolytic fibres (Fig. 4.11).

4.3.3   Routes of ATP generation in skeletal muscle

The major pathways for generation of ATP in muscle are illustrated in Fig. 4.12. Skeletal muscle uses both stored fuel (glycogen and triacylglycerol) and substrates (glucose and fatty acids) taken up from the blood. The fatty acids may be either plasma non-esterified fatty acids, or esterified fatty acids carried in the form of triacylglycerol in lipoproteins.

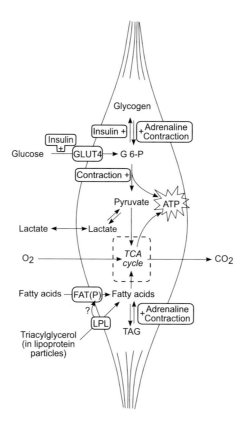

Fig. 4.12 Energy (ATP) generation in skeletal muscle. Only major pathways are shown: each arrow may represent one or more steps in a pathway. The major sites of regulation are shown: a plus sign indicates stimulation. FAT(P) represents a possible fatty acid transporter but it is not clear which might be most important in skeletal muscle (see Table 2.4). It is also possible that fatty acids released by lipoprotein lipase (LPL) (situated in the capillaries) might be transported into the cell by this means. TAG, triacylglycerol; TCA cycle, tricarboxylic acid (Krebs) cycle. The way in which muscle contraction is coordinated with metabolism is discussed in Section 8.4.3.

4.3.3.1 Glucose metabolism in skeletal muscle

Glucose uptake is mainly mediated by the insulin-sensitive glucose transporter, GLUT4 (see Box 2.2). GLUT1 is also expressed in skeletal muscle and may play a role in uptake of a glucose at a 'basal' rate. Glucose uptake by GLUT4 has certain characteristics which are relevant. The K_m is within the physiological range of plasma glucose concentrations. In the presence of low concentrations of insulin the maximal activity (V_{max}) of glucose uptake is low. Raising the insulin concentration brings more transporters into action at the cell membrane (see Fig. 2.5), and hence increases the V_{max}. Insulin thus increases the rate at which muscle takes up glucose from the blood. This glucose may be used for glycogen synthesis or metabolism via the pathway of glycolysis.

 As in the liver, insulin stimulates the enzyme glycogen synthase in muscle, and inhibits the enzyme glycogen phosphorylase. Thus, when the plasma insulin concentration is high after a meal, glucose will be stored as glycogen in skeletal muscle. However, the isoforms of the enzymes for glycogen metabolism expressed in muscle have some different regulatory properties from those in the liver. Muscle glycogen synthase has sites that can be phosphorylated by protein kinase-A, which are lacking in the liver isoform. This would give adrenaline a particular ability (acting through cAMP and PKA) to switch off glycogen synthesis in muscle whilst stimulating glycogen breakdown by the means described for the liver (Box 4.1). In addition, muscle glycogen phosphorylase is allosterically activated by AMP and inhibited by glucose 6-phosphate. These will play a role in stimulating glycogen breakdown when the energy status of the muscle cell is low (use of ATP for contraction will be accompanied by some conversion to AMP). In skeletal muscle, there is also a specific mechanism (not understood) for stimulation of glycogen synthesis after exercise when the glycogen store has been depleted. This will be illustrated later (Section 8.4.7).

4.3.3.2 Fatty acid metabolism in skeletal muscle

Fatty acids are also taken up by muscle, particularly in the oxidative fibres. These are either the plasma non-esterified fatty acids, which have arisen from stored triacylglycerol in adipose tissue, or fatty acids carried as triacylglycerol in lipoprotein particles.

It is probable that non-esterified fatty acids are taken up across the cell membrane by a specific transport mechanism (Table 2.4). The activity of the transporter may be regulated as discussed in Section 2.2.1.3, for instance with recruitment of FAT/CD36 to the cell membrane during exercise. However, under resting conditions the rate of fatty acid uptake is usually closely related to the concentration of non-esterified fatty acids in the plasma. Similarly, within the cell fatty acids are oxidised in accordance with their rate of uptake. During exercise there is clearly a need to increase the rate of delivery of substrates for oxidation. In the case of fatty acids, this is brought about by increasing the rate of blood flow through muscle (the rate of delivery from adipose tissue is also increased; see Section 4.5.3.2 below). The rate at which blood flows through any particular muscle increases several-fold when that muscle is exercising, resulting in the delivery of more fatty acids to the muscle. Experiments with perfused muscle preparations in which the delivery of fatty acids is altered either by altering their concentration or by altering the blood flow show that the rate of fatty acid uptake is largely determined by the delivery rate (i.e. blood flow × concentration).

Apart from the situation of exercise, increased uptake of fatty acids by muscle will occur when the plasma non-esterified fatty acid concentration is raised – for instance, during fasting. Under these conditions the muscle will not need to use so much glucose. Mechanisms by which the use of one fuel is regulated in response to the availability of another will be considered again in a later section (Section 6.4). However, one mechanism by which this is achieved in muscle has already been described above, for the liver. This is the inhibition of fatty acid oxidation when glucose utilisation is stimulated, via the effect of malonyl-CoA on CPT-1. It should be noted that skeletal muscle does not express fatty acid synthase, so there is no pathway of fatty acid synthesis: but it does express acetyl-CoA carboxylase to produce malonyl-CoA. Since this is not required for fatty acid synthesis, we have to conclude that it is produced solely in order to regulate the rate of fatty acid oxidation. The isoform of CPT-1 expressed in muscle is actually more sensitive to inhibition by malonyl-CoA than is the liver isoform. In addition, there are two isoforms of acetyl-CoA carboxylase, ACC1 and ACC2 (sometimes called α and β). The ACC1 isoform is generally expressed in tissues where there is an active pathway of fatty acid synthesis such as liver and adipose tissue, so we may imagine that it is feeding malonyl-CoA into this pathway. The ACC2 isoform is expressed more in tissues such as skeletal muscle, where the role of the malonyl-CoA that it produces must be purely regulatory. ACC1 is a cytosolic enzyme, whereas ACC2 is associated with mitochondria, in keeping with its role in providing malonyl-CoA to regulate CPT-1. In skeletal muscle this mechanism would presumably restrict fatty acid oxidation during the period after a meal when glucose and insulin levels are high, and it may be that it then diverts fatty acids into triacylglycerol synthesis.

Plasma triacylglycerol cannot be taken up directly. The fatty acids must first be released by the action of an enzyme, *lipoprotein lipase*, which is present in the capillaries. This process is therefore similar to the absorption of triacylglycerol from the intestine, and indeed lipoprotein lipase and pancreatic lipase belong to the same family of lipolytic enzymes. Lipoprotein lipase is also present in other tissues, especially adipose tissue. Since more is known about its action in adipose tissue, it will be described in more detail in a later section (Section 4.5.3.1; Fig. 4.15). The fatty acids it releases from triacylglycerol in the capillaries enter the muscle cells, probably by the same means as do plasma non-esterified fatty acids. Thereafter their fate may be either oxidation or re-esterification to replenish the muscle triacylglycerol store.

4.4   The heart

Here we will be concerned with the metabolism of the muscular walls of the chambers of the heart – the *myocardium*. These muscular walls are responsible for pumping blood through the lungs, and around the rest of the body. It is clearly important that they maintain their activity under all conditions. Blood is supplied to the heart muscle via arteries which branch from the aorta as it emerges from the left ventricle. These arteries encircle the heart rather like a crown; hence their name – the *coronary arteries*. If these arteries become blocked by a blood clot (a *coronary thrombosis*), then some of the myocardium will be starved of blood and hence of its supply of fuel and oxygen, and the heart will have difficulty in pumping blood around the body. This situation is a heart attack or *myocardial infarction* (infarction meaning blockage).

From the description of skeletal muscle metabolism above, it will be clear that the myocardium is an extreme example of a muscle which must be able to keep contracting over long periods; in other words, a red or oxidative muscle. It has striations under the microscope which are not dissimilar from those of skeletal muscle, and the contractile mechanism is the same.

The fuels used by the heart have been studied by threading a fine tube (*catheterisation*) into the great coronary vein which carries venous blood away from the myocardium. The blood in this vein can then be compared with blood in the arteries to see what has happened to it during passage through the myocardium. The heart is able to use a number of fuels, which it takes up from the blood. These include fatty acids, glucose and ketone bodies. The fatty acids come both from the plasma non-esterified fatty acid fraction and from plasma triacylglycerol, since the heart expresses lipoprotein lipase at relatively high levels compared with skeletal muscle. It can also take up lactate and oxidise it, via lactate dehydrogenase and the tricarboxylic acid cycle.

Its use of the different fuels depends to a large extent upon their concentrations in blood, although its uptake of glucose, by the insulin-sensitive glucose transporter GLUT4, is stimulated by insulin. In 'fed' conditions (high insulin concentrations) the myocardium therefore tends to use carbohydrate rather than fat. There must be mechanisms for regulating fuel usage according to availability. Like skeletal muscle (Section 4.3.3.2), the myocardium expresses acetyl-CoA carboxylase but not fatty acid synthase, implying that the malonyl-CoA inhibition of CPT1 mechanism will restrict fatty acid oxidation when glucose and insulin levels are high. In addition, it has long been known that the reverse is true: when fatty acids are available, there is an inhibition of glucose uptake and oxidation. This is part of a metabolic mechanism known as the glucose–fatty acid cycle, that will be described fully in Section 6.4.1.2.

4.5   Adipose tissue

Adipose tissue has a number of functions in the body which include mechanical cushioning (e.g. in the buttocks, and around some internal organs) and thermal insulation, but its main role from a metabolic point of view is that of storing chemical energy in the form of triacylglycerol, and releasing it in the form of non-esterified fatty acids when it is needed by other tissues. However, recent years have seen an explosion of interest in adipose tissue as an endocrine organ as well as a metabolic one. It is now recognised that adipose tissue secretes a number of substances, some of which are true hormones, others that may act locally, and that this capability gives adipose tissue an especially important role in metabolism.

There are several cell types in adipose tissue. We will concentrate upon the cells that store fat, the *adipocytes*. Other cells include pre-adipocytes (small cells that can differentiate into mature adipocytes when there is a surplus of fat to be stored), endothelial cells (lining blood vessels) and macrophages. Some of these other cells play a role in the secretory activities of the tissue, although not to any great extent in its 'energy metabolism'.

4.5.1   White and brown adipose tissue

There are two types of adipose tissue that can be distinguished by their gross characteristics, by their appearance under the microscope and by their metabolic pattern. These are *brown adipose tissue* and *white adipose tissue* (Fig. 4.13). Brown adipose tissue gets its colour from the presence of large numbers of mitochondria in the cytoplasm. Under the microscope, the major difference between white and brown fat cells is in the way that triacylglycerol is stored. In brown fat cells (*brown adipocytes*), the stored lipid is present in multiple droplets. In white fat cells (*white adipocytes*), it is stored as one droplet which typically almost fills the cell; the cytoplasm, mitochondria and nucleus are confined to a thin 'crust' around the outside. In function, the similarity is that both types of cell store triacylglycerol and may release fatty acids. The difference is that brown fat cells have a much higher oxidative capacity, and may oxidise a large proportion of the fatty acids released from storage.

4.5.2   Brown adipose tissue and the concept of 'uncoupling'

Brown adipose tissue has a unique metabolic feature. Like most other tissues, it can oxidise substrates, via the tricarboxylic acid cycle, in its mitochondria; unlike in any other tissue, this process can be 'uncoupled' from the generation of ATP when the tissue is stimulated by the sympathetic nervous system (Fig. 4.14).

In all tissues that have mitochondria, the electron transport chain pumps hydrogen ions (protons) out of the mitochondrial matrix (the inside of the mitochondrion) into the space between the two mitochondrial membranes, creating a 'proton gradient' across the mitochondrial inner membrane. This is a way of temporarily storing the energy released in oxidation of substrates. The proton gradient is discharged by a flow of protons back into the mitochondral matrix through an enzyme complex known as ATP synthase, which, as its name suggests, synthesises ATP from ADP and inorganic phosphate. In brown adipose tissue mitochondria this process is uncoupled by a specific *uncoupling protein* (UCP) (formerly known as *thermogenin*), which allows the proton gradient across the mitochondrial inner membrane to be dissipated or 'short-circuited'. UCP is related to other proteins that transport substrates across the inner mitochondrial membrane but has become specialised as a 'proton channel'. Discharge of the proton gradient results in the liberation of heat from oxidation of substrates without trapping the free energy in high-energy compounds, and indeed the role of brown adipose tissue is specifically to generate heat. It does not do this all the time; it can be activated via the sympathetic nervous system,

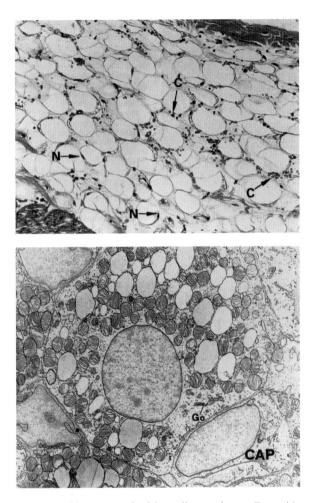

Fig. 4.13 Appearance of brown and white adipose tissue. Top, white adipose tissue under the light microscope. Each cell consists of a large lipid droplet (white) surrounded by a narrow layer of cytoplasm. The nucleus (N) can be seen in some cells, and some of the capillaries are marked (C). The picture represents a width of 0.2 mm although large human fat cells can themselves approach 0.1 mm diameter. From Burkitt, H.G., Young, B. & Heath, J.W. (1993) *Wheater's Functional Histology,* 3rd edn. Edinburgh: Churchill Livingstone. With permission of the publisher. Bottom, an electron micrograph of brown adipose tissue. In this high-powered view, one adipocyte nearly fills the picture. Unlike the white adipocytes shown above, it has multiple lipid droplets (white areas) and many mitochondria (white adipocytes also have mitochondria, but not so densely packed). CAP is a capillary adjacent to the cell, Go the Golgi apparatus. The picture represents a width of about 14 μm (i.e. it is about 14 times more enlarged than the upper picture). From Cinti (2001) with permission of the author.

bringing about both an increase in the liberation of fatty acids from the stored triacylglycerol, and a large increase in the flow of blood through the tissue. It is very highly vascularised; that is, it has many capillaries per unit cross-sectional area. The increased blood flow on stimulation brings an increased supply of oxygen, and carries away the heat produced to the rest of the body.

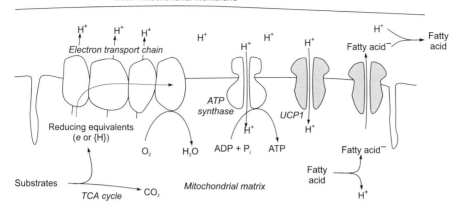

Fig. 4.14 Uncoupling of respiration in brown adipose tissue, and potentially other tissues. The electron transport chain (proteins and other molecules associated with the inner mitochondrial membrane) transfers reducing equivalents (which can be envisaged either as electrons, shown as e, or as hydrogen atoms, shown as {H}) to molecular oxygen. In the process hydrogen ions (protons) are pumped from the mitochondrial matrix to the space between the inner and outer mitochondrial membranes. The proton gradient is usually discharged by a flow of protons through the ATP synthase complex, which synthesises ATP from ADP. Thus, the free energy available from oxidation of the substrate is trapped in ATP. In brown adipose tissue, uncoupling protein-1 (UCP1) allows the proton gradient to dissipate without synthesis of ATP: therefore metabolic energy is lost as heat. UCP1, like other putative uncoupling proteins, is a member of the family of mitochondrial transporters and has six trans-membrane domains. The right-hand scheme shows how an uncoupling protein may actually facilitate the transfer of a fatty acid anion (Fatty acid⁻) out of the mitochondrial matrix. Because the anion has the possibility of combining with a proton on either side, the net effect is the same as the inward transfer of a proton. This may be the real physiological function of the 'novel' UCPs expressed outside brown adipose tissue.

Brown adipose tissue is important in animals that have a particular need to generate heat, for instance hibernating mammals. During hibernation the body temperature falls and metabolism slows, to preserve fuel stores. Awakening from hibernation is helped by the generation of heat in brown adipose tissue. Large adult mammals such as humans do not usually have a problem in generating heat, since the ratio of body mass (in which heat is generated) to body surface area (through which heat is lost) is in favour of generating too much heat, and instead adult humans have a variety of means of losing excess heat – sweating and dilation of blood vessels in the skin, for example. Correspondingly, there is no good evidence that adult humans have significant amounts of brown adipose tissue. In contrast, infants have a different surface area to body mass ratio and have a need for a mechanism to generate heat, and in infant humans brown adipose tissue has a clear role. It is lost during development. There is considerable controversy over whether it can be 'reawakened' in adults, or whether white adipose tissue can ever be converted into brown.

Since the process of uncoupling dissipates metabolic energy, there has been great interest in this process in relation to regulation of body weight: if we could

Table 4.2 'Uncoupling' proteins (UCPs).

Name	Tissue distribution	Comments
UCP1 (thermogenin)	Brown adipose tissue	Function is definitely to generate heat
UCP2	Widely expressed	Up-regulated during fasting
UCP3	Mainly skeletal muscle	
UCP4	Brain	Function unknown

There are also uncoupling proteins expressed in plants, whose function may be to warm tissues before germination.

stimulate uncoupling generally (and safely) it would be a wonderful way of regulating body weight. This interest led in 1997 to the discovery of a protein closely related to brown adipose tissue UCP. Brown adipose tissue UCP was then renamed UCP1 and the new protein called UCP2. The interesting part of the discovery was that UCP2 is expressed in many tissues, not just brown adipose tissue. We now know that there is a family of related proteins (Table 4.2). However, there is still considerable controversy over their metabolic role. UCP2 and UCP3 are both up-regulated when the flux of fatty acids is high, for instance during starvation. Since the body needs to conserve metabolic energy in starvation, what could be the 'point' of up-regulating a pathway that dissipates energy? Perhaps the most consistent explanation is the following. The newer UCPs may induce uncoupling, but their real role is as transporters of fatty acids (in their ionised form – fatty acid anions) out of the mitochondrial matrix. Fatty acids might tend to accumulate in the mitochondrial matrix when fatty acid oxidation is high (if they become detached from CoA they cannot enter the β-oxidation pathway). Thus it could be important to up-regulate a pathway that exports them. But outward transport of a fatty acid anion is equivalent to inward movement of a proton (Fig. 4.14), so uncoupling is really a byproduct. This is a very active area of research at present – not least because any possibility of up-regulating uncoupling, especially in a large tissue like skeletal muscle, offers considerable possibilities for weight loss.

4.5.3   White adipose tissue metabolism

In the adult human, adipose tissue is virtually all 'white'.[3] Its major metabolic role is the controlled storage and release of fat, stored in the form of triacylglycerol and released to the rest of the body in the form of non-esterified fatty acids. Adipose tissue is sometimes described as an inert tissue metabolically. This is true in one restricted sense only: it has a very low consumption of oxygen. But the flow of fatty acids in and out of adipose tissue represents a large proportion of the energy metabolism of the body, and this is controlled on a minute-by-minute basis.

It is worth here re-emphasising the point that lipid fuels – triacylglycerol and non-esterified fatty acids – are not water-soluble, and their presence in the plasma is dependent upon specialised transport mechanisms. Excess concentrations of lipid fuels in the plasma can have adverse consequences, outlined in Box 4.4. Therefore, the regulatory role of white adipose tissue is essential to normal health as well as to the coordination of fat metabolism in everyday life, responding to meals and overnight fasting.

Box 4.4   Adverse consequences of excessive concentrations of lipids in the circulation

Prolonged exposure of the blood vessels to high concentrations of cholesterol and triacylglycerol can lead to the build-up of fatty deposits, *atheroma*, in arterial walls – the process known as *atherosclerosis* (see Section 9.4.1 for more details).

Excessive release of non-esterified fatty acids can also have adverse effects. This can occur in stressful situations (see Section 7.3.3.2). Excessive fatty acid concentrations have adverse effects on the heart, and may predispose it to irregular patterns of contraction and, in severe cases, to *ventricular fibrillation*, an uncoordinated fluttering in which the pumping of blood effectively ceases. This is a possible link between an acutely stressful situation and a heart attack. In addition, elevated non-esterified fatty acid concentrations lead to increased hepatic secretion of triacylglycerol in the very-low-density lipoproteins, thus exacerbating any tendency to atherosclerosis. (See Oliver & Opie (1994) for a review of this topic.) Elevated non-esterified fatty acids acting over a long time impair the sensitivity of tissues to insulin and may impair insulin secretion from the pancreatic β-cell. Some prospective studies, in which participants are followed over several years, have shown that elevated plasma non-esterified fatty acids are associated with an increased risk of subsequently developing type 2 diabetes mellitus, and also of dying suddenly from a heart attack (the latter is probably related to the adverse effects on heart rhythm mentioned above). Potential adverse effects of chronically elevated concentrations of non-esterified fatty acids are discussed by Frayn *et al.* (1996).

One dramatic (although unusual) example of excessive lipid concentrations is *fat embolus*. If excess fat, usually in the form of triacylglycerol, is liberated into the plasma, then droplets of fat will circulate and may block blood vessels. This can occur after injury, when long bones such as the femur are fractured. Loosely connected fat cells are present in bone marrow, and if the bone fractures, the cells, their triacylglycerol contents, and some intact cells can be liberated in an entirely uncontrolled manner into the bloodstream. Globules of this fat may block blood vessels, particularly in the lung, leading to difficulties with breathing.

These features of excessive concentrations of lipid fuels in the circulation highlight the need to regulate their entry to and removal from the bloodstream. White adipose tissue plays an essential role in these processes.

Two distinct aspects of the metabolism of white adipose tissue will be considered: the storage of triacylglycerol when there is an excess of nutrient energy present in the circulation (as after a meal), and the liberation of fatty acids – *fat mobilisation* – when other tissues in the body require it, for instance during exercise, or after an overnight fast. Although it is simplest to consider these separately, both are actively regulated all the time; if fat storage is occurring, then fat mobilisation is suppressed, and vice versa (similar to glycogen synthesis and degradation).

The major pathways of metabolism in white adipose tissue are illustrated in Fig. 4.15.

4.5.3.1 Fat storage

The triacylglycerol droplet within an adipocyte represents a very concentrated form of energy storage, usually accumulated over a period of some years. Metabolic pathways exist for 'laying down' triacylglycerol by two major routes: (1) uptake of triacylglycerol from plasma, and (2) *de novo lipogenesis*, the synthesis of lipid (triacylglycerol) from other sources, particularly glucose. Both will be outlined, although there is no doubt that in humans – at least on a typical Western diet in which there is no shortage of fatty acids – the uptake of triacylglycerol from the plasma is by far the more important.

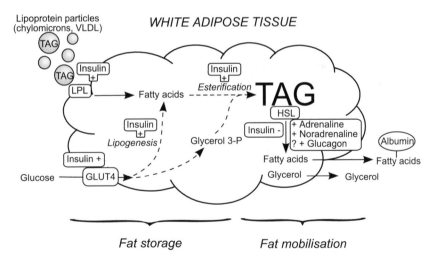

Fig. 4.15 Overview of fatty acid and glucose metabolism in white adipose tissue. The body's main store of chemical energy is in the form of triacylglycerol (TAG) in white adipose tissue. *Fat storage* is the process of deposition of TAG; *fat mobilisation* (or *lipolysis*) is the process of hydrolysis of the stored TAG to release *non-esterified fatty acids* into the plasma (bound to the carrier protein albumin), so that they can be taken up by other tissues. LPL, lipoprotein lipase; HSL, hormone-sensitive lipase; glycerol 3-P, glycerol 3-phosphate; VLDL, very-low-density lipoprotein. The major pathways and main sites of hormonal regulation are shown: a plus sign indicates stimulation, a minus sign inhibition. Dashed lines show multiple enzymatic steps.

Triacylglycerol in the plasma is present in the *lipoprotein* particles (covered fully in Chapter 9). The largest of these particles, which carry most of the triacylglycerol, are too big to escape from the capillaries into the interstitial fluid; therefore, the adipocytes cannot take them up directly. There is an interesting mechanism to overcome this difficulty. Adipocytes produce the enzyme *lipoprotein lipase*, which hydrolyses the triacylglycerol in lipoprotein particles to release fatty acids, which can then diffuse into the interstitial space and so reach the adipocytes. Since lipoprotein lipase must act in the capillaries, it is exported from the adipocytes to the endothelial cells lining the capillaries of adipose tissue. Here it is attached by chains of the complex amino-glycan *heparan sulphate*, a carbohydrate with highly negatively charged sulphate groups to which the enzyme molecules attach through a charge interaction. Lipoprotein lipase can thus come into contact with, and act upon, passing lipoprotein particles (Fig. 4.16). It acts on them to hydrolyse their triacylglycerol, thus releasing fatty acids. These fatty acids diffuse a short distance through the interstitial space towards the adipocytes, which take them up.[4] The fatty acids are mainly taken up into the cells by a carrier-mediated process involving FAT/CD36 (Table 2.4), although this is an area of current research. The diffusion of the fatty acids from the site of lipoprotein lipase action into the cells is probably regulated by concentration gradients. The concentration gradient from capillary to cell will be produced, after a meal, by the activation of lipoprotein lipase, stimulation by insulin of the esterification pathway, and the suppression of the release of fatty acids from the triacylglycerol store within the cell.

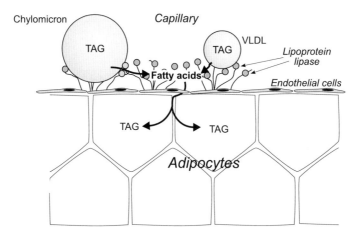

Fig. 4.16 The action of lipoprotein lipase in white adipose tissue. Lipoprotein lipase is attached to the branching glycosamino-glycan chains that form the *glycocalyx* (a fuzzy surface lining the capillary, attached to the endothelial cells). It acts on lipoprotein particles in the capillaries which contain triacylglycerol (TAG), hydrolysing this TAG to release fatty acids which are taken up into adipocytes and re-esterified for storage as TAG. More than one molecule of the enzyme acts on a lipoprotein particle at once.

Once inside the cells, the fatty acids are esterified to form triacylglycerol which joins the lipid droplet for storage. The pathway of esterification is the usual one in which the fatty acids are firstly activated by formation of CoA derivatives, then linked to glycerol 3-phosphate (the *phosphatidic acid pathway* – see Fig. 3.8). The glycerol 3-phosphate is formed through glycolysis; it is in equilibrium with dihydroxyacetone phosphate, an intermediate in glycolysis, their interconversion being catalysed by the enzyme *glycerol-3-phosphate dehydrogenase.*

The activity of lipoprotein lipase in adipose tissue is stimulated by insulin, secreted in response to an elevation in the blood glucose concentration. Since we rarely eat fat alone, this means that after a typical meal containing both fat and carbohydrate, the uptake of fat into adipose tissue will be stimulated. The activation of lipoprotein lipase by insulin is rather complex, because of the rather complicated 'life cycle' of this enzyme. The effect of insulin involves increased transcription, altered processing of the enzyme within adipocytes and probably increased export to the endothelial cells. It is therefore not a rapid process and takes a matter of 3–4 hours. This time-course will be highly relevant when we consider the coordination of metabolism in different tissues by insulin (Chapter 6). Within adipose tissue, the esterification of fatty acids is also stimulated by the production of glycerol 3-phosphate through glycolysis, increased by insulin (Fig. 4.15). Thus, insulin stimulates both the uptake and storage in adipose tissue of fat circulating as triacylglycerol in the plasma.

The other potential pathway of fat deposition in adipose tissue is that of *de novo lipogenesis*. The pathway is the same as that in the liver (Box 4.3). It is stimulated by insulin at multiple points. Thus, again, insulin acts to promote fat storage in adipose tissue.

4.5.3.2 Fat mobilisation

The mobilisation of fat results in the liberation of fatty acids from the stored triacylglycerol; these fatty acids are released into the plasma as non-esterified fatty acids bound to albumin, and so are made available to other tissues. Since the mobilisation of fat involves the hydrolysis of stored lipid, it is also called *lipolysis*. The breakdown of triacylglycerol is catalysed by a lipase, although this enzyme is necessarily situated within the adipocytes, in contrast to lipoprotein lipase which is exported to the capillaries. It is known as *hormone-sensitive lipase*, because its responsiveness to hormones was recognised before that of lipoprotein lipase. (It is better, perhaps, to think of this enzyme as the intracellular lipase.) It acts at the surface of the triacylglycerol droplet, and catalyses the hydrolysis of the ester bonds of two fatty acids. Another enzyme, a *monoacylglycerol lipase*, present in high activity, is responsible for removal of the third fatty acid. Thus, three fatty acids and one glycerol molecule are produced from each molecule of stored triacylglycerol. The fatty acids for the most part leave the cells and enter the plasma non-esterified fatty acid pool. The glycerol also leaves the cell; it cannot be utilised for esterification of fatty acids since adipose tissue almost completely lacks the enzyme glycerol kinase which would be necessary for this.

The activity of hormone-sensitive lipase must clearly be regulated very precisely, such that it is inactive when insulin levels are high. Hormone-sensitive lipase is regulated by phosphorylation in a manner similar to glycogen phosphorylase in the liver: this was discussed in Chapter 2 (Box 2.4). Phosphorylation is brought about by elevation of the cellular level of cAMP, in response to a number of regulators. It is probable in humans that the most important of these are adrenaline (in the plasma) and noradrenaline (released by sympathetic nerves). Glucagon has a potent effect in isolated fat cells in the laboratory, but appears not to affect fat mobilisation in humans *in vivo*. Equally important is the inactivation of hormone-sensitive lipase by dephosphorylation in response to insulin. This is a very potent effect – it responds to relatively low concentrations of insulin – and very rapid, occurring within a matter of minutes of raising the insulin concentration. Thus, insulin not only promotes fat storage, but it restrains fat mobilisation.

Phosphorylation of hormone-sensitive lipase appears to do more than simply change its conformation. It appears that, in its dephosphorylated, inactive form, hormone-sensitive lipase is present in the cytosol of the cell. When it is phosphorylated, it moves (translocates) to the surface of the lipid droplet and begins hydrolysing the stored triacylglycerol. Another protein is involved in this process: perilipin. Perilipin is an abundant protein in white adipocytes, and seems to coat the lipid droplet. Perilipin is also a substrate for phosphorylation with a signal chain similar to that for hormone-sensitive lipase (Box 2.4). When it is phosphorylated, it moves, or curls up, away from the lipid droplet, allowing hormone-sensitive lipase access.

Insulin has a further effect in restraining fat mobilisation. The fatty acids released by the action of hormone-sensitive lipase are available for esterification by the phosphatidic acid pathway already described. Insulin, as we have seen, stimulates this pathway by increasing the provision of glycerol 3-phosphate. Thus, insulin both inhibits the activity of hormone-sensitive lipase and 'mops up' any fatty acids it may liberate by increasing their re-esterification. These two actions are illustrated in Fig. 4.17.

4.5.3.3 Adipocyte differentiation and longer-term regulation of fat storage

We have seen above how adipocytes will take up excess fatty acids in the short term, for instance in the period following a meal that contains both carbohydrate (to stimulate insulin) and fat. Normally the uptake of fatty acids after meals will be balanced by fat mobilisation in the postabsorptive state (e.g. during the night-time fast) and during exercise, so that in many people the size of the fat stores remains relatively constant over long periods. We all know, however, that there are situations in which there is a gradual excess of fat deposition over mobilisation, or, of course, vice versa. Adipose tissue has well-developed

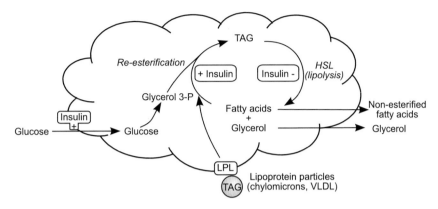

Fig. 4.17 Suppression of fat mobilisation by insulin. Insulin restrains fat mobilisation by two mechanisms: suppression of the activity of hormone-sensitive lipase (HSL), and stimulation of the re-esterification of fatty acids within the adipocytes. (The same process of esterification will also be simultaneously incorporating fatty acids from circulating triacylglycerol, released by lipoprotein lipase (LPL), into stored triacylglycerol.)

regulatory mechanisms to cope with these situations. If there is a long-term situation of positive energy balance, SREBP-1c expression will be increased by insulin and the PPARγ system will be activated by the excess availability of fatty acids (Sections 2.4.1.1, 2.4.2.2). Between them, these two systems will up-regulate expression of the key enzymes involved in fat storage (Table 4.3). Each fat cell will increase in size as it stores more fat. Activation of these systems has another important effect: it is the stimulus for the differentiation of fat cell precursors, or preadipocytes, into new adipocytes. SREBP-1c was discovered independently in adipocytes as a factor causing adipocyte differentiation, and it is also called adipocyte determination and differentiation factor-1 (ADD-1). As Table 4.3 shows, SREBP-1c is itself a stimulus to increased expression of PPARγ, which is another adipocyte differentiation factor. Thus, a long-term positive energy balance will result in both an increase in adipocyte size (hypertrophy) and an increase in the number of fat cells (hyperplasia).

Table 4.3 Some genes whose expression in adipose tissue will be increased during long-term energy excess.

SREBP-1c	PPARγ
Acetyl-CoA carboxylase	Lipoprotein lipase
Fatty acid synthase	Fatty acid transport protein
Glycerol phosphate acyl transferase	Acyl-CoA synthase
Lipoprotein lipase	GLUT4
PPARγ	

Only genes with relevance to increasing lipid storage are listed.

Small fat cells seem to be more metabolically active than big, fat-full cells, and may be particularly avid in taking up excess fatty acids. This may be the key to understanding the action of the new antidiabetic drugs, the thiazolidinediones (TZDs), which are PPARγ activators (Section 2.4.2.2). If the TZDs stimulate the proliferation of new fat cells, which are very active in 'trapping' fatty acids, then circulating fatty acid concentrations may fall and removal of metabolic competition may allow glucose utilisation by other tissues to increase – but this will be at the expense of additional fat deposition. In fact, prominent features of TZD action are a reduction in circulating non-esterified fatty acid concentrations, an increase in body weight, and an improvement in the ability of other tissues to metabolise glucose. We will revisit this topic in a later chapter (Chapter 10).

4.5.3.4 Adipose tissue as an endocrine organ

Several decades ago it was recognised that adipose tissue could produce certain steroid hormones, including oestrogens (female sex hormones). This is because cells within adipose tissue (probably mainly cells other than the adipocytes) express the enzymes to interconvert steroid hormones. Oestrogens (such as oestradiol) can be produced from androgens (such as androstenedione) that are produced by the adrenal cortex (Section 5.5.1). This has important ramifications. In obesity, when there is an excess of adipose tissue, more oestrogens may be produced. That has some beneficial effects: obese postmenopausal women (whose ovaries no longer produce oestrogens) are somewhat protected from osteoporosis, compared with lean women, because of this. The hormone cortisol is also produced from the inactive precursor cortisone. That may have untoward effects in obese men, adding to a metabolic 'stress' state.

The real impetus to this field came, however, in 1994 with the recognition that adipose tissue secretes a peptide hormone, now called leptin (from the Greek *leptos*, thin). The story of leptin will be further developed in the next chapter (Section 5.6) when we consider adipose tissue with other hormone-secreting organs, and in Chapter 11 (see Section 11.2) when we consider energy balance.

Along with leptin, which is certainly a true hormone, we now recognise adipose tissue to produce a number of other proteins, many of which are relevant to energy metabolism. One, of course, is lipoprotein lipase (see Section 4.5.3.1 above). Others include apolipoprotein E and cholesteryl ester transfer protein (both relevant to lipid metabolism: see Chapter 9), a number of cytokines (peptides that signal between cells and may play a role in inflammatory responses), proteins involved with blood clotting, and a number of components of the complement pathway involved in immunological defences. The complement story is interesting. Some years ago adipocytes were found to express in large quantities a protein that was called (for want of a better name) adipsin. Later, adipsin was found to be identical to factor D, a component of the so-called alternative complement pathway. Now we know that adipocytes produce several factors involved in this pathway and that these may interact, somewhere outside the fat cell, to produce a fragment known as acylation stimulating protein (ASP). ASP is a potent stimulator of fatty acid esterification in adipocytes. Thus, adipocytes seem to act locally to regulate their own fat storage.

4.6   The kidneys

4.6.1   General description

The two kidneys sit fairly high up towards the back of the abdomen. Strictly speaking, they are not in the abdominal cavity; they are behind the *peritoneum*, the membrane which surrounds the other abdominal organs such as the liver and intestines. The kidneys weigh about 150 g each in the adult.

The adjective *renal* (from the Latin *renes*, the kidneys) is used to describe the properties and functions of the kidneys. The kidneys are supplied with blood through the *renal arteries* which branch off the aorta, and the blood is returned to the inferior vena cava through the *renal veins*. The major purpose of the kidneys is to produce urine. This is a vehicle for excretion of (1) those products of metabolism that the body needs to dispose of; and (2) regulated amounts of water, in order to maintain the correct osmolarity of the body fluids.

The details of renal physiology are outside the scope of this book, although a brief outline is necessary in order to understand the energy requirements of the kidneys. Blood flows through a series of complex structures known as the *glomeruli*, where 'tangles' of blood vessels are surrounded by a cup-shaped structure, the *glomerular capsule* or *Bowman's capsule*. The endothelium of these blood capillaries is highly fenestrated (see Section 1.3.1) to allow ready passage of molecules out of the blood, into the capsule: this process is known as *glomerular filtration*. It is aided by the fact that the blood in the glomerular capillaries is under higher pressure than usual in capillaries. Thus, some of the plasma water, together with its complement of the smaller molecules dissolved in plasma, is lost into the capsule. The capsule is the termination of a tube, the *renal tubule*; the complete assembly of glomerular capsule and tubule is called a *nephron*, of which there are about half a million in each human kidney. The fluid thus entering the renal tubule is the beginning of urine. However, before the urine is fully formed, much of the water and many of the solutes filtered at the glomerulus will be *reabsorbed* into the blood. In contrast to filtration, reabsorption is a very selective process and much of it involves active transport – energy-requiring transport of substances up a concentration gradient back into the plasma. The renal tubule forms a long loop, the *loop of Henle*, with *descending* and *ascending* limbs, following it in order from the glomerular capsule towards its end, where it joins a larger duct collecting urine from a number of tubules. These *collecting ducts* merge and eventually form the *ureter*, the tube carrying fully formed urine from the kidney to the bladder.

4.6.2   The scale of kidney function

About 1 litre of blood passes each minute through the glomeruli, or almost 800 litres each day. Of this, about 20% is filtered through into the nephrons, producing almost 200 litres of filtrate each day. About 99% of the volume of this filtrate is reabsorbed, so that only 1–2 litres leaves the body as urine.

Water-soluble substances in the plasma are filtered along with the plasma water. Consider glucose as an example. A typical concentration of glucose in the plasma is about 5 mmol/litre, or 0.9 g/litre. Thus, almost 1000 mmol (180 g) of glucose are lost into the glomerular filtrate each day. Since the body does not 'want' to excrete glucose, virtually all of this is reabsorbed from the renal tubule.

Reabsorption of glucose has many similarities to the absorption of glucose from the intestine, discussed in Chapter 3. The epithelial cells lining the tubules have microvilli, like the intestinal mucosal cells, increasing their absorptive surface area. At least in the first part of the tubule, glucose is carried into the cells by the sodium-glucose co-transporters SGLT-1, SGLT-2 and SGLT-3 and leaves – into the interstitial fluid and thus the venous plasma – by the facilitated transporter *GLUT2* (as in the enterocyte, illustrated in Fig. 3.7). Thus, the energy for glucose reabsorption again comes from a gradient of concentration for sodium ions, which is maintained by the activity of the Na^+-K^+-ATPase, and ultimately from hydrolysis of ATP.

4.6.3   Energy metabolism in the kidney

Given the very large quantities of solutes other than glucose which also have to be reabsorbed, it should not surprise us to learn that the kidneys have a high demand for energy. In fact they consume about 10% of the total oxygen consumption of the body at rest, although they contribute less than 0.5% of body mass. However, this metabolic activity is not spread evenly throughout the kidney.

In cross-section, the kidney can be seen to be formed of three fairly distinct parts. There is an outer lighter coloured layer, the *renal cortex*, surrounding a darker centre, the *renal medulla*. In the concave part of the 'bean' shape is the *renal pelvis*, the area where the collecting ducts gather together and form the ureter. The glomeruli are situated in the cortex, and some nephrons are completely contained in the cortex. Others have their loops 'dipping down' into the medulla; but most of the energy-requiring reabsorption of solutes goes on in the cortex. The cortex has a high blood supply and it has a correspondingly aerobic pattern of metabolism; it oxidises glucose, fatty acids and ketone bodies to provide its metabolic energy. The medulla, on the other hand, is much less well supplied with blood and derives its metabolic energy from the anaerobic metabolism of glucose. This is illustrated in Fig. 4.18.

During starvation, the kidney becomes a relatively important site of gluconeogenesis. This process seems to take a few days of starvation to adapt, but may then contribute up to half the body's need for glucose. The development of gluconeogenesis in the kidney is also related to mechanisms for excretion

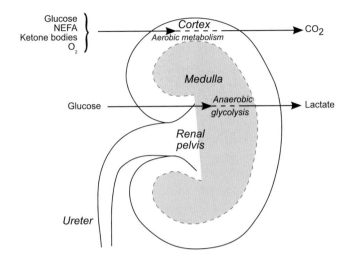

Fig. 4.18 Schematic view of energy metabolism in different regions of the kidney.
The *cortex* (outer layer) is well supplied with blood, has a high energy demand and is largely
aerobic; the *medulla* has a poor blood supply and is largely anaerobic. It may derive its
glucose by reabsorption from the tubules.

of hydrogen ions to assist maintenance of acid–base balance (see later, Section 8.3.2.4).

4.7   Endothelial cells and other cell types

4.7.1   The endothelium – a large organ distributed throughout the body

Blood vessels are lined with a single layer of flat cells, endothelial cells: this lining is called the endothelium (Fig. 4.19). The whole endothelium in humans is large, weighing around 1.5 kg, with an area similar to that of a football pitch. Endothelial cells provide a smooth lining that reduces resistance to blood flow, but they are also very active in a number of ways. They regulate the contraction or relaxation of blood vessels (by sending signals to the muscle surrounding the

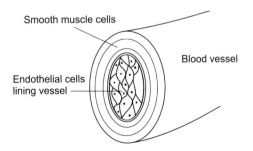

Fig. 4.19 The endothelium, a smooth single-celled lining of blood vessels.

vessel), they provide a (regulatable) barrier to prevent cells and large molecules leaving the circulation and entering the surrounding tissue, and they also prevent blood clotting (unless there is damage to the vessel wall). We will consider the first of these functions since it is relevant to metabolism. It was recognised in 1980 that endothelial cells could produce a substance that caused blood vessels to dilate (by relaxation of the smooth muscle layer of the vessel). This substance was called endothelial-derived relaxing factor (EDRF). The discovery in 1987 that EDRF is the gas nitric oxide (NO) led to a Nobel Prize for three American pharmacologists, Robert Furchgott, Louis Ignarro and Ferid Murad (and also recognition of the part played by the British scientist Salvador Moncada whom many thought should have shared the prize). Now some people believe that hydrogen peroxide (H_2O_2) is also released by endothelial cells and has similar properties. NO is produced by the enzyme nitric oxide synthase, of which there are several isoforms. The one we are concerned with here is called endothelial NO-synthase, often abbreviated eNOS. NO is synthesised from arginine (Fig. 4.20). eNOS is activated by various stimuli, including stretching of the blood vessel: thus, if blood flow is tending to increase, for instance because the heart is pumping more blood, the vessels will respond (via NO production) by relaxing to allow the blood to flow freely. This is a mechanism for preventing undue increases in blood pressure. In some tissues, in particular skeletal muscle, eNOS is activated by insulin. Muscle blood flow will increase after a meal. Some people in the field believe (although this is controversial) that this assists in increasing glucose delivery to muscle cells so that glucose utilisation can increase following a meal.

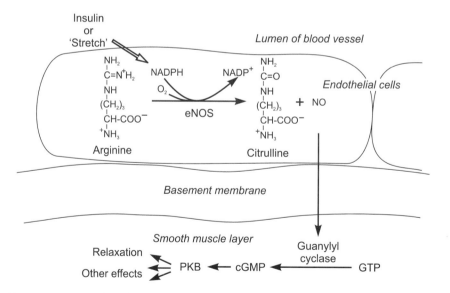

Fig. 4.20 Generation of nitric oxide (NO) from arginine in endothelial cells leads to relaxation of the underlying smooth muscle. eNOS, endothelial nitric oxide synthase; cGMP, cyclic GMP; PKG, cGMP-dependent protein kinase or protein kinase G.

4.7.2   Rapidly dividing cells

Some cells in the body normally divide rapidly, or may be called upon to do so in certain circumstances. Epithelial cells of the small intestine, or enterocytes, fall into the former category. New cells are continually being formed at the base of each crypt (between the villi – see Section 3.2.3.1). They move up towards the tip of the villus as they age, and then are shed from the tip. The average life of a small-intestinal epithelial cell is 2–5 days. Some cells of the immune system may need to divide rapidly in times of (for instance) bacterial invasion, when lymphocytes producing antibodies that react against the foreign proteins are selected and multiply. A common feature of these cells seems to be a dependence on glutamine as a metabolic fuel. This may be because glutamine can act as a nitrogen donor in the synthesis of the purine and pyrimidine bases needed for nucleic acid synthesis and cell division. In the course of glutamine degradation in the intestinal mucosa, alanine is formed and may be transported to the liver in the hepatic portal vein as a substrate for gluconeogenesis (Section 6.3.2.3).

4.7.3   Macrophages

Macrophages (from the Greek for 'large eaters') are phagocytic cells that can ingest foreign organisms, and are found in many tissues. They often have specific names according to the tissue in which they are found: for instance, Kupffer cells in the liver, microglia in the brain. There are many macrophages in the lining of blood vessels. They arise from circulating white blood cells called monocytes, which attach to the endothelium, and then migrate through it. Once in the sub-endothelial space they may grow considerably. Macrophages have several roles relevant to metabolism, but we will concentrate on their ability to take up, or ingest, not just bacteria but also lipoprotein particles (explained more fully in Chapter 9). These lipoprotein particles are taken up by specific receptors, again described more fully in Chapter 9. Related to their lipid metabolic activities, macrophages express some proteins that we will meet again when we consider lipoproteins in Chapter 9 including the enzyme lipoprotein lipase, and apolipoprotein E. They are also a source of cytokines, peptides that signal between cells, and are particularly involved in organisation of the immune defence and bodily repair systems.

4.8   Further reading

Regulation of glucose and glycogen metabolism (liver, heart, skeletal muscle)

Lawrence, J.C.J. & Roach, P.J. (1997) New insights into the role and mechanism of glycogen synthase activation by insulin. *Diabetes* 46: 541–547.

Bollen, M., Keppens, S. & Stalmans, W. (1998) Specific features of glycogen metabolism in the liver. *Biochem J* 336: 19–31.

Depré, C., Rider, M.H. & Hue, L. (1998) Mechanisms of control of heart glycolysis. *Eur J Biochem* 258: 277–290.

Nordlie, R.C., Foster, J.D. & Lange, A.J. (1999) Regulation of glucose production by the liver. *Annu Rev Nutr* 19: 379–406.

Okar, D.A. & Lange, A.J. (1999) Fructose-2,6-bisphosphate and control of carbohydrate metabolism in eukaryotes. *BioFactors* 10: 1–14.

El-Maghrabi, M.R., Noto, F., Wu, N. & Manes, N. (2001) 6-phosphofructo-2-kinase/fructose-2,6-bisphosphatase: suiting structure to need, in a family of tissue-specific enzymes. *Curr Opin Clin Nutr Metab Care* 4: 411–418.

van Schaftingen, E. & Gerin, I. (2002) The glucose-6-phosphatase system. *Biochem J* 362: 513–532.

Regulation of fatty acid and triacylglycerol synthesis and oxidation

Smith, S. (1994) The animal fatty acid synthase: one gene, one polypeptide, seven enzymes. *Faseb J* 8: 1248–1259.

Hellerstein, M.K., Schwarz, J.-M. & Neese, R.A. (1996) Regulation of hepatic de novo lipogenesis in humans. *Annu Rev Nutr* 16: 523–557.

Kim, K.H. (1997) Regulation of mammalian acetyl-coenzyme A carboxylase. *Annu Rev Nutr* 17: 77–99.

Hegardt, F.G. (1999) Mitochondrial 3-hydroxy-3-methylglutaryl-CoA synthase: a control enzyme in ketogenesis. *Biochem J* 338: 569–582.

Ruderman, N.B., Saha, A.K., Vavvas, D. & Witters, L.A. (1999) Malonyl-CoA, fuel sensing, and insulin resistance. *Am J Physiol* 276: E1–E18.

Zammit, V.A. (1999a) Carnitine acyltransferases: functional significance of subcellular distribution and membrane topology. *Prog Lipid Res* 38: 199–224.

Zammit, V.A. (1999b) The malonyl-CoA-long-chain acyl-CoA axis in the maintenance of mammalian cell function. *Biochem J* 343: 505–515.

Coleman, R.A., Lewin, T.M. & Muoio, D. (2000) Physiological and nutritional regulation of enzymes of triacylglycerol synthesis. *Annu Rev Nutr* 20: 77–103.

Kerner, J. & Hoppel, C. (2000) Fatty acid import into mitochondria. *Biochim Biophys Acta* 1486: 1–17.

Regulation of lipid metabolism

Goldberg, I.J. (1996) Lipoprotein lipase and lipolysis: central roles in lipoprotein metabolism and atherogenesis. *J Lipid Res* 37: 693–707.

Fielding, B.A. & Frayn, K.N. (1998) Lipoprotein lipase and the disposition of dietary fatty acids. *Br J Nutr* 80: 495–502.

Holm, C., Osterlund, T., Laurell, H. & Contreras, J.A. (2000) Molecular mechanisms regulating hormone-sensitive lipase and lipolysis. *Annu Rev Nutr* 20: 365–393.

Skeletal muscle metabolism

Vock, R., Weibel, E.R., Hoppeler, H., Ordway, G., Weber, J.-M. & Taylor, C.R. (1996) Design of the oxygen and substrate pathways. V. Structural basis of vascular substrate supply to muscle cells. *J Exp Biol* 199: 1675–1688. *The paper by Vock et al. (1996) is one of a series of contiguous papers. They have wonderful electron micrographs of skeletal muscle. They prompt one to think very carefully about issues of substrate and O₂ diffusion across tissues.*

Gordon, A.M., Homsher, E. & Regnier, M. (2000) Regulation of contraction in striated muscle. *Physiol Rev* 80: 853–924.

Wyss, M. & Kaddurah-Daouk, R. (2000) Creatine and creatinine metabolism. *Physiol Rev* 80: 1107–1213.

Gordon, A.M., Regnier, M. & Homsher, E. (2001) Skeletal and cardiac muscle contractile activation: tropomyosin 'rocks and rolls'. *News Physiol Sci* 16: 49–55.

Uncoupling proteins

Ricquier, D. & Bouillaud, F. (2000) The uncoupling protein homologues: UCP1, UCP2, UCP3, StUCP and AtUCP. *Biochem J* 345: 161–179.

Dulloo, A.G. & Samec, S. (2001) Uncoupling proteins: their roles in adaptive thermogenesis and substrate metabolism reconsidered. *Br J Nutr* 86: 123–139.

Notes

1   It is more correct to say that glucokinase has a low affinity for glucose: the term K_m implies strict Michaelis-Menten kinetics, which is not true. Although it is not inhibited by glucose 6-phosphate at concentrations found in the cell, it is regulated by another hexose phosphate, fructose 6-phosphate, acting as an inhibitor via binding to a specific regulatory protein. See Cornish-Bowden & Cárdenas (1991) and Further Reading at the end of this chapter.

2   In certain conditions, the hepatic fat content can become much greater and result in the pathological condition known as *fatty liver* (characterised, as its name suggests, by large fat deposits seen under the microscope). This happens in alcoholism. Fat can build up to the extent that it disrupts the normal functioning of the liver.

3   In fact, it is distinctly yellow, because fat-soluble pigments are stored along with the triacylglycerol; these include carotenoids – derivatives of vitamin A – and some breakdown products of haemoglobin.

4   Because the fatty acids are not water-soluble, the term 'diffuse' here may include some sort of structured pathway in which the fatty acids bind to albumin, or to an extension of the cell membrane.

5

Important Endocrine Organs and Hormones

5.1   Endocrine glands and hormones

A *gland* is an organ which produces a secretion, such as a hormone which may enter the bloodstream, a juice which enters the digestive tract or a substance such as sweat which enters the external environment. Other terms used in this connection are the adjectives *endocrine* and *exocrine*, endocrine referring to internal secretions or hormones, and exocrine to the production of juices to be delivered to the outside world. The tube of the intestine is regarded as the outside world, since it connects with it at either end.

The term *hormone* comes from the Greek *hormao*, meaning to urge on or excite. Hormones are released into the bloodstream from one tissue, and cause an effect in another. But the way in which they exert their effect must be distinguished from that of a metabolite – the ketone body, 3-hydroxybutyrate, for example. This substance is also produced in one organ (the liver) and causes an effect (uptake and oxidation) in another – e.g. skeletal muscle. But the essence of hormone action is that the hormone affects substances other than itself, typically by causing regulation of a metabolic pathway. Hormones consist of a variety of types of chemical: peptides, glycoproteins, steroids and other small molecules, mostly derivatives of amino acids. At their *target tissue* they act by binding to a specific *receptor*, itself a protein (Section 2.3). For peptide and protein hormones this receptor is usually an integral protein of the cell membrane. For steroid hormones and thyroid hormones it is within the cell; the hormone/hormone receptor complex enters the nucleus (or is formed in the nucleus) and affects DNA transcription, and thus synthesis of specific proteins.

The endocrine and exocrine glands are not in themselves major consumers of energy relative to other tissues in the body. But clearly their products have important effects in regulating energy supply and storage in the body. Here the

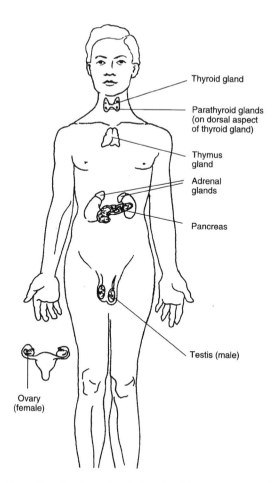

Fig. 5.1 The location of endocrine glands involved in energy metabolism.

major hormone-producing glands, and some exocrine tissues, relevant to energy metabolism will be considered. The location of the glands to be discussed is shown in Fig. 5.1.

5.2   The pancreas

5.2.1   General description of the pancreas and its anatomy

The pancreas is a fish-shaped organ, about the size of a medium herring, lying under the liver (Fig. 5.1). It has a distinct head and a narrow tail, and the head end is wrapped around the small intestine. The pancreas is a complex organ since it contains both exocrine and endocrine tissues. The exocrine function of the pancreas consists of the liberation of digestive juices into the small intestine: the endocrine function consists of the production and secretion of hormones into the bloodstream, most importantly insulin and glucagon.

The vast majority of cells in the pancreas are exocrine. These cells produce an alkaline digestive juice containing a number of enzymes, particularly amylase, pancreatic lipase and the proteases, trypsin and chymotrypsin. This juice is collected into small ducts which merge to form one main *pancreatic duct*. This is joined by the common bile duct just before it enters the duodenum; thus, bile salts and pancreatic enzymes are liberated together into the small intestine. The digestive function of the pancreas, and its regulation, were discussed in Chapter 3 (see Table 3.2).

Scattered amongst the exocrine tissue are little groups of cells, appearing like islands under the microscope. They were first described by a German medical student, Paul Langerhans, in 1869 and are known as the *Islets of Langerhans* (Fig. 5.2). These are the endocrine cells. There are around a million islets in the adult pancreas, although they constitute only 1–2% of the total mass of the pancreas. Within the islets there are three types of endocrine cell: the α-*cells* or A cells, which secrete *glucagon*, the β-*cells* or B cells which secrete *insulin* and the δ-*cells* or D cells which secrete *somatostatin*. The β-cells occupy about 60% of the volume of the islet. Somatostatin in the pancreas probably has a local regulatory role, affecting the secretion of insulin and glucagon, but this is not entirely clear, and it will not be considered further here. Each islet is supplied with blood by a branch of the *pancreatic artery*, and venous blood leaves the islet in tiny veins (venules) which merge to form the *pancreatic* and *pancreatico-duodenal veins*. As discussed in Section 4.1.1, they discharge their

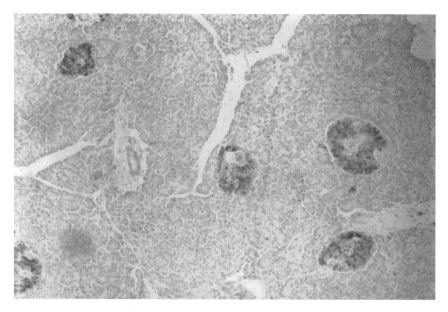

Fig. 5.2 Islets of Langerhans in the pancreas. The pancreatic tissue has been immuno-stained to show the presence of insulin (and hence the islets). Courtesy of Dr Anne Clark.

contents into the hepatic portal vein, so the liver is in a unique position as re-
gards its exposure to the pancreatic hormones.

5.2.2   Insulin

Insulin is a peptide hormone. It consists of two peptide chains, the A and B
chains, linked to each other by disulphide bonds: the A chain contains 21
amino acids, and the B chain 30 amino acids. It is synthesised within the β-
cells as a single polypeptide chain (proinsulin), and the connecting peptide or
C-peptide is removed by proteolytic action before secretion (Fig. 5.3).

Clearly, for insulin to have a useful signalling function, its rate of secretion
into the plasma must vary according to the metabolic or nutritional state. The
most important regulator of the rate of insulin secretion is the concentration of
glucose in the plasma. The β-cell is similar to the hepatocyte in that it expresses
the GLUT2 transporter and the hexokinase IV isoform (glucokinase). As in the
liver (Section 4.1.2.1), these give the β-cell the ability to act as a 'glucose sensor'.
As the external (plasma) glucose concentration rises, so glucose flows into the
cell and is phosphorylated, and then enters the glycolytic pathway. This leads
to generation of ATP, which regulates events at the cell membrane (Fig. 5.4).

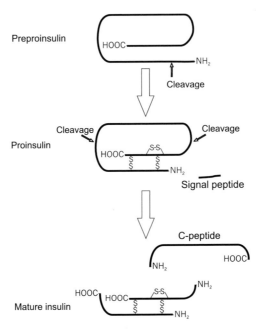

Fig. 5.3 Synthesis of insulin. Insulin is first synthesised as one long polypeptide, preproinsulin. The N-terminal portion is a 'signal sequence' that directs preproinsulin into the
secretory vesicles. It is then removed (arrows show sites of proteolytic action). Three disulphide bonds are formed between cysteine residues. (These will hold the mature protein in
a particular folded structure.) Further proteolytic cleavage releases the connecting peptide,
or C-peptide, to produce mature insulin. Insulin and C-peptide are secreted in equimolar
amounts from the β-cell. Some proinsulin is also secreted into the plasma.

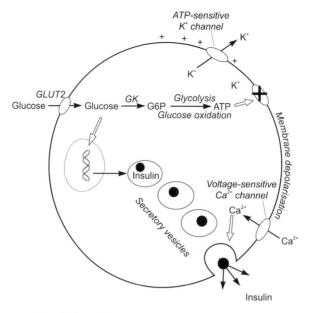

Fig. 5.4 Glucose-stimulation of insulin secretion in the pancreatic β-cell. Glucose enters the cell via the transporter GLUT2 (but see below) and is phosphorylated by glucokinase (GK) (hexokinase IV). These steps are similar to glucose utilisation in the liver and allow the β-cell to 'sense' the plasma glucose concentration. Generation of ATP from glucose utilisation closes ATP-sensitive K+ channels in the cell membrane, stopping the outward flow of K+ ions that normally maintains the resting membrane potential (see Box 7.1 for full description of this). This leads to membrane depolarisation and opening of voltage-sensitive Ca^{2+} channels. Insulin is present in multiple secretory vesicles in the cell, as a crystalline complex in the centre of the vesicle. An inward flux of Ca^{2+} ions causes exocytosis of the insulin-containing secretory vesicles, and hence insulin secretion. Glucose also stimulates synthesis of new insulin (see Section 2.4.2.1). Although this scenario is true in rodent islets, there is some question over the presence of GLUT2 in human β-cells and it may be that GLUT1 and GLUT3 give the human β-cell sufficient glucose transport capacity (for discussion, see Schuit 1997).

Insulin, which is synthesised within the cell and stored in secretory granules, is released by exocytosis of these granules – the granule membrane fuses with the cell membrane and its contents are discharged into the extracellular space. The synthesis of new insulin is also stimulated (via the transcription factor PDX1, see Section 2.4.2.1), and if the stimulus (elevated glucose concentration) persists, insulin secretion will be maintained by increased synthesis.

The response of the β-cells to the surrounding glucose concentration may be studied by isolating pancreatic islets and incubating them in medium containing different concentrations of glucose. The characteristic sigmoid dose–response curve for insulin secretion rate against glucose concentration is shown in Fig. 5.5. Insulin secretion is not much increased until the glucose concentration rises above 5 mmol/l, which (by no coincidence) is the normal concentration of glucose in plasma. In other words, an elevation of the concentration of glucose in the plasma above its normal level will result in increased secretion of insulin.

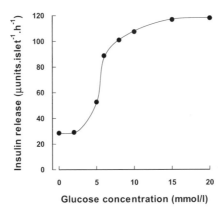

Fig. 5.5 Dose–response curve for the effects of glucose concentration on the secretion of insulin from isolated human islets of Langerhans, studied *in vitro*. Insulin secretion is stimulated as the glucose concentration rises above about 5 mmol/l (a typical concentration of glucose in the plasma). Based on Harrison, D.E., Christie, M.R. & Gray, D.W.R. (1985) Properties of isolated human islets of Langerhans: insulin secretion, glucose oxidation and protein phosphorylation. *Diabetologia* 28: 99–103. Copyright Springer-Verlag, with permission.

Glucose is not the only stimulus to insulin secretion. Insulin secretion is also responsive to most amino acids (to somewhat differing extents), so that after a meal containing protein there is a stimulus for net protein synthesis. Ketone bodies also (somewhat) stimulate insulin secretion that is stimulated by glucose: this could be seen as a mechanism for restraining ketone body concentrations, since increased insulin secretion will inhibit fatty acid release from adipose tissue and ketogenesis in the liver.

There has been considerable interest recently in the effects of fatty acids on insulin secretion. It now seems that fatty acids are essential for normal glucose-stimulated insulin secretion, and that an increase in the fatty acid concentration for a period of one or two hours will potentiate insulin secretion in response to glucose. It is suggested that a fatty acid derivative, perhaps acyl-CoA, is involved in some way in the insulin secretory pathway. However, if elevated fatty acid concentrations are maintained for more than a few hours, the opposite is seen: there is an impairment of insulin secretion. This seems to relate to an accumulation of triacylglycerol within the β-cell. The mechanism is not understood.

Insulin secretion is also modulated by the nervous system, in ways that will be discussed in more detail in Chapter 7.

Insulin circulates free in the bloodstream; it is not bound to a carrier protein. It affects tissues by binding to specific *insulin receptors*, proteins consisting of four subunits (two α- and two β-chains), embedded in cell membranes (see Boxes 2.3, 2.4). Signal chains linking the binding of insulin to its receptor and an intracellular change in metabolism were covered briefly in Chapter 2.

Insulin is removed from the circulation after binding to the cell surface insulin receptors. These, with their bound insulin, become *internalised* (i.e.

taken up into the cell) and eventually the insulin is proteolytically degraded. The process of internalisation may have some role in bringing about insulin's actions, but this is not clear. It is also not clear whether some insulin is removed from the bloodstream by processes that do not result directly in metabolic effects. However, what is clear is that about 70% of the insulin reaching the liver is removed in its 'first passage'. This means that the liver is exposed to much higher concentrations of insulin than other tissues or organs. It also means that swings in insulin concentration are to some extent 'damped down' by the time the insulin reaches the general circulation. This emphasises the special relation between endocrine pancreas and liver.

5.2.3   Glucagon

Glucagon is a single polypeptide chain of 29 amino acids. Like insulin, it is synthesised initially as a larger protein (a *prohormone*) called *proglucagon*. Proteolytic cleavage gives rise to glucagon. (The large proglucagon molecule can be cleaved to release different peptides in the endocrine cells of the small intestine; see Section 5.7). In contrast to insulin, glucagon's major action is to elevate the blood glucose concentration. In fact, it was first discovered as a contaminant of preparations of insulin made from animal pancreases, which caused some batches to have the opposite of the desired blood glucose-lowering effect.

Its secretion from the pancreatic α-cells, like that of insulin from the β-cells, responds to both glucose and amino acids. However, unlike insulin, glucagon secretion is suppressed rather than stimulated by a rise in glucose concentration (although it is stimulated by amino acids). Thus, a rise in the plasma glucose concentration will lead to an increased ratio of insulin to glucagon secretion, and a fall in the plasma glucose concentration will lead to an increased ratio of glucagon to insulin. Again, some glucagon is removed on its first passage through the liver, although probably rather less than for insulin (animal experiments suggest around 5–10%). Nevertheless, glucagon probably has no important metabolic effects in any tissue other than the liver.

Glucagon also produces its effects on intracellular metabolic pathways by binding to receptors in the cell membrane. These receptors are coupled, via G-proteins, to adenylyl cyclase, and intracellular effects of glucagon are mediated via cAMP (see Box 2.4).

5.3   The pituitary gland

The pituitary gland, about the size of a pea, is situated on the under-surface of the brain (Fig. 5.1), attached through a little stalk to the area of the brain known as the *hypothalamus*. The pituitary gland is also known as the *hypophysis*, or 'growth underneath'; removal of the pituitary gland is the operation called hypophysectomy. The hypothalamus, which itself lies under the thalamus, is the seat of integration of incoming signals from nerves with specialised 'sensing' functions, and outgoing nervous activity, particularly in the sympathetic nervous system; it will be discussed in more detail in Section 7.2.1.1. The location of the pituitary gland in close proximity to the hypothalamus is no mere chance.

The pituitary gland has two major parts, or lobes: the *anterior pituitary* – also called the *adenohypophysis* – and the *posterior pituitary*, or *neurohypophysis*. The adenohypophysis contains cells which manufacture and secrete hormones. Regulation of the synthesis and secretion of its hormones is controlled, however, by other signals (local hormones) coming down a system of blood vessels in the stalk from the hypothalamus. The neurohypophysis is composed mainly of nerve cells that have their cell bodies in the hypothalamus. It is not a true endocrine organ; rather, the hormones which it releases are synthesised in the hypothalamus, transported along axons and stored temporarily before being secreted in response to nervous stimuli from the hypothalamus. Thus, the hypothalamus controls both nervous signals and hormonal signals to the rest of the body.

The hormones produced by the pituitary gland and their target organs are shown in Fig. 5.6.

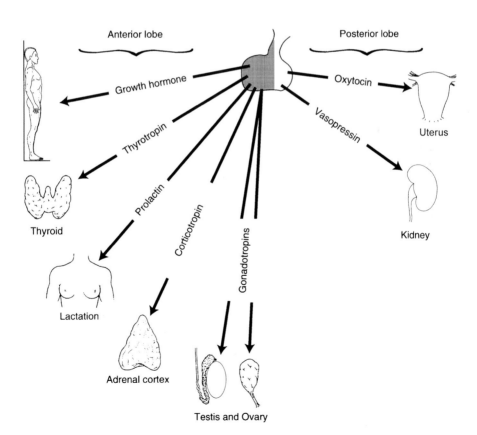

Fig. 5.6 Pituitary hormones and their target organs.

5.3.1   Hormones of the anterior pituitary (adenohypophysis)

The anterior pituitary secretes at least six distinct peptide and glycoprotein hormones. Several act on other hormone-producing organs to influence the secretion of further hormones: they are known as *tropic* (or *trophic*) *hormones*. Of these, *follicle-stimulating hormone* (FSH) and *luteinising hormone* (LH) (known together as *gonadotrophins*) have functions in the reproductive system that will not be considered further.

Adrenocorticotrophic hormone (ACTH) – sometimes called *cortico-trophin* – is a peptide hormone (of 39 amino acids) which acts on the adrenal cortex to stimulate release of glucocorticoids, particularly cortisol. ACTH is (like insulin) synthesised as a prohormone, but in this case a very large one called pro-opiomelanocortin (often abbreviated POMC). POMC is cleaved proteolytically to generate several biologically active peptides including β-endorphin and met-enkephalin (natural ligands of the receptors for cocaine, and involved in feelings of well-being, e.g. in response to exercise), α-, β- and γ-melanocyte-stimulating hormones (acting on melanocytes to influence pigmentation) and ACTH. (The melanocyte-stimulating hormones may also have a role in appetite regulation; see Box 11.1.)

ACTH is released in response to stress. It also has an important circadian rhythm (24-hour cycle); it is at its highest, as is cortisol secretion, in the morning at about the time of waking. There is feedback control of ACTH secretion: high levels of cortisol suppress ACTH secretion.

Thyroid-stimulating hormone (TSH) – sometimes called *thyrotropin* – acts on the thyroid gland to stimulate the production of thyroid hormones and to stimulate growth of the gland (discussed further below, Section 5.4). Again there is a feedback system, so that in thyroid deficiency, for example, TSH levels in blood are high; this is usually a clearer diagnostic test than direct measurement of thyroid hormone levels themselves.

Two more hormones secreted by the anterior pituitary act on other tissues that are not endocrine: *prolactin* and *growth hormone*. *Prolactin* stimulates milk production in the mammary gland and will not be considered further.

Growth hormone is a peptide hormone (of 190 amino acids in humans), sometimes called *somatotropin* because of its major role in regulating growth and development (*somato-* referring to the body). It does not do this directly. Growth hormone stimulates the production in the liver of other peptide hormones known as the *insulin-like growth factors*, IGF-1 and IGF-2, formerly known as the *somatomedins* since they mediate the effects of somatotropin. As their name implies, the insulin-like growth factors have structural similarities with insulin. They exert stimulatory effects on growth, whilst growth hormone has no direct effect. Even in adults, however, growth hormone is secreted. This occurs mainly overnight, in discrete bursts during sleep. It has some direct metabolic functions, although their importance in adults is not fully understood. The most important is probably a stimulation of fat mobilisation. This is not a rapid effect (unlike the effects of adrenaline or noradrenaline acting through the cAMP system – see Fig. 2.4.3). After a single injection of growth hormone, there is a stimulation of lipolysis after 2–3 hours. Growth hormone also has an effect on hepatic glucose production, probably involving stimulation of both gluconeogenesis and glycogenolysis. Again, this is probably not an effect of short-term importance. Adults who have had their pituitary gland removed surgically (usually because of a tumour) are usually not given growth hormone replacement, as it is expensive, and has not until recently been thought necessary. Recently, a number of trials of growth hormone replacement have shown that such treatment results in a loss of body fat and an increase in lean body mass, including muscle, reflecting a combination of the lipolytic and anabolic (growth-promoting) effects. It may also result in a feeling of well-being which is thought to reflect in part increased availability of fuels for physical work – i.e. non-esterified fatty acids and glucose in the plasma.

5.3.2   Hormones of the posterior pituitary (neurohypophysis)

The anterior pituitary secretes two structurally similar 9-amino acid peptide hormones, *oxytocin* (causing the uterus to contract) and *vasopressin*, also called *antidiuretic hormone*. The last name (ADH) suggests an obvious function in regulating urine production (more specifically, in regulating urine concentration), but the name vasopressin shows that this hormone also has a potent effect in constricting certain blood vessels. It may also, under certain conditions (particularly stress states), have a role in metabolic regulation; it has been suggested that vasopressin can stimulate glycogen breakdown in the liver. This is brought about by a change in the cytosolic Ca^{2+} concentration rather than through an increase in cAMP. An interesting relationship between the different effects of vasopressin may be seen. We have already seen that glycogen is stored with about three times its own weight of water; the liver glycogen store of about 100 g is accompanied by 300 g water. Mobilisation of glycogen therefore liberates water into the circulation. In a severe stress state brought about by loss of blood, for example, vasopressin might have multiple actions: further loss of water through the kidney is prevented by its antidiuretic action; extra water is mobilised along with glycogen; fuel (glucose) is provided for the organism to help deal with the stress (e.g. to provide energy to run away from an aggressor); and the vasoconstrictor action helps maintain blood pressure despite the loss of blood.

5.4   The thyroid gland

The thyroid gland weighs about 25 g and is made up of two lobes joined by a bridge, situated on either side of the trachea (windpipe) in the throat (Fig. 5.7). It has a rich blood supply. It is responsible for secretion both of the thyroid hormones themselves, and the protein, thyroglobulin, which carries them in the circulation. The thyroid hormones are iodinated amino-acid derivatives;

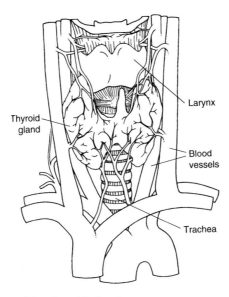

Fig. 5.7 The anatomy of the thyroid gland.

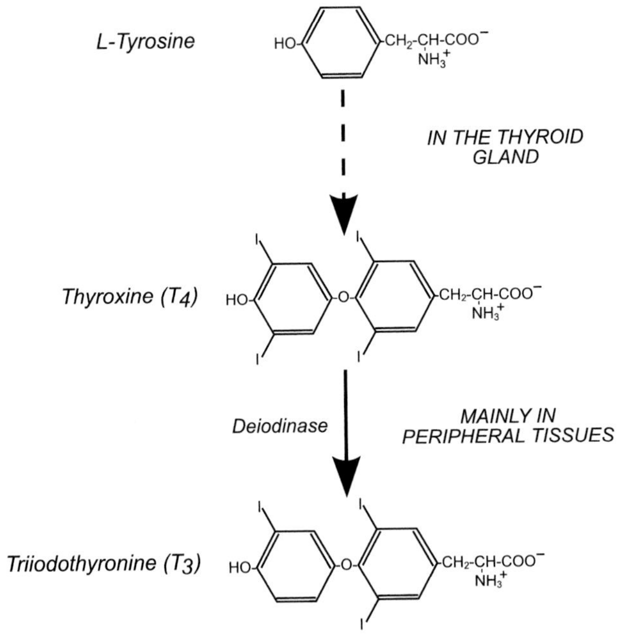

L-Tyrosine

IN THE THYROID
GLAND

Thyroxine (T4)

Deiodinase

MAINLY IN
PERIPHERAL TISSUES

Triiodothyronine (T3)

Fig. 5.8 Biosynthesis of the thyroid hormones. Thyroxine (T_4) and triiodothyronine (T_3) are synthesised in the thyroid gland from tyrosine residues in the protein thyroglobulin. The conversion of T_4 to T_3, the active hormone, occurs mainly in peripheral tissues.

they are formed from tyrosine residues within thyroglobulin, and iodine which is taken up avidly by the gland from the blood (Fig. 5.8). There are two thyroid hormones, known as *thyroxine* or T_4 (with four iodine atoms per molecule) and *triiodothyronine* or T_3 (with three iodine atoms). Both are secreted by the gland and present in blood, although it appears that T_3 is the active hormone. Most tissues express the enzyme necessary to convert T_4 to T_3.

Synthesis and secretion of the thyroid hormones are regulated by the pituitary-derived thyroid-stimulating hormone (TSH: see Section 5.3.1). TSH also increases thyroid size. In thyroid deficiency due, for instance, to lack of iodine in the diet, thyroid hormone levels in the blood are low. As discussed above (Section 5.3.1), this leads to an increase in TSH secretion in order to stimulate more thyroid hormone production. It also leads to enlargement of the thyroid gland, sometimes to a massive growth on the neck known as a *goitre*; hence the apparent paradox of an enlarged gland and a deficient hormone.

Most of the hormones which regulate metabolism do so in a very rapid manner; their secretion is regulated on a minute-to-minute basis and their effects on metabolic pathways are similarly rapid, or sometimes somewhat slower if effects on protein synthesis are involved. The thyroid hormones, however, seem to set the general level of metabolism in a long-term way. In parallel with this, the thyroid gland is unusual in storing a large amount of hormone – enough for around three months' secretion.

Some specific effects of thyroid hormones on metabolism will be covered in later chapters, particularly their effect on muscle protein metabolism (Section 6.3.3). For the most part, however, the thyroid hormones play a 'modulating' role, affecting the level of response to other hormones. In particular, they regulate the sensitivity of metabolic processes to catecholamines (adrenaline and noradrenaline): thus, an excess of thyroid hormones has many similarities to an excess of adrenaline or noradrenaline. An excess of thyroid hormones is characterised by an increase in the overall metabolic rate; a deficiency is characterised by a depression of metabolic rate.

5.5   The adrenal glands

The two adrenal glands sit like cocked hats over each kidney (Fig. 5.9) (hence their name – additions to the renal organ, or kidney). Each gland has an inner core and an outer layer of cells, the *adrenal medulla* and *adrenal cortex* respectively. The cortex (outer layer) makes up about nine-tenths of the bulk of the gland; its cells under the microscope are rich in lipid. The medulla stains darkly for microscopy with chromic salts, showing the presence of so-called *chromaffin* cells, characterised by the presence of *catecholamines* (such as adrenaline and noradrenaline).

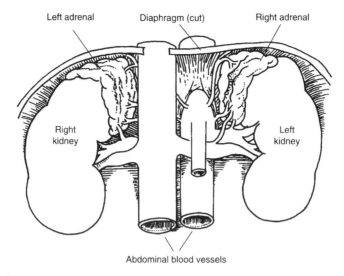

Fig. 5.9 The anatomy of the adrenal glands.

5.5.1   The adrenal cortex: cortisol secretion

The adrenal cortex secretes a number of steroid hormones which are synthesised from cholesterol. Some of these affect mainly mineral metabolism (salt and water balance) and are known collectively as the *mineralocorticoids*; some affect intermediary metabolism (glucose, fatty acid and amino acid metabolism) and are known as the *glucocorticoids*. The most important of these in humans is *cortisol*.[1]

As we have seen, the synthesis and secretion of cortisol are regulated by ACTH from the anterior pituitary. Cortisol has metabolic effects on a number of tissues. They are both short-term and longer-term. Even the short-term effects are for the most part mediated by changes in protein synthesis and therefore take a matter of hours rather than minutes. These include: a stimulation of fat mobilisation in adipose tissue, by increased activity of the enzyme hormone-sensitive lipase (this probably involves synthesis of additional enzyme protein); a stimulation of gluconeogenesis (again via synthesis of key enzymes; see Box 4.2); inhibition of the uptake of glucose by muscle (mechanism not clear); and an increase in the breakdown of muscle protein (see Section 6.3.3).

These effects of cortisol are often difficult to demonstrate in isolated tissues, and it is thought that many of cortisol's effects are more *permissive* than direct. A permissive effect means that a process cannot occur (or activation by another hormone cannot occur) in the absence of the 'permitting agent' – in this case cortisol – but the actual level of the permitting agent is not important. Thus, in people or animals whose adrenal cortex has been removed, some effects of adrenaline, for instance, do not occur (particularly stimulation of glycogen breakdown). Responsiveness to adrenaline can be reinstated by giving a glucocorticoid hormone such as cortisol, but the level achieved is not important

– just its presence. This is certainly an oversimplification for most of cortisol's effects, but it is probably true that cortisol 'sets the tone' of response to other hormones.

5.5.2   The adrenal medulla, adrenaline secretion and adrenaline action

The adrenal medulla develops as part of the nervous system. It is supplied with nerves that are part of the sympathetic nervous system. (They are preganglionic fibres whose neurotransmitter is acetylcholine; this will be discussed in detail in Section 7.2.2.1.) Its secretory activity is controlled directly by the brain through these nerves, and not by substances in the blood. It secretes the hormone *adrenaline* (named, of course, after the adrenal gland; in American literature this hormone is called *epinephrine*). More will be said about adrenaline and the related compound *noradrenaline* (*norepinephrine* in American) in a later chapter (Section 7.2.3.1); for now, it is satisfactory to think of them as having similar effects, although noradrenaline is almost entirely liberated as a neurotransmitter from sympathetic nerve terminals, and is therefore not a true hormone, whereas adrenaline is a hormone in every sense. They are both referred to as catecholamines because they are amine derivatives of the catechol nucleus. Their structures and the route of synthesis are shown in Fig. 5.10.

Adrenaline and noradrenaline act on *adrenergic receptors* (or *adrenoceptors*), found in the plasma membranes of most tissues. The adrenoceptors are 7-transmembrane domain (or serpentine) G-protein coupled receptors (see Box 2.3). There are different types of adrenergic receptor, first recognised because of the different potencies of adrenaline-like substances in bringing about various effects in specific tissues. Broadly, they may be divided into the α- and β-*receptors*, which are themselves subdivided into α_1, α_2, and β_{1-3} subtypes; the β_3 subtype is probably confined in humans to brown adipose tissue. The subtypes of adrenergic receptors are summarised in Table 5.1.

Binding of adrenaline and noradrenaline to adrenergic receptors brings about a variety of effects. From the point of view of energy metabolism, we will divide these into two groups: circulatory effects, and direct metabolic effects. The two are not independent, as will become clear in later sections.

β-*Adrenergic receptors* are linked, via the stimulatory G_s proteins, to the membrane-bound enzyme adenylyl cyclase which produces cyclic adenosine $3',5'$-monophosphate (cAMP) from ATP (see Box 2.3). Binding of adrenaline or noradrenaline to a β-adrenergic receptor thus causes an increase in cytosolic cAMP concentration, and activation of the *cAMP-dependent protein kinase* (also known as *protein kinase-A*; see Box 2.3). This may lead (directly or through other protein kinases) to phosphorylation of a key regulatory enzyme: glycogen phosphorylase and hormone-sensitive lipase are two examples (see Box 2.4). Thus, catecholamines acting through β-adrenergic receptors tend to lead to breakdown of stored fuels, triacylglycerol and glycogen. The circulatory effects of β-adrenergic receptors are mainly stimulatory, especially

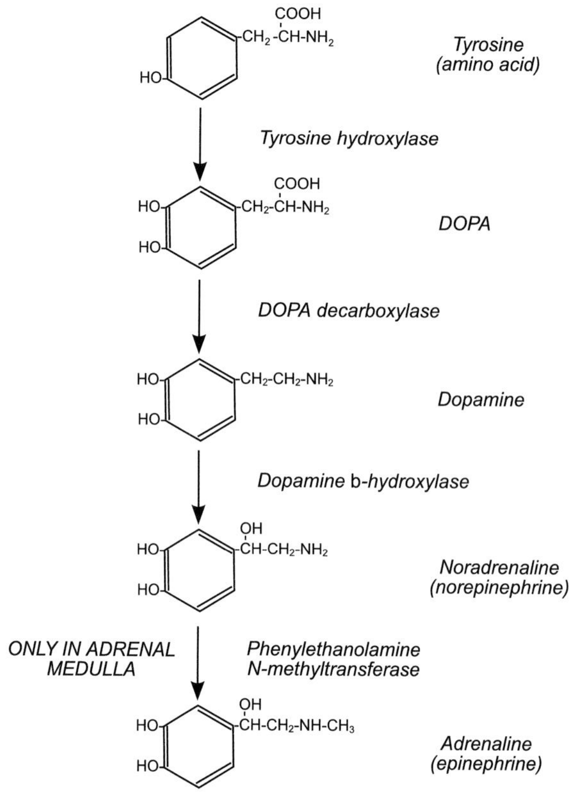

Fig. 5.10 Biosynthesis of the catecholamines. *Noradrenaline* is released from sympathetic nerve terminals, whereas *adrenaline* is a true hormone, released into the bloodstream from the adrenal medulla.

Table 5.1 Adrenergic receptors and their effects.

Receptor type	β	α_1	α_2
Second messenger system	Adenylyl cyclase/ cAMP	Phospholipase C/ intracellular Ca^{2+}	Inhibition of adenylyl cyclase
Metabolic effects	Glycogenolysis; lipolysis	Glycogenolysis	Inhibition of lipolysis
Circulatory effects	Increased heart rate and force; dilation of blood vessels	Constriction of blood vessels	Constriction of blood vessels

Note that the β-adrenergic receptors have not been subdivided here: see text, Section 5.5.2.

stimulation of the heart to beat both more rapidly (the *chronotropic* effect) and more strongly (the *inotropic* effect). Broadly, β_1 receptors mediate the effects on the heart and on lipolysis, β_2 those on blood vessels and on glycogenolysis. In rodents, lipolysis is stimulated mainly by a third type known as the *atypical β-receptor* or simply the β_3-receptor. In humans the significance of the β_3-receptor is still unclear. Its one certain role is in stimulation of thermogenesis in brown adipose tissue.

α-Adrenergic receptors may produce similar or opposite effects, depending upon the tissue. α_1-*Receptors* are linked to the second messenger system that involves hydrolysis of phosphatidylinositol $(4',5')$-bisphosphate (see Box 2.3). One of the products of this is inositol $(1',4',5')$-trisphosphate (IP_3), which causes the release of calcium ions from intracellular stores into the cytoplasm. This is involved, for instance, in an alternative route for the activation of glycogen breakdown by adrenaline: an increased cytosolic Ca^{2+} concentration will directly activate phosphorylase kinase (see Fig. 2.4.2 in Box 2.4, and also Fig. 8.8 later). α_2-*Receptors* are linked to adenylyl cyclase through the inhibitory G_i proteins, and thus adrenaline binding to such receptors will reduce the production of cAMP and oppose effects caused by its binding to β-receptors. α_2-Receptors are important in adipocytes and seem to exert a 'moderating influence' on the activation of fat mobilisation brought about by adrenaline acting on β-receptors. α-Receptors (especially α_1) also mediate the constriction of blood vessels and this has some repercussions on metabolism in stress states.

This sounds a complex system, and indeed it is. The net effect will depend upon the relative abundance of the different types of adrenergic receptor in a tissue, as well as on the concentrations of other hormones. To put it into perspective, if adrenaline or noradrenaline is injected or infused (given as a slow injection, over perhaps an hour) into human volunteers to raise the level in the blood to the upper limit of levels seen in normal everyday life, the major changes noted are an increase in heart rate and a rise in the concentrations of glucose and non-esterified fatty acids in the blood; thus, the net metabolic effect of catecholamines appears to be mobilisation of the stores of glycogen and triacylglycerol. There is also an increase in oxygen consumption, reflecting a general increase in metabolism. If very high levels are infused, then somewhat different changes may be observed, with restriction of blood flow in certain tissues and some inhibition of metabolic processes. These probably reflect the effects (which may be at least as important) of the catecholamines on blood flow in different tissues.

5.6   Adipose tissue

As mentioned earlier (Section 4.5.3.4), white adipose tissue is now recognised as an important endocrine organ, as well as a tissue involved in fat storage and mobilisation. Some the various products secreted by adipose tissue were covered in that section. Here we will discuss the secretion of one particular hormone, *leptin*.

The discovery of leptin is a fascinating story. In the 1950s, two animal breeders noticed a mutation in their mouse colony that led the affected animals to become naturally very obese. This mutation was the result of a change in one gene, which became known as the *ob* (for obese) gene. Mice heterozygous for the defective *ob* gene were normal. Only homozygous mutant mice (*ob/ob* mice) developed this spontaneous obesity. The question was, which single gene could so dramatically affect the body weight of an adult animal? Answering that question eventually required the techniques of molecular biology. In 1994 Jeff Friedman and colleagues at Rockefeller University (New York) showed that the single mutation leading to gross obesity in these mice was in a gene coding for a previously unknown protein, now known as leptin, and expressed only in white adipose tissue. The larger an adipocyte, the more leptin it produces and secretes, and of course the more adipocytes that are present in the body, the more leptin is produced. Leptin signals through receptors in the hypothalamus to restrict energy intake (i.e. to reduce appetite). In small animals it also signals to increase energy expenditure through activation of the sympathetic nervous system. The system is illustrated in Fig. 5.11 (and more details of appetite regulation by leptin and other signals will be given later, in Box 11.1). Leptin can be produced in bacteria by recombinant DNA techniques. When this recombinant leptin is injected into *ob/ob* mice, they become normal (they reduce their food intake and their energy expenditure increases).

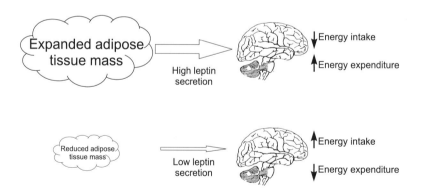

Fig. 5.11 The leptin system and regulation of fat stores. Leptin is produced in, and secreted from, adipose tissue according to the extent of the fat stores. Leptin signals to the brain (hypothalamus) to (1) reduce energy intake, and (2) increase energy expenditure (the latter has only been shown convincingly in small animals). When fat stores are depleted, low leptin levels signal to the brain to (1) increase energy intake, and (2) reduce energy expenditure. The system was discovered in the spontaneously obese *ob/ob* mouse, which has a defective leptin gene. Therefore the brain of the *ob/ob* mouse 'thinks' that it is connected to a small fat mass and increases energy intake, while in fact the fat mass expands and expands.

This story, as it emerged in 1994 and soon after, is now recognised to be an oversimplification. Leptin is produced in small amounts by other tissues including the stomach and placenta, and leptin receptors are found in many tissues. When leptin is injected into animals, there is an increase in glucose metabolism, probably implying effects in skeletal muscle. Leptin is also an important signal to the reproductive system. The *ob/ob* mouse is infertile, but becomes fertile when treated with leptin. It seems that low levels of leptin, implying low fat stores, signal to the reproductive system that the body does not have adequate energy reserves to embark upon child-bearing and rearing.

Leptin is a single-chain polypeptide hormone (16 kDa, 167 amino acids in humans). There are various isoforms of the leptin receptor, but one, known as OB-Rb or the long-form leptin receptor, seems to be the active form with an extracellular hormone-binding region and an intracellular signalling domain. Other, short-form leptin receptors may be involved with leptin transport. For instance, leptin must cross the blood–brain barrier to act on the long-form receptors expressed in the hypothalamus, and short-form receptors expressed in the choroid plexus (part of the blood–brain barrier) may facilitate this.

5.7   The intestine

We have already seen that the intestinal tract, including the stomach, is the source of several hormones that regulate intestinal motility and secretions involved in digestion (Chapter 3). The small and large intestines are also the source of hormones that affect metabolism in the rest of the body, especially through an indirect route, because they affect insulin secretion. Glucose given either orally or intravenously will stimulate insulin secretion. It was observed in the 1960s that if the amounts of glucose were chosen so that the same 'excursion' in plasma glucose concentration were achieved, then considerably more insulin was secreted following oral than intravenous glucose. The suggestion was that hormones secreted from the gut in response to glucose ingestion amplified the effect of glucose on the pancreatic β-cell. These hormones have become known as *incretins* (Fig. 5.12). There are probably several but one of the most important is *glucagon-like peptide-1* (GLP-1). This is secreted from cells known as enteroendocrine L-cells scattered amongst the epithelial cells of the intestinal wall. Like several other hormones we have met in this chapter, GLP-1 is a fragment of a larger prohormone, actually proglucagon, the precursor of pancreatic glucagon (Section 5.1.3). Cleavage of proglucagon in the enteroendocrine cells gives rise to two active products, known as GLP-1 and GLP-2. They get their name because they are similar in sequence to (pancreatic) glucagon, although not identical (approximately 50% amino acid identity). GLP-1 has a number of actions that include inhibition of gastrointestinal motility, but in addition it has a specific effect on the pancreatic β-cell, 'amplifying' glucose-stimulated insulin secretion. There are probably other incretins, including gastric inhibitory

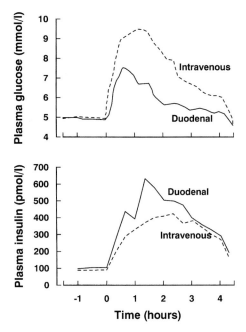

Fig. 5.12 The idea of 'incretins' (gut-derived hormones that augment insulin secretion). Volunteers received either an infusion of glucose directly into their duodenum, or an equal infusion into a vein. The plasma glucose concentration (top panel) rose considerably more with the intravenous infusion. But the response of plasma insulin (lower panel) was considerably greater, despite the lower plasma glucose concentration, with the duodenal glucose infusion. Therefore some factor associated with glucose in the small intestine must augment glucose-stimulated insulin secretion. As discussed in the text, the major incretins seem to be glucagon-like peptide-1 and gastric inhibitory polypeptide (GIP) (which was studied in this paper). Adapted from McCullough, A.J., Miller, L.J., Service, F.J. & Go, V.L.W. (1983) Effect of graded intraduodenal glucose infusions on the release and physiological action of gastric inhibitory polypeptide. *J Clin Endocrinol Metab* 56: 234–241. With permission of the Endocrine Society.

polypeptide (also known as glucose-dependent insulinotrophic polypeptide) (Section 3.2.3.2).

5.8   Further reading

General reading

Aranda, A. & Pascual, A. (2001) Nuclear hormone receptors and gene expression. *Physiol Rev* 81: 1269–1304. *This review gives more information on the action of intracellular/nuclear hormone receptors, beyond the information given in this chapter and in Chapter 2.*

Ashcroft, F.M. & Ashcroft, S.J.H. (1992) *Insulin: Molecular Biology to Pathology.* Oxford: Oxford University Press.

Bliss, M. (1983) *The Discovery of Insulin*. Edinburgh: Paul Harris. *A wonderful read, giving a feel for the excitement – and competition – of scientific research.*

Insulin secretion and insulin action

Kido, Y., Nakae, J. & Accili, D. (2001) The insulin receptor and its clinical targets. *J Clin Endocr Metab* 86: 972–979.

Rutter, G.A. (2001) Nutrient-secretion coupling in the pancreatic islet β-cell: recent advances. *Mol Aspects Med* 22: 247–284.

Schuit, F.C., Huypens, P., Heimberg, H. & Pipeleers, D.G. (2001) Glucose sensing in pancreatic β-cells: a model for the study of other glucose-regulated cells in gut, pancreas, and hypothalamus. *Diabetes* 50: 1–11.

Growth hormone and the insulin-like growth factors

Langford, K.S. & Miell, J.P. (1993) The insulin-like growth factor-I/binding protein axis: physiology, pathophysiology and therapeutic manipulation. *Eur J Clin Invest* 23: 503–516.

Butler, A.A. & Le Roith, D. (2001) Control of growth by the somatropic axis: growth hormone and the insulin-like growth factors have related and independent roles. *Annu Rev Physiol* 63: 141–164.

Catecholamines and metabolism

Macdonald, I.A., Bennett, T. & Fellows, I.W. (1985) Catecholamines and the control of metabolism in man. *Clin Sci* 68: 613–619.

Flatmark, T. (2000) Catecholamine biosynthesis and physiological regulation in neuroendocrine cells. *Acta Physiol Scand* 168: 1–17.

Nonogaki, K. (2000) New insights into sympathetic regulation of glucose and fat metabolism. *Diabetologia* 43: 533–549.

Other hormones

Kushner, J.P. (1996) Thyroid hormone effects on nutrient and energy metabolism. *Endocr Metab* 3: 219–234.

Holst, J.J. (1997) Enteroglucagon. *Annu Rev Physiol* 59: 257–271.

Falkenstein, E., Tillmann, H.-C., Christ, M., Feuring, M. & Wehling, M. (2000) Multiple actions of steroid hormones – a focus on rapid, nongenomic effects. *Pharmacol Rev* 52: 513–556.

Drucker, D.J. (2001) Minireview: the glucagon-like peptides. *Endocrinology* 142: 521–527.

Yen, P.M. (2001) Physiological and molecular basis of thyroid hormone action. *Physiol Rev* 81: 1097–1142.

Leptin

Friedman, J.M. & Halaas, J.L. (1998) Leptin and the regulation of body weight in mammals. *Nature* 395: 763–770.

Coleman, R.A. & Herrmann, T.S. (1999) Nutritional regulation of leptin in humans. *Diabetologia* 42: 639–646.

Harris, R.B. (2000) Leptin – much more than a satiety signal. *Annu Rev Nutr* 20: 45–75.

Kieffer, T.J. & Habener, J.F. (2000) The adipoinsular axis: effects of leptin on pancreatic beta-cells. *Am J Physiol Endocrinol Metab* 278: E1–E14.

Note

1   Cortisol is also known as hydrocortisone. The latter name is more commonly used when referring to a medicinal product; but chemically they are identical. In rodents the principal glucocorticoid is the related compound, corticosterone.

6

Integration of Carbohydrate, Fat and Protein Metabolism in the Whole Body

In previous chapters we have looked at carbohydrate, fat and amino acid metabolism in some individual tissues. In this chapter the aim is to show how metabolism in the different tissues is integrated in the whole body. The hormonal system plays an important part in this integration.

Numerical examples will be used to illustrate the turnover of substrates in the blood. These all involve approximations, and should be taken as illustrative only. For most purposes a fairly typical person of 65–70 kg body weight will be assumed.

6.1   Carbohydrate metabolism

Glucose is always present in the blood. It is not static; glucose molecules are continually being removed from the blood and replaced by new glucose molecules, so that the concentration remains relatively constant, at close to 5 mmol/l in humans (Fig. 6.1). In fact, amongst all the energy substrates circulating in the blood, the concentration of glucose is by far the most constant. One reason for this is that it is necessary to provide a constant source of energy for those tissues in which the rate of glucose utilisation is regulated primarily by the extracellular glucose concentration. For instance, we have seen that in the brain the rate of glucose utilisation is fairly constant over a range of glucose concentrations, but will decrease considerably – with adverse consequences – if the glucose concentration falls below about 3 mmol/l. Furthermore, consistently elevated concentrations of glucose in blood – above about 11 mmol/l – have harmful effects, although these may take a matter of years to develop; this topic will be considered later in the consideration of diabetes mellitus (Chapter 10).

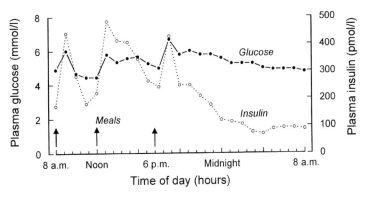

Fig. 6.1 Relative constancy of blood glucose concentrations during a typical day, compared with the relative variability of plasma insulin concentrations. For a mechanical analogy, see Fig. 6.2. Based on Reaven *et al.* (1988). Copyright © 1988 American Diabetes Association. From *Diabetes*, Vol. 37, 1988; 1020–1024. With permission of the American Diabetes Association.

Glucose enters the bloodstream in three major ways: by absorption from the intestine, from the breakdown of glycogen in the liver and from gluconeogenesis in the liver. (Remember that muscle glycogen breakdown does not liberate glucose into the blood, since muscle lacks glucose-6-phosphatase.) The relative importance of these routes will differ according to the nutritional state. Glucose leaves the blood by uptake into tissues. In normal life very little escapes into the urine; although glucose is filtered at the glomerulus, it is virtually completely reabsorbed from the proximal tubules (see Section 4.6.2).

During a typical day the average person on a Western diet eats about 300 g of carbohydrate (see Table 3.1). We can look at this in relation to the amount of free glucose in the body at any one time. The volume of blood is about 5 litres and the glucose concentration about 5 mmol/l, so the amount of glucose in the blood is about $5 \times 5 = 25$ mmol or ($\times 180$, the M_r [relative molecular mass]) 4.5 g. More correctly, we should look at the amount of glucose in all the extracellular fluid (about 20% of body weight – say 13 litres), i.e. about 12 g. Thus, in 24 hours, we eat enough to replace our 'glucose in solution' about 25 times. This illustrates the need for coordinated control; even a single meal (say 100 g carbohydrate) could elevate the glucose concentration about 8-fold if there were not mechanisms both to inhibit the body's own glucose production, and to increase the uptake of glucose into tissues.

The constancy of blood glucose concentration is brought about by coordinated control of various aspects of glucose metabolism. It will already be clear that insulin plays a major role in this coordination. The relationship between blood glucose and insulin concentrations is illustrated in Fig. 6.1, which shows the relative constancy of glucose compared with the variability of insulin. This is typical of many systems in which one component is varying in order to keep another constant. A useful analogy is with a thermostatically controlled water tank. At its simplest, a thermostat dips into the water. When the water temperature falls below a certain limit – for instance, 2° below the desired temperature or 'set-point' – an electrical switch is triggered and the heating element is switched on. When the temperature reaches an upper limit – perhaps 2° above the set-point – the switch cuts out. The water temperature (the *controlled variable*) stays constant within quite narrow limits (4° in this case), whereas the electrical current through the switch and heater (the *controlling variable*) varies between wide extremes (Fig. 6.2). We will reconsider, and improve upon, this analogy at the end of this chapter.

6.1.1   The postabsorptive state

The phrase *postabsorptive state* implies that all of the last meal has been absorbed from the intestinal tract, but not much further time has elapsed or the beginnings of starvation would be apparent. In humans, it is typically represented by the state after an overnight fast before breakfast is consumed.

In the postabsorptive state the blood glucose concentration is usually a little under 5 mmol/l. The concentration of insulin in plasma varies widely between individuals, but is typically around 60 pmol/l. The concentration of glucagon will be about 20–25 pmol/l. (There are difficulties in giving typical glucagon concentrations. Firstly, the methods used to measure it in different laboratories tend to give varying results. Secondly, the point has already been made that glucagon exerts its metabolic effects mainly, if not entirely, in the liver, and the relevant concentration is that in the hepatic portal vein; this is not easy to measure in normal volunteers.)

The rate of turnover of glucose in the postabsorptive state is close to 2 mg of glucose per kg body weight per minute, or 130 mg glucose per minute entering

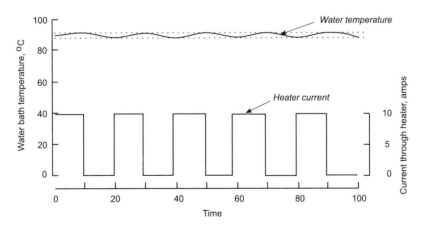

Fig. 6.2 An analogy for metabolic regulation. The temperature in a thermostatically controlled water bath (the *controlled variable*) is relatively constant with only small variations around the *set-point* (the desired temperature), whereas the electrical current flowing through the heater (the *controlling variable*) varies between much wider extremes.

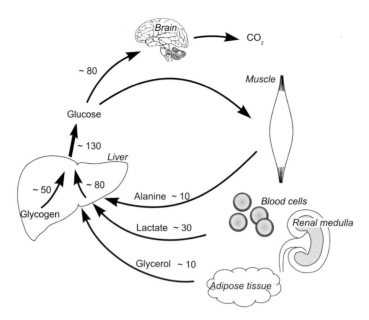

Fig. 6.3 The pattern of glucose metabolism after an overnight fast. The numbers are approximations only, in mg per min, for a typical person of 65 kg body weight. Much of the glucose delivered to peripheral tissues (muscle, adipose tissue, blood cells, etc.) is 'recycled' as lactate, which returns to the liver as a substrate for gluconeogenesis. However, a large proportion is oxidised, especially in the brain, and this constitutes an irreversible loss from the body's store of carbohydrate. Note that this picture shows only glucose metabolism: muscle and other tissues (e.g. renal cortex) will also be oxidising non-esterified fatty acids from the plasma.

and leaving the circulation. Where is it coming from, and where does it go? The pattern of glucose metabolism after an overnight fast is illustrated in Fig. 6.3.

Glucose enters the blood in the postabsorptive state almost exclusively from the liver, and of this a proportion arises from glycogen breakdown and a proportion from gluconeogenesis. These proportions vary a lot according to how much glycogen there was the evening before – which in turn depends on previous diet and other factors like the amount of exercise taken. Also, there is debate in the literature according to what method is used to measure these two contributions. But a reasonable estimate seems to be that about one-third is from glycogen breakdown – say 50 mg glucose per minute. The stimulus for glycogen breakdown (in contrast to the situation after the last meal the previous evening, when glycogen was being stored) is a decreased insulin/glucagon ratio – a little less insulin, a little more glucagon. The remainder of glucose entry (say 80 mg/min) must result from gluconeogenesis.

What are the substrates for this gluconeogenesis? Lactate will constitute a little over a half, and alanine (largely from muscle) and glycerol (from adipose tissue lipolysis) most of the remainder. The lactate arises from a variety of tissues. First, it comes from those tissues that use glucose almost entirely by anaerobic glycolysis, such as the red blood cells and renal medulla. Note that this constitutes a recycling of glucose; red blood cells, for example, use about 25 mg glucose/min, and return that amount of lactate to the liver for synthesis of new glucose. Secondly, there will be some breakdown of muscle glycogen releasing lactate from anaerobic glycolysis. The stimulus for gluconeogenesis (again, comparing with the previous evening when it was suppressed after a meal) is again mainly the decreased insulin/glucagon ratio.

On the disappearance side, the brain uses about 120 g glucose per day (see Section 4.2) or about 80 mg/min, more than half of the total glucose utilisation. The remainder is used by a number of tissues including red blood cells (about 25 mg/min), skeletal muscle, renal medulla and adipose tissue.

6.1.2   Breakfast

The postabsorptive state usually only lasts a few hours before it is interrupted by the arrival of a meal. The first meal of the day gives the most dramatic switch from 'production' to 'storage' mode and we will consider here how this comes about. For simplicity, we will consider a breakfast containing mostly carbohydrate – for instance, cereals and skimmed milk.

The carbohydrate of the meal is digested and absorbed from the intestine as described in Chapter 3. An increase in the concentration of glucose in the blood can be detected within about 15 minutes, and continues to a peak at around 30–60 minutes after a moderate breakfast (Fig. 6.4). (The exact timing depends upon factors such as the size of the meal and the amount of complex carbohydrate, fibre and simple sugars in the meal.) As the concentration of blood glucose rises, the endocrine pancreas responds: insulin secretion is stimulated and the concentration of insulin in plasma rises (Fig. 6.4). The glucagon concentration in 'peripheral' blood (e.g. taken from an arm vein) may fall a little after a typical meal, although we do not know directly what happens to glucagon secretion or to the glucagon concentration in the portal vein. Nevertheless, the insulin/glucagon ratio in plasma rises. How does this affect metabolism in individual tissues?

6.1.2.1   Carbohydrate metabolism in the liver after breakfast

The liver receives the blood draining the small intestine in the hepatic portal vein, and so it sees the largest change in blood glucose concentration. This leads to an inflow of glucose into hepatocytes via the transporter GLUT2. The elevation of intracellular glucose concentration in hepatocytes, together with the change in insulin/glucagon ratio, leads to inactivation of glycogen phosphorylase and activation of glycogen synthetase, and thus a switch from glycogen breakdown to glycogen storage (see Box 4.1).

We might expect that the pathway of gluconeogenesis would be inhibited by this hormonal switch, but this does not occur in practice. There is always an elevation of the blood lactate concentration after ingestion of carbohydrate (Fig. 6.4). This probably represents the effect of a switch to partially anaerobic glucose metabolism in a number of tissues including muscle and adipose tissue.

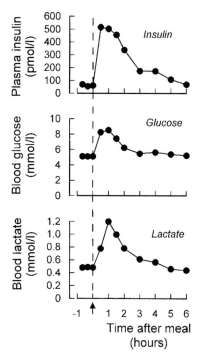

Fig. 6.4 Concentrations of insulin, glucose and lactate in blood after an overnight fast and following a single meal. The meal, shown by the arrow, contained 96 g carbohydrate and 33 g fat. Mean values for 8 normal subjects are shown; based on data in Frayn et al. (1993).

The increase in blood lactate concentration is probably sufficient in itself to maintain the activity of the pathway of gluconeogenesis. The overall effect is that some of the glucose arriving in the blood is used by tissues, released into the blood as lactate, taken up by the liver and converted to glucose 6-phosphate and then glycogen – the 'indirect pathway' of glycogen deposition (discussed in Section 4.1.2.1). It is important to note, however, that unlike gluconeogenesis after an overnight fast, this gluconeogenic flux does not lead to release of glucose into the blood: the glucose 6-phosphate is instead directed into glycogen synthesis. The direction of lactate into glycogen in the liver can all be seen as part of an intense drive to store as much as possible of the incoming glucose, even if it supplies some energy to other tissues first.

   The rate of glucose release from hepatocytes (i.e. release of glucose from glycogen and from gluconeogenesis) falls dramatically, almost to zero, within 1–2 hours after a glucose load or carbohydrate meal. This is, of course, yet another mechanism tending to reduce the increase in blood glucose concentration that might otherwise occur. At the same time, hepatocytes will take up glucose arriving in the portal vein. Total glucose release into the circulation through the hepatic veins, however, increases because of exogenous (dietary) glucose coming from the small intestine (Fig. 6.5).

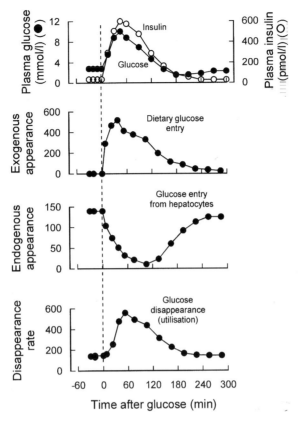

Fig. 6.5 Rates of glucose release from liver, from exogenous (dietary) and endogenous (gluconeogenesis + glycogenolysis) sources, in normal subjects before and after drinking 75 g glucose in water. The rate of glucose disappearance from the circulation (i.e. utilisation by all tissues) is also shown. All rates are in mg/min. The measurements were made by radioactive tracer techniques. Labelled [H^3]-glucose was infused into the circulation at a constant rate; the extent to which it was 'diluted' with unlabelled glucose was used to estimate the rate of entry of glucose into the circulation ('total glucose appearance'). In addition, the glucose drink was labelled with [^{14}C]-glucose, so that the rate of entry of exogenous glucose into the circulation could be measured. The 'endogenous' glucose production was then calculated by difference. Total glucose entry into the circulation (the sum of exogenous and endogenous appearance) increased after the glucose drink, and hence the blood glucose concentration rose – top panel. Release of endogenous glucose from hepatocytes was markedly suppressed. The rate of disappearance of glucose from the circulation also increased, stimulated by the increased insulin concentration. Based on Fery, F.D., Attellis, N.P. & Balasse, E.O. (1990) Mechanisms of starvation diabetes: study with double tracer and indirect calorimetry. *Am J Physiol* 259: E770–E777. With permission of the American Physiological Society.

6.1.2.2   Carbohydrate metabolism in other tissues after breakfast

Other tissues respond to the increase in insulin concentration. In skeletal muscle and adipose tissue, glucose uptake will be stimulated by the rise in insulin through increased numbers of GLUT4 transporters at the cell membrane, and by increased disposal of glucose within the cell. At the same time, the plasma

concentration of non-esterified fatty acids falls because fat mobilisation in adipose tissue is suppressed; this will be discussed in more detail below. Therefore
tissues such as skeletal muscle, which can use either fatty acids or glucose as
their energy source, switch to utilisation of glucose. Not all the glucose taken
up by muscle is oxidised under these conditions; insulin also activates muscle
glycogen synthase and glycogen storage will replenish muscle glycogen stores
(Fig. 6.6). Thus, after a meal containing carbohydrate, there is a general switch
in metabolism to the use of glucose rather than fatty acids, but there is also a
major switch to the storage of glucose as glycogen. The pattern of postprandial
glucose metabolism, and some important regulatory points, are illustrated in
Fig. 6.7.

6.1.2.3   Disposal of glucose after a meal

As we have discussed, the amount of glucose in the meal (typically 80–100 g)
would be enough to raise the concentration of glucose in the plasma about 8-
fold. In fact, in a normal healthy person, the peak glucose concentration after
such a breakfast will be about 7–8 mmol/l (Fig. 6.4), a rise of only 60% at most
from the postabsorptive value of 5 mmol/l. On the other hand, the insulin concentration may have gone from around 60 pmol/l to perhaps 400–500 pmol/l
(Fig. 6.4), a very much bigger percentage change; this illustrates the relationship between 'controlling' and 'controlled' variables discussed earlier (see
Fig. 6.2). The glucagon concentration in 'systemic' (mixed) blood plasma may
change less, but there will be a change in the insulin/glucagon ratio, probably

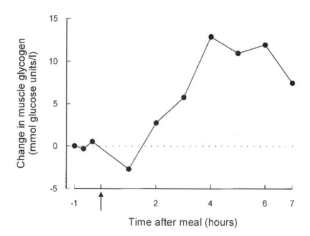

Time after meal (hours)

**Fig. 6.6 Concentrations of muscle glycogen after a single meal in normal sub-
jects, studied by the technique of nuclear magnetic resonance.** The meal, shown
by the arrow, contained 290 g carbohydrate and 45 g fat. Redrawn from Taylor, R., Price,
T.B., Katz, L.D., Shulman, R.G. & Shulman, G.I. (1993) Direct measurement of change in
muscle glycogen concentration after a mixed meal in normal subjects. *Am J Physiol* 265:
E224–E229. With permission of the American Physiological Society.

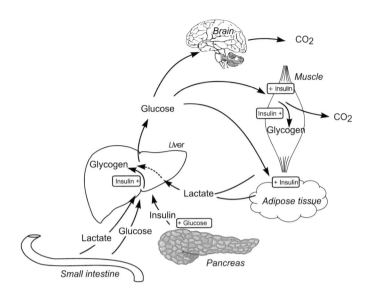

Fig. 6.7 The pattern of glucose metabolism after a carbohydrate breakfast. The *direct pathway* of glycogen storage is shown (glucose from small intestine going to liver glycogen), as is the *indirect pathway* (glucose forming lactate in the small intestine or in peripheral tissues, lactate then being used for liver glycogen synthesis): see Section 4.1.2.1.

greater still in the hepatic portal vein – i.e. in the concentrations of hormones reaching the liver.

By the end of the absorptive period – about 5 hours after the meal – approximately 25 g of the 100 g of carbohydrate ingested will have been stored and 75 g oxidised. Thus, although glucose oxidation in tissues was increased after the meal, the 'drive' for glucose storage is such that around one-quarter of the glucose in such a meal is stored for later use.

What happens towards the end of the absorptive period depends, of course, on what the subject decides to do. Most likely, another meal will be taken, and glucose storage will increase further; but exercise and other factors (e.g. stress, illness) if they occur, will influence the disposition of the nutrients. These factors will be considered in later chapters.

6.2   Fat metabolism

Whilst there is one major form of carbohydrate (glucose) circulating in the blood, and its concentration is relatively constant, there are various forms of fat and their concentrations may vary considerably throughout a normal day. In this section we will consider mainly the regulation of non-esterified fatty acid metabolism in the whole body, along with the fate of fat we eat in the form of triacylglycerol. The transport of triacylglycerol in the blood is closely linked with that of cholesterol, and these aspects will be considered again in more detail in Chapter 9.

Both triacylglycerol and non-esterified fatty acids are always present in the plasma and, like glucose, they are constantly turning over – being used and replaced. Non-esterified fatty acids turn over very rapidly; if an injection of a radioactively labelled fatty acid is given, the radioactivity disappears from the blood with a half-life of a few minutes. Triacylglycerol is present in various forms. The form in which it enters the blood after a meal, chylomicron-triacylglycerol, also has a high rate of turnover with a half-life of 5–10 minutes. Other forms of triacylglycerol in plasma have half-lives of several hours or days.

6.2.1   Plasma non-esterified fatty acids

Non-esterified fatty acids enter the plasma only from adipose tissue. The process of fat mobilisation is catalysed by the enzyme hormone-sensitive lipase (Section 4.5.3.2). Thus, control of this enzyme, and of the opposing process of esterification of fatty acids in adipose tissue, has a major effect on the plasma concentration of non-esterified fatty acids. The overall rate of utilisation of non-esterified fatty acids from the plasma does not appear to be directly controlled (although it may be so in individual tissues, e.g. via activity of fatty acid transporters at the cell membrane). It depends almost entirely on the plasma concentration of non-esterified fatty acids: the higher the concentration, the higher the rate of utilisation. The relationship is close to proportional over a wide range of concentrations – i.e. utilisation of plasma non-esterified fatty acids is essentially a first-order process (Fig. 6.8). Thus, the concentration of non-esterified fatty acids in the plasma reflects their rate of release from adipose tissue, and this in turn determines the rate of non-esterified fatty acid utilisation in other tissues.

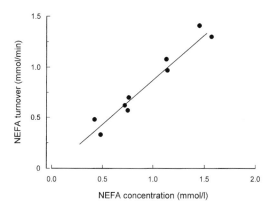

Fig. 6.8 Relationship between the concentration and the turnover of non-esterified fatty acids (NEFA) in plasma. Y-axis: rate of turnover of plasma non-esterified fatty acids measured by infusion of a radioactively labelled fatty acid; X-axis, plasma concentration of non-esterified fatty acids, in normal subjects who had fasted for various periods, from 14 h (left-most points) to 72 h (highest points). Based on Issekutz, B., Bortz, W.M., Miller, H.I. & Paul, P. (1967) Turnover rate of plasma FFA in humans and in dogs. *Metabolism* 16: 1001–1009. With the permission of W.B. Saunders Co.

Non-esterified fatty acids are not water-soluble, and they are carried in plasma bound to the plasma protein albumin. The plasma concentration of albumin is around 40 g/l and its M_r (relative molecular mass) is 66 000, so the concentration is about 0.6 mmol/l. Each molecule of albumin has binding sites for around three fatty acid molecules. (These binding sites are not as specific as, for instance, a hormone receptor binding a hormone. Albumin acts as a carrier for a number of hydrophobic substances including certain drugs and the amino acid tryptophan. Non-esterified fatty acids, tryptophan and drugs compete for binding, presumably to the same sites.) Thus, about 0.6×3, or say 2 mmol/l of non-esterified fatty acids can be comfortably accommodated. There is always an equilibrium between fatty acids bound to albumin and a very small concentration (less than 1 µmol/l) unbound, free in solution. If the plasma concentration of non-esterified fatty acids rises above about 2 mmol/l the concentration of unbound fatty acids rises considerably, and this may have adverse effects, particularly on the heart (see Box 4.4).

The plasma non-esterified fatty acid concentration during a normal day is an inverse reflection of the plasma glucose and insulin; when the body is relatively 'starved' – for instance after overnight fast – the concentrations of glucose and insulin are at their lowest and the concentration of non-esterified fatty acids is at its highest. It can fall dramatically after a carbohydrate meal (Fig. 6.9). Situations such as exercise or illness may disturb this relationship; exercise will be considered in Chapter 7.

6.2.2   Plasma triacylglycerol

Triacylglycerol is also water-insoluble and is carried in the plasma in specialised particulate structures, the lipoproteins (we have already met the largest of these, the *chylomicrons*, which transport triacylglycerol absorbed from the

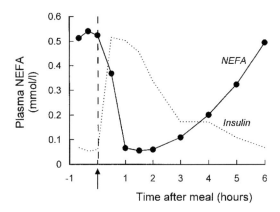

Fig. 6.9 Plasma non-esterified fatty acid (NEFA) concentrations after an overnight fast and following a meal. The meal was the same as described in Fig. 6.4. The plasma insulin concentration (expressed in nmol/l) is shown as a dotted line. Mean values for eight normal subjects are shown; data taken from Frayn *et al.* (1993).

small intestine; see Section 3.3.3). The total concentration of triacylglycerol in plasma varies widely between different people (even apparently quite healthy people), depending greatly upon fitness, body build and genetic influences – but a typical figure after an overnight fast is around 1 mmol/l. It should be borne in mind that, since each triacylglycerol molecule contains three fatty acids, this is equivalent in terms of energy delivery to a concentration of 3 mmol/l of non-esterified fatty acids. For now, we shall just consider the triacylglycerol in chylomicron particles. The concentration of chylomicron-triacylglycerol also varies widely between people, but it is close to zero in the overnight-fasted state, and rises after meals to (typically) 0.4–0.6 mmol/l. (This figure will depend, of course, on the amount of fat in the meal.)

6.2.3   The postabsorptive state

After an overnight fast, the concentration of non-esterified fatty acids in plasma is around 0.5 mmol/l, and the total triacylglycerol concentration (variable between people) around 1 mmol/l. The chylomicron-triacylglycerol concentration will be close to zero – usually less than 0.05 mmol/l.

Note that the lipid fuels (non-esterified fatty acids and triacylglycerol) circulate, for the most part, in lower concentrations than glucose (whose concentration is around 5 mmol/l in this state). But it is interesting to think in terms of 'energy yield'. Some calculations are given in Box 6.1. The box shows that lipid fuels are potentially a more important source of energy than might appear from their concentrations, and that non-esterified fatty acids constitute an important energy source in the postabsorptive state.

The turnover of non-esterified fatty acids in the postabsorptive state involves their liberation from adipose tissue and their uptake by a number of tis-

---

Box 6.1   Glucose and lipids as energy sources

Glucose and lipid fuels in the plasma are compared in terms of their potential yield of energy in the postabsorptive state. First, we will use typical concentrations in the plasma (given in the text) and look at the potential yield of energy per litre of plasma.

Substrate	Typical concentration (mmol/l)	Energy yield on complete oxidation (kJ per g)	Relative molecular mass	'Energy concentration' in plasma (kJ per litre)
Glucose	5	17	180	14
NEFA	0.5	38	280	5
TAG	1	40	850	34

Thus, lipid fuels carry more energy than more might appear from their molar concentrations; this is partly because they consist of bigger molecules than glucose, and partly because, per gram, they yield more energy on oxidation.

Even this is still not a fair comparison, however, because the bulk of triacylglycerol turns over relatively slowly in plasma, whereas plasma non-esterified fatty acids turn over very rapidly. Because triacylglycerol is so heterogeneous in plasma, we shall just compare glucose and non-esterified fatty acids in terms of 'energy turnover', or transport of energy to tissues, in the postabsorptive state.

	Glucose	Non-esterified fatty acids
Rate of turnover (μmol kg body weight^{-1} min^{-1})	10	6
Rate of turnover (mg kg body weight^{-1} min^{-1})	2	1.7
Turnover in mg/min for a 65 kg person	130	112
Energy yield* (kJ/g)	17	38
Energy value of turnover (kJ/min)	2.2	4.3
Energy value of turnover per day (kJ)	3200	6100
Percentage contribution to total energy accounted for	34%	66%

*These figures assume complete oxidation whereas, as discussed in the text, this is not completely true for either glucose or non-esterified fatty acids.

Glucose turnover delivers about one-third, and non-esterified fatty acid turnover about two-thirds, of the energy delivery to tissues calculated in this way. Even this overemphasises the contribution of glucose, since a proportion of that glucose (perhaps 20–30%) will not be completely oxidised, but will be returned as lactate. Thus, we see that non-esterified fatty acids contribute an important energy source in the postabsorptive state.

sues, predominantly skeletal muscle and liver (Fig. 6.10). As we have seen, the rate of liberation from adipose tissue reflects mainly the activity of the enzyme hormone-sensitive lipase. What is the stimulus for activation of this enzyme, in comparison with the state after last evening's supper? Unfortunately the answer is not entirely clear, but a major component is undoubtedly the fall in insulin concentration. Since insulin suppresses the activity of hormone-sensitive lipase (see Box 2.4), a fall in insulin concentration will in itself lead to activation. In addition it is probable that the enzyme is activated by the influence of adrenaline in the plasma and noradrenaline released from sympathetic nerve terminals within adipose tissue.

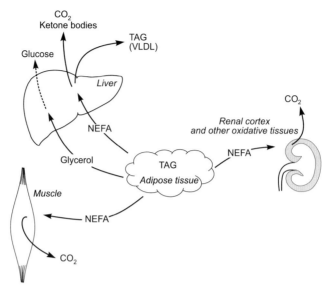

Fig. 6.10 The pattern of non-esterified fatty acid (NEFA) metabolism after an overnight fast. Fatty acids are released by the action of hormone-sensitive lipase on the triacylglycerol (TAG) stores in adipose tissue. VLDL: very-low-density lipoprotein.

The rate of non-esterified fatty acid release from adipose tissue is also regulated by the process of fatty acid re-esterification within the tissue (see Fig. 4.17). However, the process of re-esterification requires glycerol 3-phosphate produced from glycolysis, and this will be occurring at a relatively low rate, so most of the fatty acids will escape from the adipocyte. The best estimates available suggest that around 10% of the fatty acids released by hormone-sensitive lipase action are retained by re-esterification in the overnight-fasted state, but this figure falls to near zero if the fast extends another few hours.

No discussion of fat metabolism is complete without some mention of the ketone bodies. These metabolites are produced during the hepatic oxidation of fatty acids (see Fig. 4.5) and released into the blood. Their production is favoured in states of relatively low insulin/glucagon ratio. After an overnight fast their concentration in blood is low – usually less than 0.2 mmol/l for 3-hydroxybutyrate and acetoacetate combined. Their turnover is rapid, however – typically 0.25–0.30 mmol/minute per person. In 'energy' terms, oxidation of these ketone bodies would contribute around 750–800 kJ/day (if this rate of ketone body turnover were continued throughout 24 hours) or perhaps 8% of total resting energy expenditure. This contribution increases markedly during more prolonged starvation.

6.2.4   Breakfast

The effects of a meal on non-esterified fatty acid and triacylglycerol metabolism may be quite different. Initially it will be simplest, as before, to consider a mainly carbohydrate breakfast and its effects on non-esterified fatty acid metabolism. Then we shall see how a fatty meal – for instance, fried bacon and eggs – affects the responses.

6.2.4.1   Non-esterified fatty acid metabolism after breakfast

As the meal is absorbed, so the rising glucose concentration stimulates insulin secretion and the concentration of insulin in the plasma rises. This has a direct suppressive effect on the enzyme hormone-sensitive lipase. The dose–response curve for this process is such that relatively low concentrations of insulin almost maximally suppress hormone-sensitive lipase; the half-maximal suppression is seen at around 120 pmol/l of insulin, and at the peak of insulin after a typical carbohydrate breakfast (say 400–500 pmol/l) hormone-sensitive lipase will be maximally suppressed. Its activity does not appear to be completely suppressed whatever the insulin concentration, so some hydrolysis of stored triacylglycerol proceeds within adipose tissue. However, the rising glucose and insulin concentrations will also increase adipose tissue glucose uptake and glycolysis, and therefore production of glycerol 3-phosphate and re-esterification of fatty acids within the tissue (see Fig. 4.17). Thus, release of non-esterified fatty acids from adipose tissue will be almost completely suppressed after a meal, and the plasma non-esterified fatty acid concentration will fall markedly, from its postabsorptive level of around 0.5 mmol/l to less than 0.1 mol/l (Fig. 6.9). Notice that the variations in plasma non-esterified fatty acid concentration are much greater than those in plasma glucose; the organism appears to have no 'need' to regulate the plasma non-esterified fatty acid concentration more precisely, other than avoiding the hazards of particularly elevated concentrations.

The fall in plasma non-esterified fatty acid concentration affects the metabolism of tissues that use fatty acids as an oxidative fuel after the overnight fast. Skeletal muscle is a good example. As discussed earlier (Section 4.3.3.2), the rate of uptake of non-esterified fatty acids by muscle is a function primarily of fatty acid delivery – i.e. plasma concentration and blood flow. On the other hand, when glucose becomes available in the plasma after a meal, its utilisation is stimulated by the rise in insulin concentration. The muscle has no direct way of turning off fatty acid utilisation, but the coordinated control of metabolism in the whole body leads instead to its supply being cut off.

Along with the reduction in plasma non-esterified fatty acid concentration there is a switch in liver metabolism, also brought about by the increased insulin/glucagon ratio, leading to a reduction in the rate of ketone body formation and release. The blood ketone body concentration will therefore fall, typically from about 0.1–0.2 mmol/l after overnight fast to almost undetectably low levels – perhaps around 0.02 mmol/l. Their importance as a fuel decreases in proportion, so that ketone bodies are quite unimportant in the fed state.

As the absorptive phase declines after about 3–5 hours, so insulin concentrations begin to decline and the restraint of fat mobilisation is relaxed; plasma non-esterified fatty acid concentrations rise again (Fig. 6.9).

6.2.4.2 Triacylglycerol

If the meal contains a significant amount of fat, it will produce additional responses. However, the processing of dietary fat does not directly affect the coordinated responses of the glucose/non-esterified fatty acid insulin/glucagon system already described.

Consider a meal containing both carbohydrate and fat – say around 30 g of fat and 50 g carbohydrate – for example, a cheese sandwich. The plasma glucose and insulin concentrations will rise as described before, and the release of non-esterified fatty acids from adipose tissue will be suppressed so that their concentration in plasma falls. Dietary fat is almost entirely in the form of triacylglycerol (usually more than 95% is triacylglycerol). This is absorbed in the small intestine and processed in the intestinal cells to produce chylomicron particles, which are liberated into the bloodstream through the lymphatic system. This process is much slower than the absorption of glucose or amino acids, so that the peak in plasma triacylglycerol concentration after a fatty meal does not occur until 3–5 hours after the meal. As chylomicron-triacylglycerol enters the plasma, the large, triacylglycerol-rich particles give the plasma a 'milky' appearance (Fig. 6.11).

A typical postabsorptive plasma triacylglycerol concentration of 1.0 mmol/l might rise to 1.5 mmol/l, or perhaps 2.0 mmol/l after a particularly fatty meal (Fig. 6.12). The total amount of triacylglycerol in the plasma (volume around

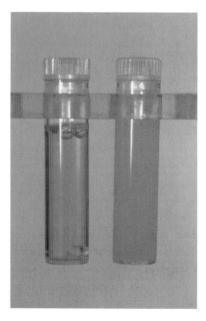

Fig. 6.11 The milky appearance of blood plasma (right) after a fatty meal, compared with its clear appearance in the fasted state (left). The turbidity is caused by the presence of the large chylomicron particles.

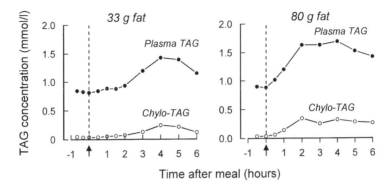

Fig. 6.12 Concentrations of triacylglycerol (TAG) in whole plasma (solid circles) and in chylomicrons (open circles) after overnight fast and after meals (shown by the arrows) containing either 33 g fat (a typical mixed meal) or 80 g fat (a high-fat meal) in groups of normal subjects. Data from Griffiths *et al.* (1994) and Coppack *et al.* (1990).

3 litres) at 1 mmol/l, with a M_r of about 900, is about $3 \times 900 = 2700$ mg or 2.7 g. Thus, again, the amount eaten (typically 30–40 g in a meal) would be sufficient to raise the plasma triacylglycerol concentration many times, but the rise is minimised by coordinated regulation of the mechanisms for its disposal.

The proportional rise in plasma triacylglycerol concentration after a meal is also lessened by the fact that only a small proportion of the plasma triacylglycerol represents that in chylomicrons. The plasma chylomicron-triacylglycerol concentration will rise from near zero to perhaps 0.3–0.4 mmol/l after a very fatty meal, a big percentage change (Fig. 6.12). The absolute rise (in mmol/l) in total plasma triacylglycerol is usually greater than the rise in chylomicron-triacylglycerol concentration because there is also an increase in concentration of other lipoproteins containing triacylglycerol, but still the proportional increase is smaller than might be expected.

The route of absorption of dietary fat means that, alone amongst nutrients, it escapes the liver on its entry into the circulation. In fact most of the triacylglycerol is removed from chylomicrons in tissues outside the liver, particularly adipose tissue and (to a lesser extent) skeletal muscle and heart. Adipose tissue contains the enzyme lipoprotein lipase in its capillaries, and this is the enzyme responsible for hydrolysis of the chylomicron-triacylglycerol (see Fig. 4.16). The activity of lipoprotein lipase is stimulated by insulin (see Fig. 4.15), so that it will be increased after the meal. Insulin stimulation of lipoprotein lipase in adipose tissue is a complex process involving both increased gene transcription and increased export of an active form of the enzyme from adipocytes to endothelial cells, and lipoprotein lipase activity in adipose tissue does not reach its peak until around 3–4 hours of insulin stimulation. It is surely no coincidence that this leads to peak lipoprotein lipase activity coinciding with the entry of chylomicron-triacylglycerol into the plasma; this represents another facet of the remarkable way in which insulin coordinates metabolism of different fuels in different tissues after a meal.

Lipoprotein lipase in adipose tissue hydrolyses the chylomicron-triacyl-glycerol, leading to the liberation of fatty acids which for the most part enter the adipocytes and are esterified to form new triacylglycerol for storage. This proc-ess is facilitated by the fact that hormone-sensitive lipase activity is suppressed after the meal, and fatty acid esterification increased by the increased insulin and glucose concentrations (and thus increased glycolytic flux, and glycerol 3-phosphate production). The concentration gradient of fatty acids will therefore be in favour of their storage rather than diffusion out of the tissue. In this way, the metabolism of triacylglycerol is influenced by the metabolism of glucose and non-esterified fatty acids.

Adipose tissue is not the only tissue that expresses lipoprotein lipase. In skeletal muscle, the enzyme is regulated in different ways. Insulin has a suppres-sive effect on muscle lipoprotein lipase, although this is fairly weak; it is also, like the stimulation of lipoprotein lipase in adipose tissue, rather slow, taking a matter of hours. Muscle lipoprotein lipase activity is influenced mainly by the fitness of the muscle for aerobic exercise. It is present at higher activity in red (oxidative) than white (glycolytic) fibres (see Table 4.1), and its activity is increased by exercise training. These features all suggest that the role of muscle lipoprotein lipase is not so much storage of fat, as utilisation of fat from plasma for energy production. The amount of chylomicron-triacylglycerol removed in skeletal muscle is not definitely known; it is likely to be rather less than the amount removed by adipose tissue in most people, but this might be very different in a fit, muscular person with less adipose tissue than average. The cellular organisation is just the same as in adipose tissue: the enzyme is present not in the muscle cells themselves, but attached to the endothelial cells lining the capillaries. It hydrolyses circulating lipoprotein-triacylglycerol (mainly chylomicron-triacylglycerol for the present discussion), liberating fatty acids which reach the muscle cells along some sort of structured diffusion pathway. Muscle is not a tissue in which triacylglycerol is stored for the rest of the body (although muscle cells do contain intracellular triacylglycerol stores) and most fatty acids entering muscle cells are oxidised. However, there is evidence, from experiments with chylomicrons containing isotopically labelled fatty acids, that chylomicron-triacylglycerol fatty acids which are taken up by muscle are largely esterified. Presumably this is how the muscle cells replenish their own local triacylglycerol store for energy production at a later time. It is only fair to say, however, that we understand very little of the regulation of lipoprotein-triacylglycerol utilisation by muscle.

The pattern of triacylglycerol metabolism after a meal containing fat is illustrated in Fig. 6.13.

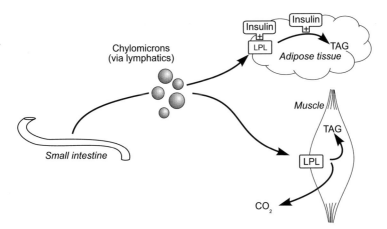

Fig. 6.13 The pattern of plasma triacylglycerol metabolism after a breakfast containing both fat and carbohydrate. Triacylglycerol (TAG) enters the circulation in the form of chylomicron particles and is hydrolysed by the enzyme lipoprotein lipase (LPL) in the capillaries of tissues (see Fig. 4.16 for more details of this process).

6.3   Amino acid and protein metabolism

6.3.1   General features

The topic of amino acid and protein metabolism is vast; twenty[1] different amino acids can be incorporated into proteins and several others exist in the body, and each has its own pathway for synthesis and degradation (except that the so-called essential amino acids are not synthesised in the human body). Furthermore, the synthesis and degradation of individual proteins (e.g. enzymes under hormonal control) is so specific that it may appear very difficult to make generalisations. The emphasis here will be on aspects that relate to energy metabolism, and on aspects of the control of protein turnover at a whole-body and tissue level where general features of hormone action can be distinguished.

Amino acids can be oxidised just as can glucose and fatty acids. In fact, very little amino acid is lost from the body intact – we shed some in skin cells, and we lose some in faeces and a tiny amount of free amino acid and some protein in the urine. But most of the amino acids we ingest are ultimately oxidised. At a whole-body level, therefore, the total oxidation of amino acids (per day) roughly balances the daily intake of protein, around 70–100 g in the typical Western diet. Amino acid oxidation contributes around 10–20% of the total oxidative metabolism of the body under normal conditions (Fig. 6.14).

The total content of amino acids in the body (present in proteins) could therefore represent a large store of energy. One important difference between amino acids and carbohydrates and fatty acids, however, is that (in mammals) amino acids are not stored simply for energy production: all proteins have some

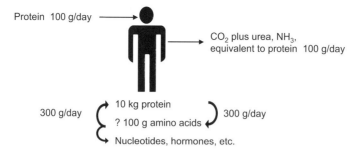

Fig. 6.14 Overview of protein and amino acid turnover in the body. We eat (very approximately) 100 g protein per day and therefore (unless we are growing) must dispose of an equal amount, mainly by oxidation of amino acids with generation of CO_2, H_2O, urea and some NH_3. Of the (approximately) 10 kg of protein in the body, there is continuous synthesis and breakdown of (about) 300 g/day (i.e. a 3% 'turnover'), although this varies greatly from tissue to tissue (Table 6.1). Some of the amino acid pool is used for synthesis of purines, pyrimidines and hormones. This may also be put in terms of nitrogen balance. Each 6.25 g protein contains about 1 g nitrogen. Therefore (in round figures) we take in about 16 g N per day. Each day, around 2 g is lost in faeces, 0.5 g in shed skin cells, etc., and the remainder of the 16 g as urea and NH_3 in urine. Reproduced from Frayn (in press).

biological function apart from storage. For this reason, body protein is largely preserved during normal conditions; the amount does not fluctuate like the glycogen store, for instance. However, unlike fatty acids, amino acids can be converted into glucose. This gives the body's protein store a special role during starvation, when the body must maintain the availability of circulating glucose despite the absence of an external carbohydrate supply. (The utilisation of protein in starvation will be considered further in Chapter 8.)

Protein is a constituent of all tissues, but some tissues play a more important role than others in amino acid metabolism. Skeletal muscle, in particular, is important mainly because of its bulk – about 40% of body weight. The liver is important for a number of reasons: because it is the first organ through which amino acids pass after absorption from the intestine; because some important links between amino acid and carbohydrate metabolism occur there; and because it is the organ where urea synthesis takes place.

Both protein and the pools of individual amino acids turn over in a constant cycle of breakdown or utilisation, and replenishment. The rate of protein turnover varies from tissue to tissue. It is normally measured in terms of percentage replacement per day. These estimations are made by studying the incorporation of isotopically labelled amino acids into protein. Usually they measure turnover of mixed proteins. More specific measurements of the turnover of individual proteins can be made (for instance, by isolating them with immunological techniques after incorporation of an isotopically labelled amino acid), and of course the turnover of some individual proteins is controlled on a very specific basis. We can generalise, however, about rates of protein turnover in different tissues (Table 6.1). The percentage replacement rates are very high in liver and the intestine, but muscle, despite a low fractional protein turnover,

Table 6.1 Protein turnover in the whole body and in various tissues.

Organ	% Replacement per day	Total protein synthesis (g/day)	% Contribution to whole body protein synthesis
Whole body	3%	300	(100)
Skeletal muscle	2%	120	41%
Liver	10%*; 7%†	80	25%
Small intestine	14%	70	23%
Large intestine	7%	8	3%
Kidneys	5%	3	1%
Heart	2%	1	0.4%

*Includes proteins synthesised for export (e.g. albumin).

†Protein retained in liver.

These figures are very approximate: they were originally based on experiments in adult (8-week-old) rats, in whom protein turnover is much more rapid than in adult humans, but they have been adjusted to give approximate human figures.

Original (rat) data based on Goldspink & Kelly (1984), Goldspink et al. (1984) and Lewis et al. (1984). Data for skeletal muscle are calculated assuming muscle to represent 40% body weight, and 'red' (soleus-type) and 'white' (anterior tibialis-type) to represent 50% each of this.

makes the greatest contribution to whole-body protein turnover because of its large protein mass.

Free amino acids (i.e. those not bound in proteins) are found both in tissues and in the blood. As we saw in Chapter 2 (Section 2.2.1.2, Table 2.2), they are taken up into tissues by specific active transport mechanisms, and their concentrations inside tissues may be many times those in blood. The concentration of amino acids in blood is therefore a poor indicator of the amount of free amino acid in the body. The body pool of free amino acids, like protein, is constantly being utilised and replaced. The amount of free amino acid within the body reflects the balance between a number of processes: input into the pool from the intestine (i.e. amino acids from food), from the breakdown of proteins and by synthesis of new amino acids; and loss by incorporation into protein, oxidation and conversion to other metabolites. There is some general control of the rates of protein synthesis and breakdown in particular tissues, and some regulation of the rates of interconversions of amino acids and conversion to non-amino acid metabolites, but little active control of amino acid oxidation. This is because the enzymes for degradation and oxidation of amino acids almost exclusively have high K_m values, and thus, when amino acids are in excess, they will be degraded and oxidised in proportion to the extent of their concentration.

One reaction that is particularly important in amino acid metabolism is transamination (Box 6.2). Pairs of amino acids can be interconverted in what is usually an equilibrium reaction, by transfer of the amino group. An amino

Box 6.2   Transamination

The reaction of transamination involves the transfer of an amino group from one amino acid (the donor) to a 2-oxoacid (the recipient), thus forming a new 2-oxoacid (from the donor) and a new amino acid (from the recipient). The enzymes are often called transaminases, but are now known as aminotransferases. The reactions are usually at near-equilibrium (and thus the direction is governed by the relative concentrations of the reactants). One partner is usually either 2-oxoglutarate/glutamic acid, or oxaloacetate/aspartic acid.

The reaction is illustrated here for pyruvate and glutamic acid.

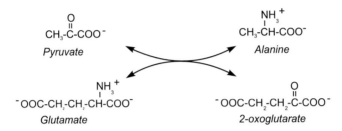

Fig. 6.2.1 A representative transamination reaction.

Some amino acids and their 2-oxoacid derivatives are listed below.

Amino acid	2-Oxoacid	Relevance to energy metabolism
Alanine	Pyruvate	End-product of glycolysis
Glutamate	2-Oxoglutarate	Intermediate in tricarboxylic acid cycle
Aspartate	Oxaloacetate	Intermediate in tricarboxylic acid cycle
Leucine	2-Oxo-3-methylvalerate	May be oxidised in muscle
Isoleucine	2-Oxo-4-methylvalerate	May be oxidised in muscle
Valine	2-Oxo-3-methylbutyrate	May be oxidised in muscle

acid from which an amino group has been removed is a 2-oxoacid (often called a keto-acid). Each amino acid has a 2-oxoacid partner. Some examples are alanine and pyruvate, aspartate and oxaloacetate, glutamate and 2-oxoglutarate (Box 6.2). The 2-oxoacids corresponding to the branched-chain amino acids are less well known, but important nonetheless: they are also listed in Box 6.2. Since the 2-oxoacid partners listed above have obvious roles in other metabolic systems (e.g. pyruvate in glucose metabolism, oxaloacetate and 2-oxoglutarate as intermediates of the tricarboxylic acid cycle), it is clear that transamination serves both as a link between amino acid and other aspects of metabolism, and as a route for oxidation of amino acids.

6.3.2   Some particular aspects of amino acid metabolism

6.3.2.1   Essential and non-essential amino acids, and other metabolically distinct groups of amino acids

The classification of amino acids into *essential* and *non-essential* was originally based upon the need for them to be supplied in the diet: the non-essential were regarded as those which could be synthesised within the body. A group of *conditionally essential* amino acids was also distinguished. In recent years tracer methodology has led to an improved understanding of the essential nature of amino acids: see Table 6.2.

The twenty different amino acids that normally form proteins occur in reasonably constant proportions in a range of proteins. In some metabolic studies, obvious differences from these proportions are seen and these observations have led to some of our knowledge of amino acid metabolism in individual tissues.

For instance, after eating a meal containing protein, amino acids appear in the portal vein. We presume that these largely reflect the composition of the meal. However, those leaving the liver in the hepatic vein after a meal show quite different proportions. In particular, they are enriched in the three *branched-*

Table 6.2 Essential and non-essential amino acids.

Essential	Non-essential
Arginine (C)	Alanine
Isoleucine	Aspartic acid
Leucine	Asparagine
Valine	Cysteine (C)
Histidine (C)	Glutamic acid
Lysine	Glutamine
Methionine	Glycine (C)
Threonine	Proline (C)
Phenylalanine	Serine (C)
Tryptophan	Tyrosine (C)

Essential amino acids are those which must be supplied in the diet (since they cannot be synthesised within the human body).

Non-essential amino acids can be synthesised directly by transamination of a 'carbon skeleton' which is a readily available metabolic intermediate (e.g. pyruvate, forming alanine).

The conditionally essential amino acids may in principle be synthesised from the essential amino acids: in nutritional terms, they may be needed in the diet under some circumstances. For instance, histidine cannot be synthesised sufficiently rapidly if none is provided in the diet, and arginine is needed by young children. Tyrosine and cysteine can both be synthesised, but from other essential amino acids (phenylalanine and methionine respectively). Thus, they become essential if other amino acids are lacking. The classification of amino acids into essential and non-essential is always controversial. For further discussion see Further Reading.

chain amino acids, valine, leucine and isoleucine. These three essential amino acids constitute about 20% of dietary protein, but represent about 70% of the amino acids leaving the liver after a meal. The implication is that other amino acids have been preferentially retained in the liver. The branched-chain amino acids are instead preferentially removed by muscle after a meal. Since muscle removes these amino acids preferentially, it cannot require them simply for protein synthesis, or they would not be matched in proportion by other amino acids. In fact, skeletal muscle has the ability to oxidise the branched-chain amino acids.

Another departure from the proportions in protein is in the pattern of amino acids leaving muscle and other non-hepatic tissues after an overnight fast; there is always a large preponderance of alanine and glutamine (Fig. 6.15), much more than their occurrence in muscle protein would suggest. Similarly, it is possible to measure the uptake of amino acids across the liver and intestine, and glutamine and alanine are found to contribute the majority of amino acids taken up (Fig. 6.15). These observations show us that individual amino acids

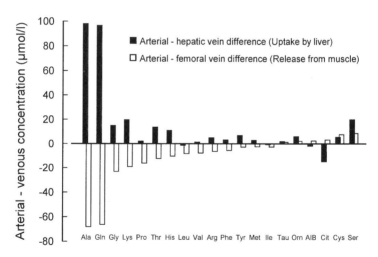

Fig. 6.15 The typical pattern of amino acid metabolism in different tissues. The diagram shows the difference in concentration between arterial blood and (1) the blood in a hepatic vein, carrying the venous blood from the liver; or (2) a femoral vein, which carries the venous blood mainly from the skeletal muscles of the leg. Thus, the solid bars represent the extent to which different amino acids are taken up across the small intestine and liver (the *splanchnic bed*), whilst the open bars show the release of amino acids from muscle into the bloodstream. These observations led to the idea that alanine (Ala) and glutamine (Gln) predominated in transferring both amino groups and carbon atoms from muscle proteolysis, to be taken up by the liver for urea synthesis and gluconeogenesis. The studies were carried out in normal subjects after an overnight fast. AIB: α-amino-isobutyric acid (a minor amino acid, not incorporated into protein). Based on Felig, P. (1975). With permission, from the *Annual Review of Biochemistry* 44: 933–955. ©1975 by Annual Reviews www.annualreviews.org.

have specific pathways of metabolism in different tissues, some of which we shall discuss.

6.3.2.2 Branched-chain amino acids and muscle amino acid metabolism

The branched-chain amino acids (leucine, isoleucine and valine) are preferentially taken up by skeletal muscle after a meal. Their uptake is not directly stimulated by insulin and increases because the blood concentration rises. The size of the pool of branched-chain amino acids within muscle reflects the balance between a number of processes: inward transport from plasma and outward release into plasma, utilisation for protein synthesis, production from protein breakdown, and loss by transamination and degradation. There is no synthesis from other amino acids, since they are essential amino acids.

Muscle possesses a specific branched-chain 2-oxoacid dehydrogenase, which is a large complex related, and similar in many ways, to pyruvate dehydrogenase (also a 2-oxoacid dehydrogenase). Thus, branched-chain amino acids in muscle may be transaminated and oxidised, providing a source of energy for the muscle. The amino group is transferred to a 2-oxoacid. It may then be 'passed around' between recipients, but usually the ultimate acceptor 2-oxoacid is either pyruvate (forming alanine) or 2-oxoglutarate (forming glutamate). In addition, amino groups may form ammonia (strictly, ammonium ions, NH_4^+) through the action of *glutamate dehydrogenase* (Fig. 4.8) which removes the amino group from glutamate as NH_4^+, producing 2-oxoglutarate again, which may again participate in transamination reactions. Glutamate and ammonia may also combine to form glutamine through the action of *glutamine synthetase* (Fig. 6.16). Thus, catabolism of branched chain and other amino acids leads predominantly to the release of glutamine and alanine (see Fig. 6.15). Alanine and glutamine are considered further in the next section. These interrelationships are shown in Fig. 6.17.

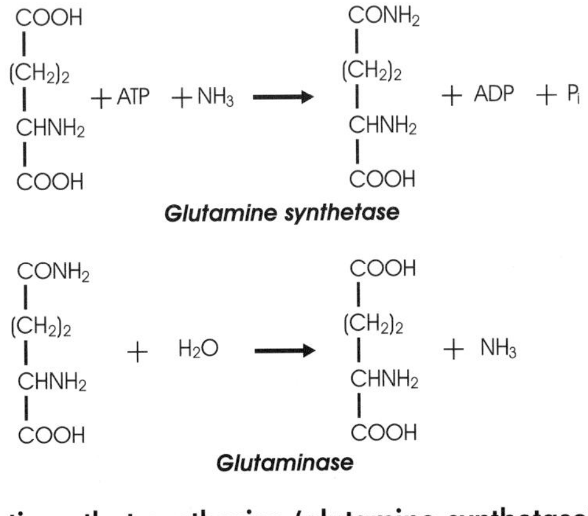

Fig. 6.16 The reactions that synthesise (glutamine synthetase) and break down (glutaminase) glutamine. (Note that, for simplicity, ionisation states are not shown correctly: e.g. NH_3 would be in the form of NH_4^+ at physiological pH.)

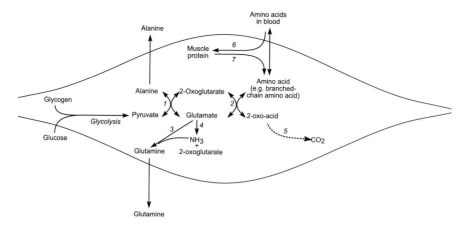

Fig. 6.17 Major amino acids interconversions in muscle. (Adipose tissue and brain may be similar.) *1,* alanine aminotransferase (also called glutamate-pyruvate transaminase); *2,* leucine, valine or other aminotransferase; *3,* glutamine synthetase; *4,* glutamate dehydrogenase; *5,* branched-chain 2-oxoacid dehydrogenase and further catabolism; *6,* muscle protein synthesis; *7,* muscle protein breakdown (*proteolysis*). For simplicity, ionisation states are not shown (e.g. NH_3 would be in the form of NH_4^+ at physiological pH).

6.3.2.3 Alanine and glutamine

These amino acids have a special place in a discussion of energy metabolism, as they provide links between amino acid and carbohydrate metabolism.

As discussed above, alanine and glutamine predominate amongst the amino acids leaving muscle. This is also true of other 'peripheral tissues', including adipose tissue and brain. Since glutamine carries two nitrogen atoms (in its amino group and its amide group), it is usually a larger transporter of nitrogen than is alanine. The preponderance of alanine and glutamine is much greater than would be expected if the amino acids leaving muscle simply reflected the composition of proteins being degraded (Fig. 6.15). Therefore, they must be synthesised in the tissues. We will consider their formation a little more deeply. The amino groups for alanine and glutamine, and the amide group of glutamine, may arise from the amino groups of other amino acids as discussed above. What, then, is the origin of their 'carbon skeletons' (i.e. the corresponding 2-oxoacids)?

For alanine, the corresponding 2-oxoacid is pyruvate, the end-product of glycolysis. Treatments which increase glycolysis (for instance, in isolated muscle preparations, addition of extra insulin or glucose) usually also increase alanine release. It is possible in principle that the carbon skeletons of some amino acids may form pyruvate, but the evidence that these routes contribute much to the carbon skeleton of alanine leaving muscle is not strong, and it is most likely that most of the carbon skeleton of the excess alanine leaving peripheral tissues (i.e. in excess of that produced by protein breakdown) arises from glycolysis.

For glutamine, the 2-oxoacid is 2-oxoglutarate, an intermediate in the tricarboxylic acid cycle. It is rather more possible that the carbon skeletons of other amino acids may contribute to glutamine than to alanine, since any amino acid whose breakdown leads to acetyl-CoA may do so. However, an intermediate of the tricarboxylic acid cycle cannot be 'tapped off' indefinitely without some topping up of cycle intermediates – or, since it is a cycle, it will stop. It may be that pairs of amino acids contribute to this process: for instance, catabolism of leucine leads to acetyl-CoA, and catabolism of valine leads to succinyl-CoA, another intermediate in the tricarboxylic acid cycle. Thus, these two amino acids together may replace the 2-oxoglutarate used in glutamine formation.

Alanine is taken up avidly by the liver, particularly under conditions of active gluconeogenesis, when its uptake is stimulated by glucagon. Within the liver, which has very active transaminases, alanine readily passes its amino group to 2-oxoglutarate, leaving its carbon skeleton as pyruvate, a substrate for gluconeogenesis.

Glutamine is not as good a substrate for hepatic uptake, but is removed particularly by the kidney and by the intestinal mucosal cells. In the kidney, the action of glutaminase (Fig. 6.16) removes the amide group (forming ammonia) and leaves glutamate; glutamate can be converted to 2-oxoglutarate by the action of glutamine dehydrogenase, again forming ammonia. It is generally believed that this ammonia is a route for urinary excretion of protons (H^+ ions), especially in conditions of excessive acidity in the body. This point is controversial, however, and will not be further discussed here. In the intestinal cells, glutamine is an important metabolic fuel (Section 4.7.2). The pathway of metabolism leads to production of alanine, which leaves in the portal vein and thus reaches the liver, again as a substrate for conversion to pyruvate and hence glucose. Glutamine is also an important fuel for other rapidly dividing cells, as discussed in Section 4.7.2.

The major pathways of amino acid flow between tissues discussed in the last two sections are outlined in Fig. 6.18.

6.3.3   The overall control of protein synthesis and breakdown

There are some generalisations that can be made about the regulation of protein synthesis and breakdown (summarised in Fig. 6.19). Two hormones have a general anabolic role (stimulating net protein synthesis) in the body: insulin and growth hormone. In people with a deficiency of insulin (insulin-dependent diabetes mellitus; see Chapter 10) there is marked loss of protein from the body – the 'melting of flesh into urine'. Treatment with insulin restores body protein. Growth hormone acts through the insulin-like growth factors IGF-1 and IGF-2, and has an important role during development. In the adult this is not of major importance; adults whose pituitaries have been removed do not need growth hormone to be replaced to lead fairly normal lives. However, growth hormone is beneficial in stimulating protein anabolism in patients who have lost protein through severe illness.

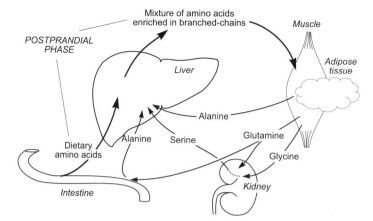

Fig. 6.18 Major pathways for amino acid flow between tissues. The pathways are discussed in the text, with the exception of serine release by the kidney. The precursor for this is probably glycine (released from peripheral tissues). In the liver, serine may be converted to D-2-phosphoglycerate (or pyruvate in some species) and thus enter the hepatic pool of gluconeogenic precursors. Based loosely on Felig (1975) and Christensen (1982): for discussion of serine metabolism see Snell (1986); Snell & Fell (1990).

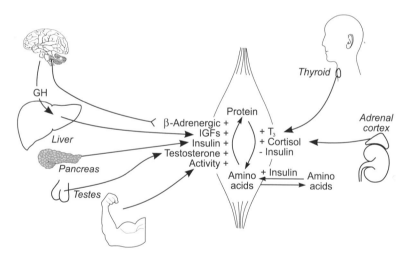

Fig. 6.19 Overall control of protein synthesis and breakdown in muscle (and other tissues). Some of the stimuli here are tissue-specific (especially physical activity, testosterone and β-adrenergic stimulation); more details are given in the text. *IGFs* are the insulin-like growth factors (IGF-1 and -2), generated in the liver in response to growth hormone (GH). *β-adrenergic* represents activation of β-adrenergic receptors, either by noradrenaline released at sympathetic nerve terminals or by adrenaline in the plasma.

The male sex hormone, *testosterone* (a steroid hormone produced in the testes), also has a role in promoting protein synthesis, particularly in muscle. This was first realised because of the difference in average muscle strength between men and women. It became clear that this was a function of testosterone. Since that time, synthetic steroids have been developed which have increased *anabolic* tendencies and less *androgenic* (masculinising) tendencies – these are the *anabolic steroids*.

In individual tissues, there are other specific controlling factors. In skeletal muscle, the level of physical activity is an obvious one. The various factors generally work in concert; the effects of exercise and anabolic steroids, for instance, are greater than either alone. Skeletal muscle protein mass is also regulated by adrenergic influences. It has long been known that if a muscle is denervated – has its nerve supply cut – then it wastes away (*atrophies*). It has been assumed that this is because it no longer contracts, and therefore there is no 'training stimulus' to growth – so-called *disuse atrophy*. Now it appears that loss of an adrenergic stimulus may also be important. Administration of adrenergic β-stimulating drugs can increase muscle bulk. It is still not clear whether these act through one of the 'classical' β-adrenergic receptors or whether some new type of receptor is involved. One such agent is *clenbuterol*, which has been used in agriculture to increase muscle bulk in cows, and misused in the sports world.

Some endocrine glands are stimulated to growth by their own *trophic* (or *tropic*) (hormone-releasing) factors. A good example is the stimulation of the thyroid gland by thyroid-stimulating hormone (TSH) from the anterior pituitary. TSH increases thyroid size as well as stimulating thyroid hormone secretion (see Section 5.3.1). However, this is not of significance for the overall protein metabolism of the body.

The overall rate of *protein breakdown* to amino acids is also under hormonal control. Insulin itself may act more by restraining protein breakdown than by stimulating protein synthesis. Since there is continual turnover of protein, the net effect is the same. In addition, two hormones are regarded as having particularly catabolic effects: cortisol and the thyroid hormone triiodothyronine (T_3).

The protein catabolic effect of cortisol does not affect all tissues equally. This is clearly seen in *Cushing's syndrome*, the disease caused by overproduction of cortisol from the adrenal cortex.[2] In this condition there is loss of protein from both muscle and bone, and one of the consequences is a liability to bone fractures. The wasting of muscle is, however, somewhat selective and affects the so-called proximal muscles – those nearer the trunk rather than on the lower limbs. It also affects primarily the Type II, fast-twitch muscle fibres.

Loss of body mass, including muscle mass, is one of the features of thyroid excess, and it is clear that the thyroid hormones have a net degradative effect on muscle protein. In experimental models, T_3 may also increase the rate of protein synthesis, but less than it increases protein degradation, so the net result is accelerated protein turnover and net loss of protein.

6.4   Links between carbohydrate, fat and amino acid metabolism

So far, the topics of carbohydrate, fat and amino acid metabolism have largely been kept separate for clarity. In reality there are many connections between them, as we shall now see.

6.4.1   Carbohydrate and fat metabolism

6.4.1.1   Lipogenesis

Lipogenesis means the synthesis of lipid. More strictly, the term *de novo lipogenesis* means the synthesis of fatty acids and triacylglycerol from substrates other than lipids – particularly glucose, although amino acids which can be converted to acetyl-CoA can in principle also be substrates. The pathway itself was outlined in Box 4.3. It provides a means by which excess carbohydrate can be laid down for storage as triacylglycerol (since, as we have seen, this is the most energy-dense storage compound). The pathway of *de novo lipogenesis* may occur in both liver and adipose tissue. We do not know the relative importance of these tissues in humans; both are thought to play some role, although liver is likely to be more important.

The regulation of lipogenesis illustrates some useful points about metabolic regulation and its coordination in the whole body that were first brought up in the 'metabolic regulation puzzle' in Fig. 2.3. Fatty acids are synthesised from acetyl-CoA, and the pathway is stimulated by insulin, mainly by activation of the rate-controlling enzyme acetyl-CoA carboxylase (see Box 4.3). Acetyl-CoA may be produced from the breakdown of glucose, amino acids or fatty acids. What, then, prevents simultaneous fat oxidation, producing acetyl-CoA, and lipogenesis, reconverting acetyl-CoA to fatty acids? That would represent a 'futile' and energy-wasting metabolic cycle.

The first and easiest answer is that some important tissues do not carry out both these processes. Skeletal muscle has a high capacity for fatty acid oxidation, but it does not express fatty acid synthase. Adipose tissue has the capacity for fatty acid synthesis, but it seems hardly to oxidise fatty acids. But what about the liver, where both processes can certainly take place? The answer is mainly the supply of substrate, regulated by insulin in other tissues. Under conditions when insulin might stimulate lipogenesis, it will also suppress fat mobilisation from adipose tissue; thus, the supply of fatty acids for oxidation in the liver will be diminished. In addition, under these conditions an increased concentration of malonyl-CoA will divert those fatty acids reaching the liver into esterification rather than oxidation (via inhibition of CPT-1 – see Fig. 4.3). Thus, several different regulatory points act together to direct metabolism in appropriate ways.

The pathway of lipogenesis, although of interest from the point of view of metabolic regulation, is probably not of major importance as a route of fat deposition in humans on a Western type of diet. The evidence for this is reviewed in Box 6.3.

Box 6.3   The physiological importance of de novo lipogenesis in humans on a Western diet

The occurrence of *net* lipogenesis in the body – that is, a rate of lipogenesis which exceeds the rate of fat oxidation in the body as a whole – can be detected by measuring the consumption of O_2 and production of CO_2 by the body (indirect calorimetry). *Net* lipogenesis results in a ratio (mole for mole) of CO_2 production to O_2 consumption which is greater than 1.00; this is mainly because pyruvate (3-carbon) has to be converted to acetyl-CoA (2-carbon), and for each mole of pyruvate used, one mole of CO_2 is thus liberated. In contrast, the ratio of CO_2 production to O_2 consumption – called the *respiratory quotient* – for oxidation of glucose is 1.00, and that for fat is around 0.71 (discussed further in a later chapter, Box 11.2.)

    If normal volunteers are fed a large carbohydrate breakfast (600 g carbohydrate, 9.6 MJ) then studied over the next 10 hours, they continue to oxidise rather than synthesise fat in a net sense (Acheson *et al.* 1982). If they are fed a very high carbohydrate diet for several days beforehand, then net lipogenesis will occur for a few hours after a high-carbohydrate meal; it is as though continuing high insulin concentrations have 'primed' the pathway (Acheson *et al.* 1984). Similarly, if volunteers are fed more than their normal daily energy requirements (overfeeding) then net lipogenesis will occur after a day or two, exactly as we might expect because this is the pathway for conversion of excess carbohydrate into fat for storage (Aarsland *et al.* 1997).

    Another situation in which net lipogenesis is observed is in patients being fed intravenously to help them recover body mass lost during a severe illness. Sometimes these patients are given their energy almost entirely in the form of carbohydrate (glucose in solution), and then over a period of days they begin to show net lipogenesis; the carbohydrate taken in is being laid down as fat for storage (King *et al.* 1984).

    Because these are extreme situations, it seems certain that in normal conditions lipogenesis is not a way in which we lay down fat in a *net* sense, although the metabolic pathways clearly exist and can be activated under some circumstances. The situation may well be different in people eating more traditional carbohydrate-based diets in developing countries.

    In recent years novel techniques have been introduced using stable isotopic tracers to assess the contribution of *de novo* lipogenesis to hepatic triacylglycerol secretion (in VLDL particles). Note that this is not the same as *net* lipogenesis: the body as a whole might still be oxidising more fat than it is synthesising, but because of the capacity for lipogenesis in the liver, it might make a large contribution to hepatic triacylglycerol production. In fact, in almost all situations examined the absolute rate of hepatic *de novo* lipogenesis is small, and most hepatic triacylglycerol arises from hepatic uptake of fatty acids (as plasma NEFA and as triacylglycerol-fatty acids in lipoprotein particles).

6.4.1.2 Metabolic interactions between fatty acids and glucose: the glucose–fatty acid cycle

The *glucose–fatty acid cycle* refers to important metabolic interactions between glucose and fat metabolism (Box 6.4). These interactions occur in adipose tissue and in muscle; the endocrine pancreas is involved via insulin secretion. They were first observed in rat heart muscle, but there is now considerable evidence that they occur in skeletal muscle in humans.

In adipose tissue, we have already seen these mechanisms at work. When the glucose concentration in plasma is high, the plasma insulin concentration responds. Insulin suppresses fat mobilisation (the release of fatty acids from adipose tissue). Thus, a high plasma glucose concentration leads to a low plasma non-esterified fatty acid concentration. In muscle, the rate at which fatty acids are utilised from plasma is dependent almost entirely on the plasma non-esterified fatty acid concentration (and the blood flow) (see Section 4.3.3.2). Thus, when additional glucose becomes available in the plasma – after a meal, for instance – the muscle will tend to switch to the use of glucose rather than fatty acids because, firstly, glucose uptake will be stimulated by insulin, and, secondly, the plasma non-esterified fatty acid concentration will fall and remove that substrate.

On the other hand, between meals (in the postabsorptive phase), the plasma glucose concentration falls a little, insulin secretion decreases, and the plasma non-esterified fatty acid concentration rises. In this situation the body's strategy is to 'spare' the use of carbohydrate for tissues such as the brain which

---

Box 6.4   The glucose–fatty acid cycle

The glucose–fatty acid cycle integrates the utilisation of fatty acids and glucose. These interactions between glucose and fatty acid metabolism were first described in 1963 by Philip Randle and colleagues (Randle *et al.* 1963). Central to this is a mechanism whereby the oxidation of fatty acids in muscle reduces the uptake and oxidation of glucose. The metabolic interactions involved are as follows. A high rate of fatty acid oxidation, and hence acetyl-CoA formation, leads to a high rate of citrate formation (via citrate synthase). In addition, the $NADH/NAD^+$ and ATP/ADP ratios will be increased. The high acetyl-CoA/CoA and $NADH/NAD^+$ ratios inhibit pyruvate dehydrogenase (via phosphorylation, by pyruvate dehydrogenase kinase). Thus, the oxidation of pyruvate (derived from glycolysis) is suppressed. This is linked with coordinated inhibition of glucose uptake and glycolysis. Citrate (in the cytosol) is an inhibitor of the regulatory glycolytic enzyme phosphofructokinase (it potentiates the inhibition by ATP). (Box 4.3 shows how citrate can be exported from mitochondria to cytosol.) Fructose 6-phosphate and correspondingly glucose 6-phosphate build up, and glucose 6-phosphate is an allosteric inhibitor of hexokinase. Hence, the pathway of glucose breakdown and oxidation is inhibited. Accumulation of free glucose is assumed to occur within the cell, thus inhibiting the uptake of further glucose. (There is some difficulty here, since free glucose concentrations in muscle are low and difficult to measure, and never seem to approach those in plasma as would be necessary for this story to hold completely. But the evidence for operation of the glucose–fatty acid cycle is so strong that it seems likely that our understanding of free glucose concentrations is at fault rather than the theory.) These interactions are illustrated in Fig. 6.4.1. There is also evidence for a direct inhibition of glucose transport into the cell, although the mechanism of that is not understood.

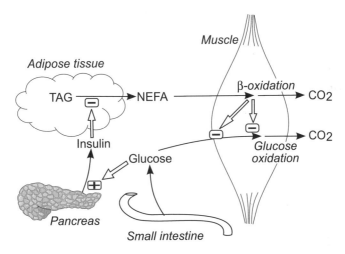

Fig. 6.4.1

   The glucose–fatty acid cycle may lead to adverse consequences in unusual situations when both non-esterified fatty acids and glucose are elevated. Some such situations will be discussed in later chapters: they include 'stress' and diabetes. This situation can also occur after a particularly large meal of both fat and carbohydrate. The muscle cannot oxidise non-esterified fatty acids *and* glucose at the rates expected from their concentrations in plasma; there is no mechanism for disposing of excess ATP, and it would clearly be wasteful of energy and of precious carbohydrate. Then the operation of the glucose–fatty acid cycle leads to an impairment of glucose uptake and metabolism, with the net effect that glucose uptake by muscle is reduced compared with that expected at given concentrations of insulin and glucose in the plasma. It appears that insulin does not stimulate glucose uptake as normal, and this is known as *insulin resistance*. Insulin resistance, perhaps better termed *reduction in sensitivity to insulin*, is a common alteration and will be covered in detail later (see Box 10.2 and Section 11.4.4).

cannot use fatty acids. This is achieved by the fact that oxidation of fatty acids in muscle suppresses the uptake and oxidation of glucose. The mechanism for this effect is described in Box 6.4, together with further consequences of the glucose–fatty acid cycle in situations of disturbed metabolism.

The glucose–fatty acid cycle is not a metabolic cycle in the normal sense – it does not involve the interconversion of glucose and fatty acids – but a series of metabolic regulatory events that coordinate glucose and fat metabolism under normal and some abnormal conditions.

The reverse of this interaction is also true and was examined in the previous section: when glucose and insulin levels are high, production of malonyl-CoA will inhibit fatty acid oxidation (this applies in both liver and skeletal muscle). This has recently been termed the 'reverse glucose-fatty acid cycle' (Sidossis & Wolfe 1996). We might see both mechanisms as providing fine tuning over the rate of utilisation of metabolic subtrates, particularly in skeletal muscle.

6.4.2   Interactions between carbohydrate and amino acid metabolism: the glucose–alanine cycle and gluconeogenesis from amino acids

It has already been mentioned that alanine released from muscle may be 'pyruvate in disguise' – pyruvate onto which has been transferred an amino group from the breakdown of another amino acid. Pyruvate is a potential precursor for gluconeogenesis. Glucose thus formed may be released into the circulation, taken up by muscle and, through glycolysis, pyruvate formed. This pyruvate may be transaminated – and so on. This has been termed the glucose–alanine cycle. It is very closely related to the glucose–lactate cycle or Cori cycle, described in the 1920s by the Coris (Carl and Gertrude Cori, husband and wife, who shared the Nobel Prize for Medicine in 1948). These two cycles are illustrated in Fig. 6.20. The glucose–alanine cycle provides a clear link between glucose and amino acid metabolism and attracted a lot of attention when it was first proposed by Philip Felig and colleagues (Felig et al. 1970). But it needs close examination. What does it achieve for the body?

There needs to be a link between amino acid and glucose metabolism. The body's store of carbohydrate is relatively limited and, as has been stressed several times, certain tissues require a supply of glucose. Much of the metabolic regulation we have been considering seems directed at preserving and storing glucose when it is available. But many amino acids can, in principle, be converted to glucose, so that the body's protein reserves – particularly the bulk of skeletal muscle – could maintain glucose production for a considerable time. Thus, there needs to be a mechanism for transporting the necessary substrates to the liver (the main site of gluconeogenesis). But the glucose–alanine cycle as just outlined does not do this: it merely recycles pyruvate, derived from glucose. It is a means by which muscle glycogen (which cannot lead directly to glucose release from muscle) may lead to release of glucose into the circulation (i.e. from the liver). It also provides a way for the muscle to export amino-nitrogen,

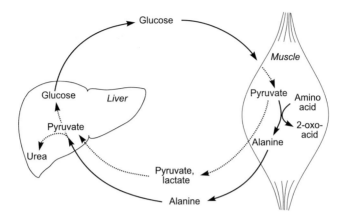

Fig. 6.20 The glucose–alanine cycle operates in parallel with the Cori (glucose–lactate) cycle. Muscle is shown, but adipose tissue also participates, and a number of tissues – e.g. red blood cells – take part in the glucose–lactate cycle.

liberated from those amino acids whose 2-oxo acids it has oxidised (e.g. the branched-chain amino acids). The nitrogen will eventually be excreted as urea, which is synthesised in the liver.

In order for the glucose–alanine cycle to function as a means of transporting amino acid *carbon* to the liver for gluconeogenesis, the 'carbon skeleton' of the alanine also needs to be formed from an amino acid, not from glucose. In fact there is not a lot of evidence that this occurs, although much effort has been devoted to attempting to demonstrate it. Glutamine may be a more likely carrier of such carbon (as discussed above, Section 6.3.2.3). Nevertheless, the cycle certainly operates, even if only as an alternative arm of the Cori cycle.

6.5   An integrated view of metabolism: a metabolic diary

The postabsorptive state provides a useful starting point in which to re-examine the patterns of carbohydrate, fat and amino acid metabolism. Some of this will be a recapitulation of the previous sections, but the aim will be to show how all facets of energy metabolism interact during two typical days which contrast substrate flow in two extreme lifestyles.

6.5.1   The postabsorptive state: waking up

Plasma concentrations of glucose and insulin are at their lowest in the normal 24-hour cycle, and plasma non-esterified fatty acids at their highest. Glucose enters the blood from the breakdown of liver glycogen and from hepatic gluconeogenesis. Of this glucose, a large proportion is taken up by the brain and completely oxidised, some is taken up by red blood cells and other obligatory glycolytic tissues, which return the carbon to the liver in the form of lactate to be recycled through gluconeogenesis. Skeletal muscle uses very little glucose, because the glucose and insulin concentrations are low, and also because concentrations of non-esterified fatty acids are high and the glucose–fatty acid cycle operates. There is net breakdown of protein in muscle, mainly because of the low insulin concentration. Some of the amino acids released – especially the branched-chain amino acids – are oxidised in the muscle and their amino groups transferred to pyruvate (resulting from muscle glycogen breakdown as well as the small amount of glucose uptake) to form alanine; this is taken up by the liver as a substrate for gluconeogenesis.

Liberation of fatty acids from adipose tissue is high because of lack of the restraint of hormone-sensitive lipase by insulin. These non-esterified fatty acids become the preferred fuel for muscle. In the liver fatty acids are taken up and the low insulin/glucagon ratio leads them into oxidation rather than esterification. The ATP formed is used to drive gluconeogenesis amongst other metabolic processes. Fatty acid oxidation is accompanied, as usual, by ketone body formation although the blood ketone body concentration is not high enough to make ketone bodies a major fuel for any tissue. The ketone bodies are taken up and oxidised by a number of tissues including muscle, brain and adipose tissue.

6.5.2   Breakfast goes down

Here we will follow two divergent stories, beginning with a lazy day on holiday – plenty of food and not much exercise. Breakfast is a substantial meal with carbohydrate, protein and plenty of fat. The time-course over which these nutrients are absorbed and enter the circulation differs: glucose and amino acids enter the portal vein and then the general circulation (via the liver) within about 15–30 minutes, although after a good meal the plasma glucose concentration will remain somewhat elevated for another 3–4 hours. As the glucose concentration in the portal vein rises, so glucose uptake into hepatocytes increases, thus 'damping down' the increase in glucose concentration in the general circulation. Nevertheless, the pancreas responds rapidly to the increasing glucose concentration and plasma insulin concentrations rise in parallel with those of glucose. Glucagon secretion into the portal vein may also be somewhat decreased.

Under the influence of the increasing glucose concentration and the insulin/glucagon ratio, hepatic glycogen metabolism switches from breakdown to synthesis. Much of the incoming glucose remains within the liver. The liver also extracts many of the amino acids arriving in the portal vein, although leaving the branched-chain amino acids which enter the general circulation.

The increasing glucose and insulin concentrations act on adipose tissue to reduce the release of non-esterified fatty acids. Because the uptake of non-esterified fatty acids by tissues is driven mostly by the plasma concentration, it decreases as the plasma concentration falls, reaching its lowest at about 1–2 hours after a meal.

The declining plasma non-esterified fatty acid concentration removes the drive for muscle to oxidise fatty acids; instead, glucose uptake is stimulated by the increasing glucose and insulin concentrations. Thus, skeletal muscle switches to glucose uptake; glycolysis increases, the output of lactate and pyruvate increase, and glucose oxidation increases. Glycogen synthesis is stimulated by insulin. Muscle also takes up amino acids, particularly the branched-chain which it may use as an oxidative fuel; but net protein synthesis is also stimulated in this state.

Increased glucose uptake by a number of tissues leads to increased lactate release into the bloodstream. Hepatic gluconeogenesis is maintained through the increased substrate supply; lactate channelled through gluconeogenesis leads to glucose 6-phosphate which is directed into glycogen synthesis rather than glucose release.

Thus, the metabolic picture within the first 1–4 hours after a meal reflects an intense switch to glucose utilisation, and particularly to glucose storage as glycogen. The body's fat stores are conserved by suppression of fatty acid release. The body is in 'storage and conservation mode'.

This is reinforced towards the end of the period by the arrival of chylomicron-triacylglycerol. At the same time, the enzyme lipoprotein lipase in adipose tissue has been increasing in activity, stimulated by the insulin response. Thus the drive is for esterification and storage of fatty acids as triacylglycerol in adipocytes.

At around 4 hours after the meal, then, intense storage of carbohydrate has been occurring for some time and fat storage is now getting into full swing. But this is a holiday, and we are not going to sit around and let ourselves get back into a postabsorptive state – it's surely time for lunch, or at least coffee and a snack.

6.5.3   Another meal follows

Insulin-stimulated processes become 'primed' by previous insulin stimulation. The probable explanation is that cellular metabolism is influenced by insulin which has left the plasma compartment and found its way to receptors on cell membranes. The effect of a second meal following on the heels of breakfast will be to considerably reinforce the pattern of substrate storage. The events described for the first meal will occur again but are likely to do so to a greater extent: the plasma non-esterified fatty acid concentration will remain suppressed, glycogen synthesis in liver and muscle will continue with little lag, and storage of triacylglycerol in adipose tissue may be almost continuous, one plasma triacylglycerol peak merging into another. It is not difficult to imagine how the body's energy stores will be increased by such events.

Suppose now that the second meal, whether elevenses or an early lunch, is followed not so many hours later by yet more food: there will hardly be a break in the storage of nutrients in the tissues. We can well see that the body's energy stores will end the day in a considerably more replete state than that in which they started. Furthermore, expression of carbohydrate- and insulin-regulated genes, particularly those for fat synthesis, will have been stimulated, so setting the scene for continued fat deposition.

6.5.4   An energetic day

Now contrast this with a different day: one in which more widely spaced meals are interspersed with some activity, requiring the use of metabolic fuels. The aim is to show how the overall storage of energy is regulated in such a way that the body's immediate needs are met, and any surplus stored; there is integration not just between different modes of substrate storage, but also between substrate storage and utilisation. Some specific details of metabolism in exercise have not yet been covered; this will be done in Chapter 8.

First, imagine that the subject for this 'thought experiment' is sufficiently health-conscious as to eat a mainly carbohydrate breakfast: cereals and semi-skimmed milk, perhaps, but no bacon and eggs. Such a breakfast is likely also to be lower in energy content than a high-fat breakfast.

The disposition of glucose and amino acids will be much as described earlier, although there may be a sharper peak in glucose (and hence insulin) concentration, depending upon the amount and type of carbohydrate eaten. Release of non-esterified fatty acids from adipose tissue will be suppressed, leading to preservation of the adipose tissue triacylglycerol store.

At about an hour after this breakfast, our health-conscious subject sets out for some exercise – nothing strenuous, perhaps a swim or brisk walk for an hour, or even cycling to work. What effects will this have on substrate flow? Clearly the skeletal muscles will require more substrate in order to produce the energy required. For relatively gentle exercise, the mechanisms involved in supplying this are basically those which have already been covered, but they are accompanied by some physiological changes: increased activity of the sympathetic nervous system increases the heart rate and strength of pumping, and blood flow through the exercising muscles increases, delivering more substrate. This in itself leads the exercising muscle to take up more glucose from the plasma. In addition, depending on how strenuous the exercise is, sympathetic nervous activity and increased adrenaline in plasma may gently switch on fat mobilisation in adipose tissue. Thus, the rise in plasma glucose concentration following the meal is diminished (or the decline from the peak concentration is accelerated), and the correspondingly lower glucose concentrations are accompanied by lower insulin concentrations and less conservation of fat stores.

Any suppression of glucagon secretion by the high glucose concentration is somewhat relieved, and glucagon concentrations may rise a little, stimulated also by the sympathetic nervous system (this will be covered in more detail in Chapter 7). The general hormonal tone is changed from one of high insulin/glucagon ratio and intense substrate storage, to one in which substrate storage is lessened and substrate is diverted instead to the working muscle.

It is probably unnecessary to labour the point by following our health-conscious subject much further. Clearly, a low-fat lunch will be superimposed on a much less storage-primed metabolic system. An afternoon walk will divert yet more substrate into oxidation rather than storage. The net result at the end of the day is that less substrate will have been stored, more oxidised. This is not in the least surprising – the *first law of thermodynamics* (the law of '*conservation of energy*') tells us that if more substrate has been oxidised, less can have been stored. But the laws of thermodynamics do not enable us to see how the body achieves this, diverting substrates into different pathways and between tissues to maximise the amount stored when nutrients are available, whilst making energy available for activity as required.

6.6   Summary: metabolic control in a physiological setting

The terms 'somewhat' and 'slightly' were used fairly liberally in the last section. This is deliberate. The hormonal regulation of metabolism is not 'on or off'; it is mostly achieved by subtle, gradual changes. An analogy was used earlier to describe control of the plasma glucose concentration by insulin, likening the glucose concentration to the temperature in a water bath which triggers a thermostat to switch a heater (the insulin concentration) on or off. By now it should be clear that a much better analogy is that of a *proportional control* system. The thermostat is not of the 'either on or off' kind. It regulates the flow of current through the heater depending on the departure of the water temperature from the desired temperature – the 'set-point'. The more the temperature falls below the set-point, the greater the current through the heater. As the temperature rises to the set point, the current diminishes to just that required to balance heat loss. If the temperature rises above the set-point, the current is further reduced in proportion to the amount of rise. Similarly, insulin and other hormones do not change in 'all or none' fashions; their concentrations are regulated in a continuous manner to achieve extremely precise control of energy metabolism.

6.7   Further reading

Glucose, fatty acid and ketone body turnover
Coppack, S.W., Jensen, M.D. & Miles, J.M. (1994) In vivo regulation of lipolysis in humans. *J Lipid Res* 35: 177–193.
Zammit, V.A. (1994) Regulation of ketone body metabolism. A cellular perspective. *Diab Rev* 2: 132–155.
Landau, B.R., Wahren, J., Chandramouli, V., Schumann, W.C., Ekberg, K. & Kalhan, S.C. (1996) Contributions of gluconeogenesis to glucose production in the fasted state. *J Clin Invest* 98: 378–385.
Hellerstein, M.K., Schwarz, J.-M. & Neese, R.A. (1996) Regulation of hepatic de novo lipogenesis in humans. *Annu Rev Nutr* 16: 523–557.

Chandramouli, V., Ekberg, K., Schumann, W.C., Kalhan, S.C., Wahren, J. & Landau, B.R. (1997) Quantifying gluconeogenesis during fasting. *Am J Physiol Endocrinol Metab* 273: E1209–E1215.

Zechner, R. (1997) The tissue-specific expression of lipoprotein lipase; implications for energy and lipoprotein metabolism. *Curr Opin Lipidol* 8: 77–88.

Zierler, K. (1999) Whole body glucose metabolism. *Am J Physiol* 276: E409–E426.

Landau, B.R. (2001) Methods for measuring glycogen cycling. *Am J Physiol Endocrinol Metab* 281: E413–E419. *In the text, I have suggested that when liver glycogen synthesis is stimulated, glycogen breakdown is inhibited and vice versa. This is certainly true, but it may not be complete: there is now substantial evidence for a degree of 'glycogen cycling' whereby there is continuous breakdown and resynthesis of liver glycogen. In this very technical review, Landau discusses the evidence that this is true. (His conclusion is that we do not know for certain in normal individuals with relatively normal glycogen levels.)*

Protein and amino acid metabolism

Krebs, H.A. (1972) Some aspects of the regulation of fuel supply in omnivorous animals. *Adv Enz Reg* 10: 397–420. *This paper by Hans Krebs is old but not out-of-date: it indicates clearly how a physiological problem (why the body tends to oxidise excess dietary protein) can be analysed by the application of biochemical knowledge (mainly the kinetic characteristics of the enzymes involved).*

Jackson, A.A. (1989) Optimizing amino acid and protein supply and utilization in the newborn. *Proc Nutr Soc* 48: 293–301.

Yeaman, S.J. (1989) The 2-oxo acid dehydrogenase complexes: recent advances. *Biochem J* 257: 625–632.

Sugden, P.H. & Fuller, S.J. (1991) Regulation of protein turnover in skeletal and cardiac muscle. *Biochem J* 273: 21–37.

Patel, M.S. & Harris, R.A. (1995) Mammalian α-keto acid dehydrogenase complexes: gene regulation and genetic defects. *FASEB J* 9: 1164–1172.

Reeds, P.J. (2000) Dispensable and indispensable amino acids for humans. *J Nutr* 130: 1835S–1840S.

Navegantes, L.C.C., Migliorini, R.H. & Kettelhut, I.C. (2002) Adrenergic control of protein metabolism in skeletal muscle. *Curr Opin Clin Nutr Metab Care* 5: 281–286.

Glutamine metabolism

Calder, P.C. (1994) Glutamine and the immune system. *Clin Nutr* 13: 2–8.

Curthoys, N.P. & Watford, M. (1995) Regulation of glutaminase activity and glutamine metabolism. *Annu Rev Nutr* 15: 133–159.

Hall, J.C., Heel, K. & McCauley, R. (1996) Glutamine. *Br J Surg* 83: 305–312.

Integration of metabolism in the fasting and fed states
Frayn, K.N. (1997) Integration of substrate flow in vivo: some insights into metabolic control. *Clin Nutr* 16: 277–282.
Frühbeck, G. & Salvador, J. (2000) Relation between leptin and the regulation of glucose metabolism. *Diabetologia* 43: 3–12.
Kelley, D.E. & Mandarino, L.J. (2000) Fuel selection in human skeletal muscle in insulin resistance: a reexamination. *Diabetes* 49: 677–683.
McGarry, J.D. (2002) Banting lecture 2001: dysregulation of fatty acid metabolism in the etiology of type 2 diabetes. *Diabetes* 51: 7–18. *Both these papers (Kelley & Mandarino 2000 and McGarry 2002) discuss how disturbances of normal metabolic regulation may lead to the condition of insulin resistance and hence diabetes. The paper by McGarry was sadly published after his untimely death. (See also Section 4.1.2.2 for a note on one of his many contributions to metabolism.)*

Notes

1   A twenty-first amino acid for which there is a transfer-RNA molecule has recently been recognised: selenocysteine. This is not a common constituent of proteins, however.
2   This disease was first described by Harvey Cushing, an American neurosurgeon, in 1932. He linked it to tumours of the pituitary gland. We now understand that these tumours may secrete excessive amounts of ACTH, leading to increased cortisol production. This is true Cushing's disease. Over-activity of the adrenal cortex for any reason produces similar changes, and the term Cushing's syndrome is used to cover the clinical effects without implying a cause.

7

The Nervous System and Metabolism

7.1 Outline of the nervous system as it relates to metabolism

7.1.1 The nerve cell

Nerve cells, also known as *neurons*, have a number of distinctive properties. They may be very long and thin (spinal cord to toe length, for instance). They are very long-lived (in many cases the lifetime of an individual) but cannot divide by mitosis; hence, if a nerve cell is destroyed, it cannot be replaced by cell division. They have a very high rate of metabolism, requiring glucose and oxygen to support this, and if deprived of oxygen for more than a few minutes will die.

All nerve cells have a *cell body*, an enlarged part in which are found the nucleus and all the biosynthetic apparatus of the cell (including rough endoplasmic reticulum), from which extend various projections. The *dendrites* are multiply branched extensions from the cell body, involved in receiving information from the environment and other nerve cells. The *axon* is a long, slender, usually unbranched projection, extending from the cell body to the point where the nerve cell will exert its effects. At the distal end (far end) the axon may branch, extending several 'feet' to the target tissue or organ (Fig. 7.1).

At the end of each 'foot' of the axon, contact is made with another neuron or with another type of cell through the structure known as a *synapse*. The synapse is formed by a swelling on the end of the axon facing, across a small space known as the *synaptic cleft*, a specialised receptor area on the cell which will receive the signal. There are two sorts of synapses. *Electrical synapses* occur between two neurons; ion channels effectively connect the cytoplasm of the two cells, and the electrical signal being transmitted along

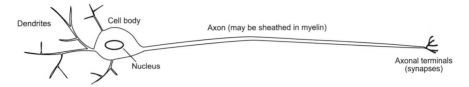

Fig. 7.1 **Basic structure of a nerve cell** *(neuron).*

one continues almost without interruption along the next. However, more relevant from the point of view of regulation of metabolism are the *chemical synapses.* At a chemical synapse, vesicles containing a *neurotransmitter substance* are stored within the swelling at the end of the axon. There are a great many neurotransmitters used by different neurons, but of particular relevance to us will be acetylcholine and noradrenaline (Fig. 7.2). When an electrical impulse arrives, the neurotransmitter substance is released into the synaptic cleft, and acts on receptors on the target cell. The nature of a nerve impulse, and the events occurring at a synapse, are discussed in Boxes 7.1 and 7.2.

A synapse may be with another neuron. Alternatively, it may be with a muscle cell, in which case it is called a *neuromuscular junction,* or with an endocrine cell, in which case it is sometimes known as a *neuroglandular junction.* The neuromuscular junction is a specialised structure, activation of which leads to muscle contraction. It will be considered in more detail later (Section 7.2.2.3).

When we speak of *a nerve* in the anatomical sense, that refers to a specialised structure containing a number of axons and associated supporting cells, together with fine blood vessels.

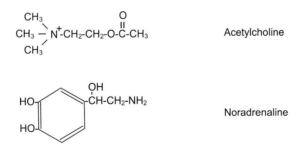

Fig. 7.2 **The structures of two important neurotransmitters, *acetylcholine* (neurotransmitter in the parasympathetic nervous system, parts of the sympathetic nervous system and in the somatic nervous system responsible for activating muscle contraction), and *noradrenaline* (neurotransmitter in the peripheral parts of the sympathetic nervous system).** The route of synthesis of noradrenaline was given in Fig. 5.10.

Box 7.1   The membrane potential and nerve impulses

An axon is a prolongation of a cell (see Fig. 7.1). As in all cells, the cytoplasmic
K^+ concentration (about 150 mmol/l) is considerably greater than that outside
(in the interstitial fluid and plasma – about 5 mmol/l). The nerve cell membrane is selectively permeable to K^+ ions, which therefore diffuse out (through
specific K^+ channels) down their concentration gradient. They take with them
positive charge – leaving the interior of the cell with a negative charge relative
to the outside. This is known as the *resting membrane potential.* It can be measured with a voltmeter in a large nerve, and is about – 70 mV. (The negative
sign is conventional, implying that the inside is negatively charged with respect
to the outside.) Na^+ ions have the opposite distribution: they are present at
higher concentration outside (about 150 mmol/l) than inside (about 15 mmol/
l). However, the membrane is less permeable to Na^+ ions than to K^+ ions, so the
potential difference is maintained. In addition, nerve cell membranes contain
the Na^+-K^+-ATPase which pumps out 3 Na^+ ions in exchange for 2 K^+ ions
from outside (and uses ATP for this). This further maintains the resting energy
potential (since there is a net outward movement of positive charge). This is
illustrated in the top panel of Fig. 7.1.1.

   The above is true for most cells. However, nerve cells and skeletal muscle
cells have the characteristic of *excitable membranes* (Fig. 7.1.1, lower panel).
They possess proteins in the membrane which are *voltage-gated sodium channels*: they have pores which can be opened to allow Na^+ ions to pass through,

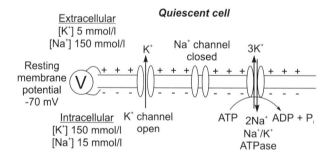

Quiescent cell

Extracellular
[K⁺] 5 mmol/l
[Na⁺] 150 mmol/l

Resting membrane potential -70 mV

K^+ channel open

Na⁺ channel closed

Intracellular
[K⁺] 150 mmol/l
[Na⁺] 15 mmol/l

ATP   2Na⁺   ADP + P_i
Na⁺/K⁺ ATPase
3K⁺

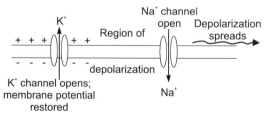

Passage of an action potential

Na⁺ channel open   Depolarization spreads

Region of depolarization

K⁺ channel opens; membrane potential restored

Na⁺

Fig. 7.1.1

but these pores are normally closed by the negative membrane potential. An *action potential* is started by depolarisation of the membrane (the negative membrane potential is lost) in a specific area. This allows the opening of voltage-gated sodium channels in adjacent parts of the membrane, so that Na^+ ions can flow in (down their concentration gradient), thus depolarising yet more of the membrane. Thus, this depolarisation spreads like a wave (the *nerve impulse*) along the length of the axon. It passes any one point very rapidly: as sodium ions flow in and the local membrane potential falls to zero (or becomes positive) the entry of further sodium ions is restricted. In addition, voltage-gated K^+ channels open a short time after the voltage-gated Na^+ channels, allowing potassium ions to leak out again. The normal resting membrane potential is therefore re-established after about 2 msec.

7.1.2   The wiring diagram

There are a great many neurons in the body, performing a wide variety of functions, although the nervous system as a whole is highly integrated, and also interacts with many other bodily systems. However, the nervous system can be subdivided in certain ways according to the general function of different groups of neurons.

The term *central nervous system* (CNS) refers to the brain and spinal cord. The *peripheral nervous system* refers to other parts of the nervous system, mainly nerves running to and from the spinal cord (*spinal nerves*) and to and from the brain (*cranial nerves*). This is a structural definition. There is also a functional classification, listed below:

(1) The *autonomic nervous system*, a system of nerves carrying impulses from the CNS to other organs and tissues. This part of the nervous system cannot be controlled voluntarily – it seems to be autonomous, and hence its name. (It is sometimes referred to as the *involuntary nervous system*.) It controls such functions as heart rate, some aspects of digestive function, and some aspects of hormone secretion and of metabolism. The autonomic nervous system can be subdivided into:
   - the *sympathetic nervous system*, which acts as though 'sympathetic' to the body's needs; it speeds up the heart when we are excited or exercising, for instance. This appears to be counteracted by:
   - the *parasympathetic nervous system* – which appears in many ways to counter the sympathetic system; for instance, it slows the heart.
(2) The *somatic nervous system* is the system of nerves which runs from the CNS to the skeletal muscles, causing them to contract. It is sometimes called the *voluntary nervous system* since we can activate specific parts of it voluntarily (e.g. lift a hand to scratch our nose).
(3) The *afferent nervous system* refers to those nerves which bring signals

Box 7.2   Synaptic transmission

A *synapse* is where an axon makes contact with another cell. When an action potential (see Box 7.1) reaches the *synaptic terminal* (or axonal terminal), it leads to opening of *voltage-gated calcium channels*, which allow extracellular Ca^{2+} ions to enter the cell; these lead (as in other secretory cells) to exocytosis of the secretory vesicles containing the neurotransmitter. Exocytosis involves the granules – each of which is surrounded by a phospholipid membrane – fusing with the synaptic membrane and discharging their contents into the space outside, the *synaptic cleft*.

The neurotransmitter molecules can then diffuse across the narrow gap of the synaptic cleft, and bind to specific receptors on the target cell membrane. Events then depend upon the nature of the target cell. It may be another neuron, in which case binding of the neurotransmitter will open ion channels and begin the passage of an action potential along the new neuron. If it is a skeletal muscle cell, the result will be increased permeability to Na^+ ions, depolarisation spreading across the membrane and the opening of Ca^{2+} channels which allow Ca^{2+} ions to enter the intracellular space; it is these calcium ions which trigger muscle contraction. On the other hand, the target cell may not be another excitable cell. If the neurotransmitter is noradrenaline, the target cell may have β-adrenergic receptors; binding of noradrenaline to these will activate (through the G-protein system) adenylyl cyclase and raise the cellular level of cAMP.

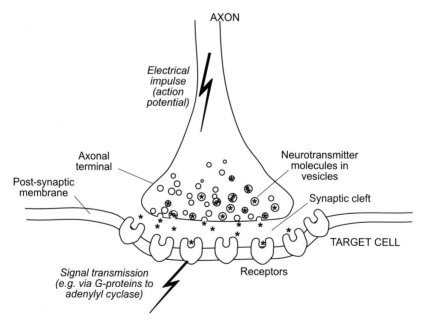

Fig. 7.2.1

from tissues and organs back to the CNS. This includes, for instance, pain receptors, chemoreceptors monitoring the pH of the blood, and receptors monitoring the presence of digestion products in the intestinal tract; we have met some examples of these under the consideration of digestion (Chapter 3).

(4) A fourth component of the nervous system is recognised, the *enteric nervous system*, regulating gastrointestinal function. This is closely connected with both the sympathetic and the parasympathetic nervous systems, but also functions to some extent autonomously, with local 'circuits' so that one part of the intestinal tract can regulate the function of another without the involvement of the CNS. It is highly complex, and will not be considered further here.

7.2   Basic physiology of the nervous system

The operation of the nervous system is highly integrated: there are interconnections between neurons so that one affects the functioning of another (in either an *excitatory* or *inhibitory* way), local 'feedback loops' and other interactions. In a simple way we can look on it as follows. The brain is the controlling centre, and for the most part nervous signals travel either towards the brain (*afferent signals*) or outwards from the brain (*efferent signals*). The brain is the great integrating centre. It receives signals from receptors all over the body: *mechanical* – pressure, stretch, etc.; *chemical* – pH, presence of food in the intestine etc.; *'noxious'* – pain, damage; *special senses* – vision, hearing, smell, etc.). It then collates and integrates them, and sends out signals via the autonomic and somatic branches of the nervous system to regulate bodily function appropriately. The nature of the afferent (incoming) nervous system is largely outside the scope of this book, although we have seen some examples, and will see more, of its relevance to metabolic regulation. We begin with a look at the organisation of the brain.

7.2.1   The brain

The brain is composed of a great many cell types, organised in a highly structured manner. It has a high rate of blood, and therefore nutrient, supply (Section 4.2). Amongst the many cell types found in the brain, neurons themselves are outnumbered approximately nine times by other cells, generally referred to as *glial* cells (from the Greek for glue). These glial cells perform many functions of mechanical support and electrical 'insulation', protection against infection and repair of damage. The most abundant type, the *astrocytes* (so-called because of their star shape, with multiple radiating projections), probably act as intermediaries between the capillaries and the neurons, regulating the supply of nutrients and also the extracellular ionic environment. In recent years it has been realised that glial cells can themselves transmit signals, in the form

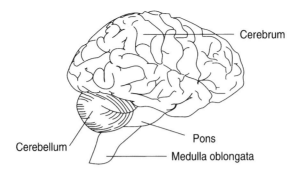

Fig. 7.3 The human brain and its main components.

of calcium waves that pass between glial cells and can also communicate with neurons. It is not yet understood what part glial cells may play in information processing within the CNS.

The brain contains both complete neurons, and the cell bodies of neurons that extend into the spinal cord and beyond. It is organised into a number of relatively discrete structural parts (Fig. 7.3). The two *cerebral hemispheres* are the most prominent part. In fact they are roughly quarter spheres, together making up about one hemisphere, but the terminology is unlikely to change. The outer layer, a few mm thick, contains many cell bodies and is referred to as *grey matter* because of its appearance when fixed with alcohol for microscopy. It forms the *cerebral cortex* and is responsible for many higher functions: receipt of information from the special senses, and motor control (control of muscles). The cerebral cortex, although only 2–4 mm thick, occupies a surprisingly large proportion of brain volume (around 40%) because of the many convolutions of the brain surface, and hence large surface area. Underlying the cortex is the *cerebral white matter* (again from its appearance when fixed with alcohol), largely composed of myelinated fibres grouped into large bundles, responsible for transmission within the brain. Amongst the white matter are found a number of local regions of grey matter, known as *nuclei*, where there are further groups of cell bodies. These nuclei have names and their functions are becoming clear, but more detailed description is beyond the scope of this book. Within the cerebral hemispheres is the central core of the brain, the *diencephalon*, a structure itself composed of three parts – the *thalamus*, underneath which is the *hypothalamus* with the *epithalamus* behind.

7.2.1.1 The hypothalamus

The hypothalamus is the region of the brain of most interest with respect to metabolic regulation. It is an integrating centre: it receives information and also sends it out. It receives information from other brain areas, but in addition the hypothalamus itself contains important sensors. It monitors the concentration of glucose in the blood, and initiates appropriate responses to maintain this close to a constant level of around 4–5 mmol/l. (This includes both autonomic responses, e.g. initiation of glycogen breakdown in response to a fall in blood glucose concentration, and regulation of dietary intake by control of appetite.) The hypothalamus also senses fluid balance by monitoring the osmolarity of the blood, and initiates appropriate measures to maintain an optimal level (both via regulation of thirst, and control of water excretion by the kidneys). It has a temperature-sensitive region, monitoring the temperature of blood flowing through it, and responding as appropriate to maintain the required body temperature. This includes elevation of the body temperature when this is seen as appropriate during infection.

The hypothalamus controls drives such as thirst and appetite by signalling to other brain areas. It regulates other bodily functions in two main ways. It is responsible for most of the output of the sympathetic nervous system. Signals from the hypothalamus are transmitted via other brain centres to the sympathetic tracts within the spinal cord, and thus to tissues and organs within the body. It also regulates the secretion of hormones by the pituitary gland. Connections between the hypothalamus and pituitary were discussed in Section 5.3. Thus, the hypothalamus is a very important part of the brain in terms of the role of the nervous system in metabolic regulation. The term *neuroendocrine system* is often used to describe the combination of nervous and hormonal systems of regulation, and the hypothalamus is at the centre of this combination.

7.2.1.2   The cerebellum and brainstem

Other parts of the brain act as further regulatory centres, and as 'relay stations'. The *cerebellum* has important functions in coordinating movement; disorders of cerebellar function can lead to uncoordinated movements, trembling, etc. The *brainstem* is the connection between higher centres of the brain and the spinal cord. In some ways it is analogous to a primitive brain, and regulates very basic functions such as heart rate, breathing and blood pressure in a 'pre-programmed', automatic manner. Thus, if the spinal cord is severed from the brainstem, these vital functions cease. On the other hand, if the brainstem remains intact after severe injury to other parts of the brain, the victim can enter a state of primitive existence in which consciousness is absent but life can be maintained so long as food is provided – the state sometimes called 'vegetative existence'.

7.2.2   The autonomic nervous system

7.2.2.1   The sympathetic nervous system

The nerves of the sympathetic nervous system are carried in the spinal cord in discrete bundles known as the *sympathetic trunks*. There are synapses between neurons arranged 'in series' (one follows another), and the cell bodies of the neurons which eventually emerge from the spine are located in the thoracic and lumbar regions of the spine (the back of the chest and the lower back). Their axons emerge from between vertebrae and reach out towards other parts of the body. At this stage the sympathetic nerves mostly make chemical synapses with other cells, using the neurotransmitter acetylcholine (Fig. 7.2). Only one branch of the sympathetic nervous system reaches its target tissue directly: that controlling the *adrenal medulla* (discussed in Section 5.5.2). Thus, the nerves regulating the adrenal medulla liberate acetylcholine to cause it, in turn, to release the hormone *adrenaline* into the blood. However, most branches of the sympathetic nervous system emerge from the spinal cord and then meet groups of cell bodies, located near the spine, called *sympathetic ganglia* (each one is called a *ganglion*). The ganglia are relay stations. The terminals of the sympathetic nerves synapse with new neurons. The fibres emerging from the spinal cord, the *preganglionic fibres*, liberate acetylcholine, and this excites the new fibres to transmit impulses. However, the neurotransmitter used by these new fibres, the *postganglionic fibres*, is not (for the most part) acetylcholine but *noradrenaline* (Fig. 7.2). Noradrenaline is usually regarded as the characteristic neurotransmitter of the sympathetic nervous system, although you will see that this only applies to transmission of signals to the target tissues. As we already know, noradrenaline can interact with receptors on other tissues, and these receptors are broadly classified as α- or β-adrenergic receptors (see Section 5.5.2).

There are some exceptions to this rule. For instance, the sympathetic nervous system controls sweat secretion via *cholinergic* fibres (i.e. using acetylcholine as their transmitter). In addition, the sympathetic nervous system has cholinergic fibres that innervate the blood vessels in skeletal muscle in order to cause relaxation of the vessels. The significance of this will be considered in more detail later (Section 8.4.5). But most aspects of metabolism that it controls involve *adrenergic* impulses (i.e. liberation of noradrenaline).

7.2.2.2   The parasympathetic nervous system

The parasympathetic nerves do not, for the most part, run in the spinal cord. Those fibres regulating functions in the head and face – e.g. salivary secretion, contraction of the pupils of the eyes – are cranial nerves. The most important branch of the parasympathetic nervous system from the point of view of metabolic regulation is a large nerve called the *vagus nerve* (from the Latin *vagus* for wandering, since it 'wanders' around the body). The vagus is also a cranial nerve; that is, it emerges directly from the brain and a branch runs down the neck close to the carotid artery. It divides and its branches run to various organs, particularly the heart and stomach, other parts of the digestive tract and the pancreas. (We saw the importance of parasympathetic regulation of the production of saliva and gastric secretions in Chapter 3.)

The neurotransmitter of the parasympathetic nervous system is acetylcholine. Thus, blockers of cholinergic transmission block its effects. One of the classic blockers is the substance *atropine* found in the deadly nightshade plant, *Atropa belladonna*. We saw in Chapter 3 that the parasympathetic nervous system stimulates the flow of saliva, and one of the effects of low doses of atropine is a dry mouth. The parasympathetic nerves usually contract the muscles controlling the size of the pupil of the eye; when this action is inhibited, the pupil dilates and becomes unresponsive to light. Eye-drops containing extracts of deadly nightshade were used by the Greeks and Romans to produce 'beautiful ladies' – hence the name *belladonna* for the plant. Larger doses of atropine block the normal restraining effect of the parasympathetic system on the heart rate; hence the heart speeds up.

7.2.2.3   The somatic nervous system

The nerves of the somatic nervous system (except those supplying the muscles of the head, neck and face) run down the spinal cord, and emerge again between the vertebrae. They do not form further synapses, but run directly to the muscles that they stimulate. Their neurotransmitter is acetylcholine. The nerve terminals meet the muscle cells at the specialised structures known as neuromuscular junctions (Fig. 7.4). Here, acetylcholine is released when the nerve is activated. The flattened, branching end of the axon is known as the *end-plate*; it makes contact with a receptive area on the muscle cell membrane (the sarcolemma) called the *sole-plate*. We will look in more detail at the effects of activation of the motor neurons supplying skeletal muscle in Section 8.4.3.

7.2.3   Neurotransmitters and receptors

There are an enormous number of neurotransmitters, including amino acids and derivatives, amines, peptides and acetylcholine. Much of the diversity of transmitters occurs within the CNS, and also within the enteric nervous system. With regard to metabolic regulation, we will be considering mainly adrenergic and cholinergic transmission.

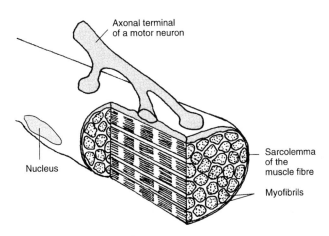

Fig. 7.4 The neuromuscular junction.

7.2.3.1   Adrenergic transmission

The pathway for synthesis of noradrenaline and adrenaline was shown in Fig. 5.10. Dopamine (the biosynthetic precursor of noradrenaline) is also a neurotransmitter in the CNS. The sympathetic nerve terminals release noradrenaline, although a small amount of dopamine (present in the secretory vesicles) is co-secreted. The adrenal medulla is, in effect, a modification of a postganglionic neuron – it is, as we have seen, stimulated by a (cholinergic) preganglionic fibre, and has evolved to secrete the hormone adrenaline into the bloodstream rather than noradrenaline into a synaptic cleft. Note from Fig. 5.10 that adrenaline is one biosynthetic step beyond noradrenaline.

Adrenaline and noradrenaline, which are similar in structure, act through the same receptors, in a molecular sense. It is probable, however, that some receptors (for instance, those on the receiving side of a synaptic cleft) will only 'see' noradrenaline, whereas others more exposed to the circulation will respond to adrenaline carried in the blood. After noradrenaline has been liberated into the synaptic cleft, it is rapidly taken up again, both back into the synaptic terminal (for recycling) and into other tissues. However, a proportion 'escapes' re-uptake and enters the extracellular fluid, and thence the plasma. The concentration of noradrenaline in the plasma is, in fact, usually higher than that of adrenaline, although it is only there through this 'spillover' effect. The concentration of noradrenaline in plasma gives an indication of the overall activity of the sympathetic nervous system in the body. (This concept can even be refined. It is possible to show release of noradrenaline from the muscle of the forearm, for instance, by measurement of the concentrations in the artery supplying, and in a vein draining this muscle. It has been shown that noradrenaline release correlates with the activity of the sympathetic nerves supplying this muscle, measured by micro-electrodes applied to the nerves.)

The two broad subtypes of adrenergic receptors, known as α and β, and the subdivisions of these receptors, were discussed in connection with adrenaline action in Section 5.5.2 and Table 5.1.

7.2.3.2   Cholinergic transmission

Acetylcholine (Fig. 7.2) is synthesised from acetyl-CoA and choline. After its release from cholinergic nerve endings, acetylcholine is rapidly degraded (into choline and acetate) by the enzyme *acetylcholinesterase*, which is present on the postsynaptic membrane. The choline is taken up again by the nerve terminal for synthesis of more acetylcholine. A large group of pesticides, the *organophosphorus esters*, act by binding to the enzyme acetylcholinesterase, and thus causing excessive accumulation of acetylcholine. They are, of course, toxic to humans by exactly the same mechanism, and lead to muscle paralysis, with death eventually from respiratory paralysis. The effects can be reversed to some extent with atropine.

Recognition that there are two main types of cholinergic receptors was one of the early triumphs of experimental pharmacology. Dale in 1914

showed that there were some actions of acetylcholine which could be mimicked by administration of *muscarine*, the active component of the poisonous
mushroom *Amanita muscaria*; these effects were abolished by small doses of
atropine. They correspond roughly to the effects of the parasympathetic nervous system. Other effects of acetylcholine were still apparent after blockade
with muscarine, and these were similar to the effects of *nicotine* (the active
component of tobacco). The effects produced by nicotine included stimulation
of the contraction of skeletal muscle, and the release of adrenaline from the
adrenal medulla. We now recognise that these effects are mediated through
two specific types of acetylcholine receptor, the *muscarinic receptor* and the
nicotinic receptor. Both nicotinic and muscarinic receptors have since been
further subdivided on the basis of cloning of homologous receptor proteins.
Cholinergic synapses within the central nervous system are nicotinic; outside
the central nervous system they are mostly muscarinic at target organs, unless
they are preganglionic fibres.

The function of the two types of receptor, together with noradrenaline, in
the central and peripheral nervous systems is illustrated in Fig. 7.5.

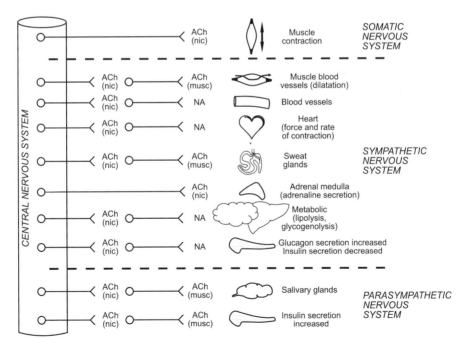

Fig. 7.5 Types of neurotransmission in the central and peripheral nervous systems.
ACh, cholinergic transmission; nic, nicotinic receptor; musc, muscarinic receptor; NA, noradrenaline. Based loosely on Rang & Dale (1991).

7.3   Major effects of adrenergic stimulation

7.3.1   Stimuli for activation of the sympathetic nervous system and adrenal medulla

The sympathetic nervous system affects many bodily functions. It would clearly be a very inefficient means of control if the whole system had to be activated at once, and this is not so: particular branches of the sympathetic nervous system are activated specifically under different conditions. This could make a complete description of sympathetic activation very complex, but for the most part it is still reasonable to think of the general effects of the whole system. Not only does the whole of the sympathetic nervous system *tend* to respond as one, but also the secretion of adrenaline from the adrenal medulla (which is effectively another extension of the sympathetic nervous system) *tends* to occur under the same conditions. This makes some generalisations possible.

The activity of the sympathetic nervous system is constantly changing, and is, in fact, changing in specific branches, regulating physiological functions such as heart rate and blood pressure; but overall (as reflected by the concentration of noradrenaline in the plasma) it is relatively constant during normal daily life. The secretion of adrenaline, similarly, is relatively constant during everyday life. When a 'stress' hits the system, on the other hand, the adrenal medulla springs into action, and there is a more general activation of the sympathetic nervous system.

The stimuli for activation of the sympathetic nervous system are generally those of '*stress*' in the most general sense. This was first clearly described by the American physiologist Walter B. Cannon, whose book *Bodily changes in pain, hunger, fear and rage*, published in 1915, summarised the role of adrenaline and of the sympathetic nervous system in stress states.

For instance, the effects of the sympathetic nervous system on the circulatory system (heart and blood vessels) are brought into play by a fall in blood pressure. This may happen quite often. Think for a moment of the hydrostatic pressure of a column of blood about 2 metres high. Then contemplate the fact that when you get out of bed and stand up, the pressure of blood available to perfuse your brain is going to drop rapidly and dramatically. This is an immediate stimulus to the sympathetic nervous system to maintain blood pressure, which it does, as we shall see in more detail below, by effects both on the heart and the blood vessels. Most people are familiar with a feeling of faintness on standing up too quickly, particularly on a hot day when blood volume may be depleted by sweating. The brain receives the information that blood pressure is beginning to fall from receptors in the great vessels, collates this in the hypothalamus and causes the appropriate responses to be set in motion.

Another type of stress is that of exercise. Even gentle exercise (running for the bus, for instance) requires both circulatory and metabolic adjustments. More substrate needs to be made available for energy production, and blood flow and oxygen delivery need to be increased. The only component over which we have voluntary control is the decision to cause our muscles to contract in a particular way. The necessary adjustments that follow are looked after by the sympathetic nervous system, triggered by changes in the circulation. For example, diversion of the blood to the muscles, brought about by local metabolic changes, will tend to cause a fall in blood pressure: the sympathetic nervous system will counteract this. Similarly, increasing acidity of the blood, caused by lactic acid production, will trigger an increased depth of breathing via *chemoreceptors* and activation of the sympathetic nervous system.

A more severe stress, rarely met in everyday life but commonly studied in laboratories (because it is a reproducible test of responses to stress, unlike, for instance, trying to frighten someone!), is a rapid lowering of the concentration of glucose in the blood to produce the state of *hypoglycaemia*. Experimentally this is brought about by an injection of insulin. Outside the laboratory it can occur in certain metabolic diseases in which gluconeogenesis or glycogenolysis are impaired, or in people with diabetes who have injected too much insulin. Glucose receptors in the hypothalamus relay the information, and there is activation both of the sympathetic nervous system generally and of adrenaline secretion from the adrenal medulla (Fig. 7.6). We will see shortly how these responses act to restore a normal glucose concentration.

Note that I have emphasised a *rapid* lowering of glucose concentration. The slow, gentle fall that occurs during early starvation (e.g. fasting overnight) is probably not a stimulus for the sympathetic nervous system. The direct role of the sympathetic nervous system and of adrenaline in metabolic regulation is most important in acute stress situations rather than normal everyday fluctuations. On the other hand, it was stated above that the sympathetic nervous system is active continuously, maintaining bodily functions such as blood pressure; these *specific* actions of the sympathetic nervous system do, of course, also affect metabolism indirectly; if blood flow to the brain is reduced, it cannot metabolise at a normal rate.

More dramatic stress states such as physical injury or severe infection are very potent stimuli for activation of the sympathetic nervous system and of adrenaline secretion from the adrenal medulla. The stimuli reaching the brain are multiple. The special senses may alert the brain to danger (you may see a bus about to hit you, for example). Loss of blood reduces the circulating blood volume; this is sensed through pressure receptors and is a particularly potent stimulus for adrenaline secretion. Lack of blood volume leads to impaired oxygen delivery and hence anaerobic glycolysis; the resulting acidity in the blood is detected by chemoreceptors and relayed to the brain. There are also afferent (incoming) impulses arriving in the nerves responding to pain, tissue damage, etc. All these afferent signals are integrated in the hypothalamus, and appropriate activation of the sympathetic nervous system and adrenal medulla is set in train from there. It is probably in such extreme situations that the sympathetic nervous system and adrenal medulla play their most vital roles.

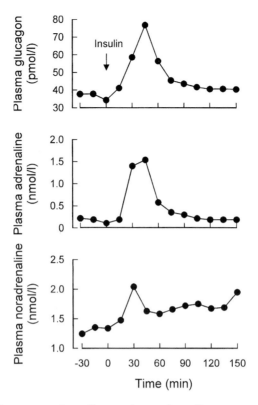

Fig. 7.6 Plasma glucagon, adrenaline and noradrenaline concentrations in re-sponse to rapid lowering of the blood glucose concentration (by injection of in-sulin). Based on Gerich, J., Davis, J., Lorenzi, M. et al. (1979) Hormonal mechanisms of recovery from insulin-induced hypoglycemia in man. *Am J Physiol* 236: E380–E385. With permission of the American Physiological Society.

It should now be appreciated that the sympathetic nervous system can in-fluence metabolism in both direct and indirect ways. The indirect ways include changes in the circulatory system. They also include effects on hormone secre-tion, which we will consider below.

7.3.2   Circulatory effects of adrenergic activation

Activation of β_1 receptors in the heart increases both the force of contraction and the rate of beating; thus, the rate of delivery of blood to the rest of the body (the *cardiac output*) is increased. This is probably an effect of noradrenaline released from sympathetic nerve endings rather than of adrenaline, except at very high adrenaline concentrations (e.g. in severe stress).

In the blood vessels, the *resistance* of particular blood vessels (the diameter of the lumen) is regulated by smooth muscle in the walls. These smooth mus-cles are regulated by the sympathetic nervous system. For the most part, this is achieved through α_1 and α_2 receptors, which bring about contraction of the muscle and *vasoconstriction* (narrowing of the vessels). This has two effects. In the body as a whole, blood pressure will be increased since the heart is pumping blood through narrower channels. In specific organs and tissues, this is a means of selectively increasing or decreasing blood flow under different conditions. In fact, in most tissues there is continuous *vasomotor tone*; the sympathetic fibres are active continuously, under the influence of the *medulla oblongata* in the brainstem (the very primitive part of the brain); variations in flow are brought about by relaxation of this tone, or further constriction.

In skeletal muscle, it was mentioned earlier that the smooth muscle of the blood vessels is innervated by cholinergic sympathetic fibres. Activation of these fibres leads to *vasodilatation* (opening up of the vessels with a consequent increase in blood flow). This is certainly true in some animals although its significance in humans has been questioned. It will be discussed again in connection with the increased skeletal muscle blood flow that is seen during exercise (Section 8.4.5).

7.3.3   Metabolic effects of catecholamines

Adrenaline and noradrenaline are both amines derived from the catechol nucleus, and the term *catecholamines* is often used to cover them both (see Fig. 5.10). It will be appreciated that the catecholamines have indirect effects on metabolism which are mediated through 'physiological' changes – heart rate, blood flow, etc. They also have indirect effects mediated through changes in hormone secretion, as well as direct effects in some tissues.

7.3.3.1   Glycogenolysis

In the liver, the catecholamines stimulate glycogen breakdown (*glycogenolysis*) through β_2 (adenylyl cyclase-linked) receptors and the 'cascade' mechanism discussed earlier (see Box 2.4). In addition, they can activate glycogenolysis through a second mechanism, via the α_1 (phospholipase C-linked) receptors (see Table 5.1) and elevation of the cytoplasmic Ca^{2+} concentration. (This was mentioned in Box 2.4; one particular situation in which elevation of intracellular Ca^{2+} concentration stimulates glycogenolysis will be covered in Section 8.4.3 and Fig. 8.8.) The degradation of glycogen, via glucose 1-phosphate, leads to production of glucose, which can be released into the bloodstream. This is a major response to *hypoglycaemia* (a fall in the blood glucose concentration) and leads to rapid restoration of the glucose concentration provided there is adequate glycogen stored in the liver. There is much experimental evidence that the liver is supplied with sympathetic nerves and that these can activate glycogenolysis directly, although adrenaline from the adrenal medulla is also released under such conditions and will certainly play a role. In humans, it has been very difficult to show directly that the sympathetic nerves are involved, but people whose adrenals have been removed can respond fairly normally to glucose deprivation, implying that at least in that situation the sympathetic nerves to the liver can play a role.

In skeletal muscle, the catecholamines are undoubtedly important for stimulation of glycogenolysis; but they are not in themselves sufficient to activate it. The activation of skeletal muscle glycogen breakdown is intimately linked with the stimulation of muscle contraction, which, as we have seen, is brought about by the cholinergic fibres of the somatic nervous system. (The links between contraction and glycogenolysis will be fully discussed in Chapter 8; see Fig. 8.8.) Glycogenolysis seems to be 'primed' by catecholamines, perhaps released in response to anticipation of the exercise. Circulating adrenaline is likely to be more important in this respect than noradrenaline from sympathetic nerve terminals, since the main (possibly the only) sympathetic supply to muscle is to the smooth muscle of the blood vessels and is responsible for regulation of blood flow.

7.3.3.2 Lipolysis

Human fat cells have both α_2- and β_1-adrenergic receptors. There are also β_3 ('atypical') receptors that are responsible for stimulation of lipolysis in rodent fat cells, although their role in humans is presently unclear.

The α_2 receptors are linked, via inhibitory G_i proteins, to adenylyl cyclase, and reduce its activity. The β_1 receptors are linked to it through G_s proteins and stimulate its activity. Activation of adenylyl cyclase will increase the cellular concentration of cAMP and activate hormone-sensitive lipase (see Box 2.4), bringing about a breakdown of the triacylglycerol stores and the release of non-esterified fatty acids into the plasma.

There is usually a balance between stimulatory and inhibitory effects, and in normal sedentary daily life it is probable that regulation of hormone-sensitive lipase by insulin predominates. However, in response to any kind of stress, including exercise, there is activation of the β_1 receptors so that lipolysis is stimulated. Blockade of the β receptors with the β-antagonist propranolol reduces, or may completely suppress, the liberation of non-esterified fatty acids into the plasma in response to exercise (Fig. 7.7). Activation of hormone-sensitive lipase can be brought about purely by mental stress. Stimulation of lipolysis is an important feature of the response to physical stresses such as surgical operations or injury. Again, it is not certain to what extent the direct innervation of adipose tissue is involved, or whether circulating adrenaline plays the major role. But, as with glycogenolysis, people without adrenals can raise their plasma non-esterified fatty acid concentration in response to lack of glucose, so the sympathetic nerves must play a role in that situation.

Not only is the rate of lipolysis regulated by the nervous system, but also the rate of blood flow through adipose tissue. This can have indirect effects on the release of non-esterified fatty acids. In very severe stress states, typified by physical injury with major blood loss, α-adrenergic effects predominate in the blood vessels of adipose tissue and cause it to constrict. Presumably the body is trying to preserve blood for more vital organs and tissues. This reduces the ability of adipose tissue to liberate fatty acids into the plasma, since the binding

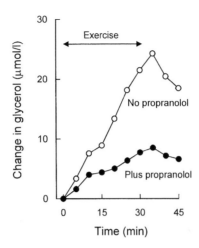

Fig. 7.7 Propranolol (a β-adrenergic blocker) inhibits lipolysis in response to exercise. The figure shows changes in the concentration of glycerol (released in fat mobilisation) in the interstitial fluid in adipose tissue, measured with a small probe. During exercise (0–30 min) the glycerol concentration rises, indicating lipolysis. When propranolol is introduced (via the probe) the rise is inhibited. In separate experiments, when phentolamine (an α-adrenergic blocker) was introduced, glycerol release was not affected. Based on Arner, P., Kriegholm, E., Engfeldt, P. & Bolinder, J. (1990) Adrenergic regulation of lipolysis in situ at rest and during exercise. *J Clin Invest* 85: 893–898. Reproduced with permission.

sites on the albumin become saturated, and fatty acids may accumulate within the tissue. Thus, after moderately severe injuries or during surgical operations, the level of non-esterified fatty acids in the plasma is usually very high, but after very severe injuries the level may be relatively normal. Although there is no doubt that lipolysis is activated, the fatty acids are unable to leave the adipose tissue as rapidly as they are released from triacylglycerol (Table 7.1). The same phenomenon may come into play to some extent during strenuous exercise (see Chapter 8).

7.3.3.3   Glucose utilisation

There is consistent evidence that elevated plasma adrenaline concentrations impair glucose utilisation by skeletal muscle. One plausible mechanism is that adrenaline stimulates glycogenolysis, so there is an accumulation of glucose 6-phosphate, which will inhibit hexokinase and reduce the entry of further glucose into the cell. This might seem odd during exercise, but in that situation other mechanisms operate to stimulate glucose entry, mainly exercise-induced translocation of GLUT4 to the cell membrane. Also, during exercise glycolysis will be rapid and so any build-up of glucose 6-phosphate probably minimised. But we can see that during hypoglycaemia, inhibition of muscle glucose utilisation by adrenaline would spare glucose for use by the brain.

However, there is also evidence for β-adrenergic receptor-stimulation of glucose uptake into muscle. This seems to be mediated by the sympathetic nervous system rather than by circulating adrenaline: effects of hypothalamic

Table 7.1 Plasma glycerol and non-esterified fatty acid (NEFA) concentrations after physical injury.

Measurement	Non-injured (after overnight fast)	Minor injuries	Moderate injuries	Severe injuries
Plasma NEFA (μmol/l)	400	740	910	680
Plasma glycerol (μmol/l)	50	90	110	140
Plasma adrenaline (nmol/l)	0.4	1.0		13
Plasma noradrenaline (nmol/l)	2.1	3.4		13

Minor injuries included, for instance, single arm bone fractures; moderate injuries included single leg bone fractures and combined injuries; severe injuries were life-threatening multiple injuries. All injured patients were studied within 12 h of injury. They were in a variety of nutritional states.

The plasma glycerol concentration may be taken as an indication of the rate of lipolysis: it increases consistently with increasing severity of injury. The plasma non-esterified fatty acid concentration, on the other hand, is not as high as expected after severe injuries (despite very high catecholamine concentrations) because of constriction of the blood flow through adipose tissue. The same phenomenon occurs during strenuous exercise, although not to such a marked extent.

Sources: Frayn (1982; 1986); Coppack *et al.* (1990).

stimulation are still seen if the adrenal medullas are removed, but not if the sympathetic nerve system is deactivated with the compound guanethidine. The physiological significance perhaps again relates to the need to stimulate glucose utilisation during exercise independently of insulin, whose concentration may be reduced (see next section).

7.4   Effects of the autonomic nervous system on hormone secretion

The pancreatic islets have both α- and β-adrenergic receptors, and are innervated by sympathetic nerves. They also receive fibres of the parasympathetic nervous system. These nerves regulate the secretion of both insulin and glucagon, as summarised in Table 7.2. These influences on pancreatic hormone secretion probably operate at the level of 'fine tuning' in normal daily life, and it is not easy to demonstrate their role. In rodents, there is undoubtedly a normal adrenergic restraint on insulin secretion, since the plasma insulin concentration rises if the adrenal medullas are removed. In humans, the effects of adrenergic blocking drugs in the whole body are very difficult to interpret because they cause such widespread changes in both circulation and metabolism. The effects of the parasympathetic innervation of the pancreatic islets are undoubtedly

Table 7.2 Adrenergic and parasympathetic effects on hormone secretion from the pancreas.

Input	Insulin secretion	Glucagon secretion
α-adrenergic	Suppresses (dominant effect)	Suppresses
β-adrenergic	Increases (only seen if α-effects blocked)	Increases
Parasympathetic	Increases	Increases

Sources: Robertson & Porte (1973); Bloom et al. (1974); Humphrey et al. (1975a, b); Brunicardi et al. (1987).

important. They mediate the 'cephalic phase' of insulin secretion in response to the sight or smell of food, mentioned in Chapter 3 (Section 3.2.1). Also, in patients whose vagus nerve is cut at surgery to reduce gastric acid secretion (a former treatment for gastric ulcers), insulin secretion in response to a glucose drink is impaired, as is glucagon secretion in response to hypoglycaemia.

However, the effects of the nervous system (particularly adrenergic influences) on pancreatic hormone secretion become of great importance in 'stress' situations such as strenuous exercise or physical injury. In these situations, there is β-adrenergically mediated stimulation of glucagon secretion, and α-adrenergic suppression of insulin secretion. These mechanisms reinforce the mobilisation of fuel stores (glycogen and triacylglycerol) and, in the case of physical injury, reinforce the resultant hyperglycaemia (elevation of the blood glucose concentration). During strenuous exercise, glucose utilisation by exercising muscle is increased greatly by insulin-independent mechanisms, so these effects may be seen as a means of maximising the availability of energy-providing substrates to the muscles without compromising glucose utilisation. (Metabolism during exercise will be covered in Chapter 8.)

7.5   Summary

The nervous system may affect metabolism in various ways: (1) through direct effects on metabolically active tissues (e.g. stimulation of lipolysis), and also on the digestive system (e.g. stimulation of salivary flow, gastric acid secretion); (2) through stimulation of muscle contraction, which is in turn linked to various metabolic adjustments; (3) through indirect effects mediated by changes in hormone secretion (especially modulation of insulin and glucagon release); and (4) through indirect effects on other bodily systems, particularly the circulatory system (e.g. changes in cardiac output and distribution of blood flow to different organs and tissues).

The indirect effects are operative continuously, maintaining normal operation of the body. The importance of the direct effects of the nervous system on metabolism in everyday life is probably a matter of 'fine tuning', but becomes more apparent in acutely stressful situations such as exercise, mental stress or physical injury. The adrenal medulla works in many ways like an extension of the sympathetic nervous system (which it is), and it is often difficult to distinguish effects of noradrenaline released at sympathetic nerve terminals from those of circulating adrenaline.

Activation of the sympathetic nervous system has a generally catabolic function, whereas the parasympathetic has a more anabolic role, although these generalisations do not hold true for all specific effects.

7.6   Further reading

Catecholamines, their receptors and metabolism

Esler, M., Jennings, G., Lambert, G., Meredith, I., Horne, M. & Eisenhofer, G. (1990) Overflow of catecholamine neurotransmitters to the circulation: source, fate, and functions. *Physiol Rev* 70: 963–985.

Nicoll, R.A., Malenka, R.C. & Kauer, J.A. (1990) Functional comparison of neurotransmitter receptor subtypes in mammalian central nervous system. *Physiol Rev* 70: 513–565.

Flatmark, T. (2000) Catecholamine biosynthesis and physiological regulation in neuroendocrine cells. *Acta Physiol Scand* 168: 1–17.

Nonogaki, K. (2000) New insights into sympathetic regulation of glucose and fat metabolism. *Diabetologia* 43: 533–549.

Hypoglycaemia and the counter-regulatory response

Amiel, S. (1991) Glucose counter-regulation in health and disease: current concepts in hypoglycaemia recognition and response. *Q J Med* 80: 707–727.

Cryer, P.E. (1993) Glucose counterregulation: prevention and correction of hypoglycemia in humans. *Am J Physiol* 264: E149–E155.

Regulation of pancreatic hormone secretion

Ahrén, B. (2000) Autonomic regulation of islet hormone secretion – implications for health and disease. *Diabetologia* 43: 393–410.

Other aspects

Kunze, W.A. & Furness, J.B. (1999) The enteric nervous system and regulation of intestinal motility. *Annu Rev Physiol* 61: 117–142.

Morrison, S.F. (2001) Differential control of sympathetic outflow. *Am J Physiol Regul Integr Comp Physiol* 281: R683–R698.

8

Coping With Some Extreme Situations

8.1 Situations in which the body needs to call on its fuel stores

So far, we have looked mainly at how the body stores nutrients when they are in excess, and releases them when required during a normal daily cycle. At the end of each day the body's fuel stores end up in more or less the same state as they started. Much of this regulation is achieved through the levels of substrates in the plasma (e.g. the plasma glucose concentration rising as carbohydrate is absorbed from the intestine), and modulation of the secretion of the pancreatic hormones, insulin and glucagon.

However, there are a number of situations in which the body needs to mobilise the fuels from its stores more rapidly, or to a greater extent. These situations include *exercise*, when the requirement for energy is suddenly increased, and *starvation*, when continued existence depends upon the use of stored fuels. This chapter will contrast the means by which fuel mobilisation is brought about in these two states. In starvation, the mechanisms seem to be largely extensions of the normal daily pattern, and are mediated through gradual changes in plasma substrate and hormone concentrations. In contrast, in the more sudden situation of exercise, more vigorous changes in metabolic regulation take place, and the role of the nervous system, particularly the sympathetic, comes into prominence. There are other situations in which body fuels are mobilised rapidly; these are various *stress states*, such as mental stress (for instance, fear or sitting an examination) and – more extreme – physical injury or severe infection. In these states, the role of the sympathetic nervous system and adrenal medulla may become dominant.

We will begin with a discussion of the body's fuel stores.

8.2   The body's fuel stores

8.2.1   Carbohydrate

The amount of free glucose in the circulation and extracellular fluid is small, as we saw in Section 6.1 – typically about 12 g. If we were able to use all of this without replenishing it, it would support the metabolism of the brain for about 2 hours. Clearly, this is not adequate even to keep us alive overnight, and hence we have stores of carbohydrate. We looked in Chapter 1 (Section 1.2.1.2) at the osmotic problems that would arise if free glucose were stored in cells, and hence humans store carbohydrate in polymeric form, as glycogen. Only two tissues, skeletal muscle and liver, have stores of glycogen which are significant in relation to the needs of the whole body, although most tissues have a small store for 'local' use. Approximately 40% of the human body is accounted for by skeletal muscle – say 25 kg on average. A typical concentration of glycogen in skeletal muscle is around 15 g/kg wet weight – i.e. each kg of muscle in its normal, hydrated state contains *around* 15 g of glycogen; thus the total muscle glycogen store is around 350–400 g.[1] This is not, of course, available directly as glucose to enter the circulation since muscle lacks glucose-6-phosphatase, although it can be exported to the liver as lactate, pyruvate and/or alanine as we saw in Chapter 6 (Fig. 6.20) for formation of glucose. On the other hand, the liver glycogen store is more directly available in the form of glucose, and undoubtedly plays the major role of a 'buffer' for changing hour-to-hour requirements. A typical liver glycogen concentration is about 50–80 g/kg wet weight, and varies during the day. The liver weighs around 1–1.5 kg, so the total liver glycogen store is around 50–120 g. You will see immediately that this is not far from '24-hours' worth' for the brain. Thus, our carbohydrate stores are sufficient to enable us to ride out periods of a day or so without food.

8.2.2   Fat

Our fat stores are usually larger by one to two orders of magnitude. This is not surprising. We looked in Chapter 1 (Section 1.2.2.2) at the considerable advantage, in weight terms, of storing excess energy in the form of hydrophobic triacylglycerol molecules, in the lipid droplets characteristic of adipocytes. A typical figure for body fat content is about 15–30% of body weight. (This figure is higher *on average* in women than in men.) Thus, a typical fat store is of the order of 10–20 kg. The energy content of fat is around 37 kJ/g, so we store the equivalent of around 500 MJ in the form of fat. A typical daily energy expenditure (to be discussed further in Chapter 11) is around 10 MJ, so we store sufficient energy for about 50 days of life; in fact more, since, as we shall see, one of the prominent aspects of the metabolic adaptation to starvation is that daily metabolic rate (energy expenditure) is reduced. This accords well with recorded times for survival of starvation victims of up to 60 days for initially normal people. A few obese people have starved, voluntarily, for therapeutic reasons for considerably longer periods. (They were closely monitored medically, and given necessary vitamin and mineral supplements.)

However, storage of most of our energy reserves in the form of fat poses a biochemical problem. As we have seen, some tissues and organs require glucose, and cannot oxidise fatty acids. Fatty acids cannot be converted to glucose in mammals because acetyl-CoA formed from fatty acids is oxidised completely to CO_2 in the tricarboxylic acid cycle and is therefore unable to contribute to the gluconeogenic pathway. Only the glycerol component of triacylglycerol can form glucose, and this is a minor component in terms of numbers of carbon atoms. As we shall see, one 'strategy' adopted by the body during starvation is an increased conversion of fatty acids into water-soluble intermediates, the *ketone bodies* (see Fig. 4.5), which can be used by tissues normally requiring glucose, particularly the brain.

8.2.3   Amino acids

The body contains around 20% by weight of protein – about 10–15 kg. Amino acids can be oxidised to provide energy, or converted to glucose and fatty acids, which can then be oxidised. Amino acids, when completely oxidised in a calorimeter, liberate around 24 kJ/g. This is not a realistic figure for metabolic oxidation, since urea is formed, which itself has a certain energy content. Amino acid catabolism to CO_2 and urea liberates about 17 kJ/g. Thus, about 200 MJ of biological energy is present in the body in the form of protein. However, we must be careful in interpreting this as an energy store. Animals do not produce any specific protein purely for storage: all proteins have some other function – as structural components, enzymes, etc. Thus, the body's content of protein is only available as an energy store at the expense of loss of some functional protein. In fact, it will become apparent in the discussion of the metabolic adaptation to starvation that body protein is conserved so far as is consistent with the body's metabolic requirements; protein is not utilised as an energy reserve in the same way that carbohydrate and fat are.

Of the 10–15 kg of protein in the body, about 5 kg are in skeletal muscle. This appears to be the main source of supply when amino acids are required. There is some loss from other organs and tissues, but presumably they are relatively 'spared' because of their vital functions. It appears that the body can only tolerate a loss of about half of its muscle protein. After this, the respiratory muscles in particular become so weakened that chest infection and pneumonia may set in (probably assisted by impaired immune function as a result of malnutrition) and death follows.

The body's fuel reserves are summarised in Table 8.1.

Table 8.1 The body's fuel stores.

Fuel	Amount (typical in 65 kg person)	Energy equivalent	Days supply if the only energy source
Carbohydrate			
Free glucose	12 g	0.2 MJ	0.02, = 30 min
Glycogen	450 g	7.65 MJ	0.77, = 18 h
Fat			
Triacylglycerol	15 kg	550 MJ	55
Protein	12.5 kg*	210 MJ	21

The numbers on this table should be taken as rough estimates only. They are discussed more in the text. Assumptions: energy produced by biological oxidation, 17 kJ/g for carbohydrate and protein; 37 kJ/g for fat; energy expenditure 10 MJ/day.

*As discussed in the text, not all the body protein can be utilised, so the numbers for protein are notional only.

8.3   Starvation

The response to absolute deprivation of food proceeds in a number of stages, leading ultimately to death: but the manner in which metabolism adapts, to postpone that final end-point as long as possible, illustrates a number of important points about the integration of metabolism in the whole body. Starvation has undoubtedly always been a threat to humans and other animals, and the metabolic responses that minimise its impact have evolved throughout the development of all living things. Because this response has evolved so directly to counteract the threat posed by lack of food, it is tempting to look on it as 'purposeful', and indeed it helps considerably in understanding it if we think in terms of the body's 'strategy'. Nevertheless, bear in mind that the use of a term such as 'strategy' does not imply anything other than a response that has evolved because it is beneficial.

There are distinctions between absolute starvation and partial starvation or undernutrition. We will consider absolute starvation, as this provides the clearest illustration of metabolic adaptation. Figure 8.1 shows a scheme for looking at the different phases of total starvation.

8.3.1   The early phase

We have already looked at the pattern of metabolism in very short-term starvation (Section 6.5.1), namely the *postabsorptive state* after overnight fast. A gentle decrease in the concentration of glucose in the plasma led to a small decrease in the ratio of insulin/glucagon, stimulation of hepatic glycogenolysis and liberation of fatty acids from adipose depots. The availability of fatty acids in the plasma leads tissues such as muscle to use fat, and spare glucose, as their major metabolic fuel.

The five phases of glucose homoeostasis

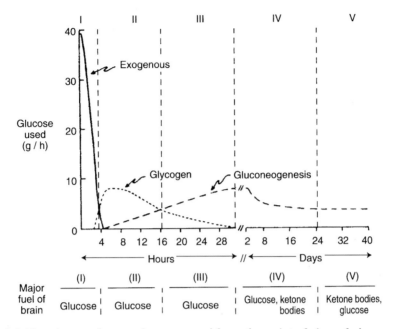

Fig. 8.1 The phases of starvation, assessed from the point of view of glucose metabolism. Reproduced from Ruderman (1975). With permission, from the *Annual Review of Medicine* 26: 245–258. ©1975 by Annual Reviews www.annualreviews.org.

The postabsorptive state leads into a phase sometimes called the *gluconeogenic phase*, lasting until the second or third day of absolute starvation. Liver glycogen stores are virtually depleted within 24 hours (Fig. 8.2), and therefore gluconeogenesis must come into operation to supply the requirements of the brain and other glucose-requiring tissues (e.g. erythrocytes). The main signal for this will again be the decrease in insulin/glucagon ratio. The concentration of another important hormonal stimulator of gluconeogenesis, cortisol, does not change systematically in starvation. In addition, the supply of substrate for gluconeogenesis will increase over this period. The falling insulin concentration will lead to net proteolysis in muscle and release of amino acids, mainly alanine and glutamine. The latter is partially converted to alanine in the intestine (see Section 6.3.2.3), and thus the liver receives an increased supply of this amino acid. Increasing lipolysis in adipose tissue releases glycerol, which is also a substrate for gluconeogenesis.

Gluconeogenesis in this early stage of starvation is therefore proceeding largely at the expense of muscle protein, a situation that is clearly not good for survival. Studies of experimental underfeeding of volunteers have shown that muscle function is impaired with surprisingly small degrees of undernutrition. Not all amino acids can be converted into alanine and glutamine, and some are oxidised, representing an irreversible loss from the body's stores. Around 1.75 g

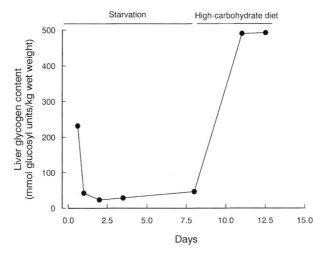

Fig. 8.2 Liver glycogen concentrations in normal human volunteers, after overnight fast, then during 2–10 days' total starvation, and then following refeeding with a carbohydrate-rich diet. The 'basal' value already includes the effects of 12–14 hours without food (a sample was not taken in the fed state). The samples were obtained with a fine needle inserted through the rib cage. Based on Nilsson & Hultman (1973).

of muscle protein must be broken down to provide each gram of glucose (since not all amino acids can be converted to glucose), and with the brain requiring around 100–120 g of glucose per day, the rate of muscle protein breakdown could be rapid. If no other adaptations took place, this would require the breakdown of around 150 g protein per day. (Some glucose is, of course, provided from glycerol.) The body's store of protein in muscle would be rapidly depleted. This is avoided by a series of interrelated adaptations to starvation, which are summarised in Table 8.2.

Table 8.2 Metabolic adaptations that lead to sparing of muscle protein in starvation.

1.	Ketogenesis increases; brain begins to use significant quantities of ketone bodies; therefore the need for glucose production is decreased
2.	Gluconeogenesis is stimulated, so other precursors are used maximally (e.g. lactate is efficiently recycled)
3.	As lipolysis increases, glycerol becomes an increasingly important substrate for gluconeogenesis
4.	Thyroid hormone concentrations fall (probably via a fall in leptin concentration); metabolic rate is decreased, thus lessening demand for energy generally
5.	Ketone bodies may exert a restraining influence on muscle protein breakdown (discussed in text; see Section 8.3.2.3).

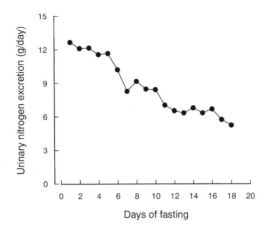

Fig. 8.3 Rate of urinary nitrogen excretion in five obese subjects during starvation.
Based on Owen, O.E., Tappy, L., Mozzoli, M.A. & Smalley, K.J. (1990) Acute starvation.
In: *The Metabolic and Molecular Basis of Acquired Disease* Vol. 1 (eds Cohen, R.D., Lewis,
B., Alberti, K.G.M.M. & Denman, A.M.), 550–570. With permission of the publisher W.B.
Saunders.

The sparing of the body's protein stores is brought about gradually. The excretion of nitrogen in the urine, a measure of the irreversible loss of amino acids, decreases steadily from the start of starvation (Fig. 8.3). At first sight, this seems to contradict the idea of increased gluconeogenesis from amino acids in the early phase of starvation. However, this is not a fair picture. We should think in terms of *nitrogen balance*. Nitrogen balance is the difference between total nitrogen intake, and total nitrogen loss. Some nitrogen is lost in faeces and shed skin cells, but most is lost in the urine in the form of urea and ammonia, and represents the catabolism of amino acids. During normal life, we are approximately in nitrogen balance on a day-to-day basis – the amount of nitrogen we take in is equal to the amount we lose, and the body store of nitrogen (mainly in amino acids and protein) stays roughly constant. At the start of starvation, nitrogen intake falls suddenly to zero, but nitrogen excretion continues at about the same level as before. Suddenly, therefore, there is a net loss of the body's protein stores. Nitrogen excretion then declines steadily, representing the sparing that is necessary for starvation to be prolonged beyond a week or two.

8.3.2   The period of adaptation to starvation
The changes listed in Table 8.2 come into place gradually over the first three weeks or so of total starvation; this is the period of adaptation.

8.3.2.1   Hormonal changes
Blood glucose concentrations fall very gradually in prolonged starvation and they are followed by the plasma insulin concentration. Glucagon concentrations, on the other hand, rise, so that the ratio of insulin/glucagon reaching the liver must change considerably from early to late starvation. The plasma leptin

concentration also falls. In longer starvation this may be due to a reduction in adipose tissue mass, but in the shorter term it also reflects a 'sensing' of energy deficit in adipose tissue, perhaps through reduced insulin concentrations (insulin will acutely stimulate leptin secretion from adipose tissue after feeding).

The onset of starvation is also marked by a decrease in the level of the active thyroid hormone, triiodothyronine (T_3, see Fig. 5.8), in the blood (Fig. 8.4). Several factors appear to cause this. The early reduction in secretion of thyroid hormones has been attributed to the fall in leptin action on the hypothalamus (reducing thyroid-stimulating hormone secretion from the anterior pituitary, and hence thyroid hormone secretion). Therefore, although this may appear to be a central effect, it arises in turn from 'peripheral' sensing of fuel shortage. There is also a shift towards production of an inactive form, *reverse triiodothyronine* (reverse T_3), at the expense of T_3 (Fig. 8.4). The effect of the fall in T_3 concentration is to reduce overall metabolic rate, and to reduce the rate of proteolysis in muscle. The reduction in overall metabolic rate leads, of course, to a decrease in the rate of depletion of the body's fuel stores. However, it is unlikely that the metabolism of the brain, usually the largest glucose consumer, is reduced significantly, so the need for glucose is still present; it is reduced, however, by the mechanisms described below.

Both the sympathetic nervous system and the adrenal medulla play some role during starvation. However, although starvation is a state in which fuel mobilisation is required, the adrenergic systems play a much lesser role than in other, more stress-driven states (such as exercise). There is some activation of both sympathetic nervous system and adrenaline secretion during the first week or so of starvation. These changes would normally cause an elevation in overall

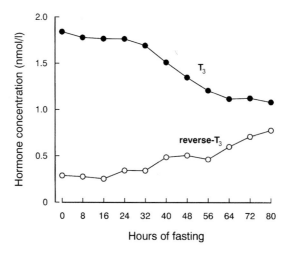

Fig. 8.4 Serum concentrations of triiodothyronine (T_3) and reverse triiodothyronine (reverse-T_3) during early starvation in normal volunteers. Based on Gardner *et al.* (1979).

metabolic rate; this is not seen, since it is outweighed by the reduction in T_3 concentration. On the other hand, the adrenergic systems are probably important in stimulation of lipolysis in adipose tissue. This latter will be reinforced by the continuing reduction in insulin concentration. Therefore, the plasma non-esterified fatty acid concentration rises during the adaptation period (Fig. 7.5).

8.3.2.2 Adaptation of fatty acid, ketone body and glucose metabolism

The elevation in plasma non-esterified fatty acid concentration leads to a number of adaptations. Skeletal muscle will use non-esterified fatty acids almost entirely in preference to glucose for its energy production. In the liver, the rate of fatty acid esterification, usually stimulated by insulin, will decrease; fatty acids will be diverted into oxidation (glucagon stimulates this pathway). This diversion is mediated in part by a decrease in hepatic malonyl-CoA concentration, a result of the decrease in insulin concentration (see Fig. 4.3). Increased oxidation of fatty acids leads to increased production of the ketone bodies, 3-hydroxybutyrate and acetoacetate (see Figs 4.3, 4.5). These can be used as an oxidative fuel by many tissues, at a rate simply depending on their concentration in the blood. Most importantly, they can be used by the brain. This is a crucial feature of the response to starvation: the brain begins to use a fuel derived from the body's fat stores, in preference to glucose. By the end of the third week of starvation, blood ketone body concentrations may reach 6–7 mmol/l, compared with < 0.2 mmol/l normally (Fig. 7.5). At this stage, ketone body oxidation can account for approximately two-thirds of the oxygen consumption of the brain. Thus, about 70–80 g per day of glucose is spared oxidation.

The body's need to form new glucose from amino acids is also reduced by the stimulation of gluconeogenesis in the liver, enabling glucose to be efficiently recycled. Glycolytic cells and tissues such as erythrocytes and the renal medulla will still need to use glucose. (They cannot use ketone bodies since they do not have the oxidative capacity.) Glycolysis in these tissues, however, leads to the release of lactate that is returned to the liver and avidly reconverted into glucose (the Cori cycle, see Fig. 6.20). Thus, the glucose that must be used by these tissues is recycled. Energy for this process comes from the increased oxidation of fatty acids in the liver, forming the NADH necessary to drive gluconeogenesis. This means that, in effect, the glycolytic tissues run on energy derived from the fat stores.

8.3.2.3 Sparing of muscle protein

By the mechanisms described above, the need to produce glucose from muscle protein is reduced, and the loss of nitrogen in the urine decreases. However, with the insulin concentration decreasing, the net stimulus would seem to be for increasing muscle protein breakdown. How is the sparing of muscle protein brought about?

The possible role of the decreasing T_3 concentration has been mentioned: T_3 usually has the effect of stimulating muscle proteolysis (see Section 6.3.3, Fig. 6.19). Another possibility is that the increase in plasma adrenaline concentration may be involved: adrenergic drugs have an anabolic effect on muscle (see Section 6.3.3), although this effect is not clearly understood, and the receptors by which it is mediated have not been delineated.

The other possible mediator is the increase in blood ketone body concentration. Some experimental studies show that elevation of the blood ketone body concentration leads to a reduction in the net breakdown of muscle protein. There is a possible mechanism. The branched-chain amino acids are catabolised in muscle by transamination, followed by the action of branched-chain 2-oxo-acid dehydrogenase (see Section 6.3.2.2). This enzyme complex has many similarities with pyruvate dehydrogenase. Like pyruvate dehydrogenase, its activity is inhibited by a high acetyl-CoA/CoASH ratio. In other words, if the muscle is plentifully supplied with other substrates for oxidation (such as fatty acids and ketone bodies, in starvation) then the oxidation of the branched-chain amino acids will be suppressed.

However, another way of looking at the fall in nitrogen loss in starvation is that it may be another facet of the general slowing down of metabolism. In this case no specific mechanism need be postulated. This has been discussed by Henry *et al.* (1988), who argue that conventional understanding of the response to starvation is heavily biased since it is based mainly on obese subjects undergoing starvation for the purpose of weight reduction.

8.3.2.4 Kidney metabolism

During this period of starvation, there are marked changes in the metabolic pattern of the kidney that will be briefly discussed here. The concentrations of lipid-derived fuels – non-esterified fatty acids and ketone bodies – are high in the plasma, as shown in Fig. 8.5. Each of these is a biological acid. Therefore, the production of hydrogen ions increases and the pH of the blood tends to fall. In order to counter this, the body must excrete excess hydrogen ions. In Section 6.3.2.3 one means for achieving this was mentioned: the kidney can excrete ammonia, which carries with it one hydrogen ion (since it will be in the form of NH_4^+). The ammonia may be derived from the action of glutaminase on glutamine, and glutamate dehydrogenase on glutamate, in the kidney (see Section 6.3.2.3). The renal uptake of glutamine increases in starvation in order to provide a means for excretion of excess hydrogen ions. Glutamine metabolism in the kidney can lead to glucose production, especially during starvation, when the kidney can become an important gluconeogenic tissue. Thus, again we see the efficiency of metabolism: a metabolic process (ammonia excretion) necessary to regulate blood pH is coupled with the conversion of a muscle-derived amino acid to glucose.

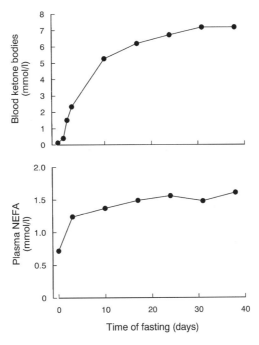

Fig. 8.5 Concentrations of non-esterified fatty acids (NEFA) and ketone bodies (the sum of acetoacetate and 3-hydroxybutyrate) in blood in obese subjects during starvation. Based on Owen, O.E., Tappy, L., Mozzoli, M.A. & Smalley, K.J. (1990) Acute starvation. In: *The Metabolic and Molecular Basis of Acquired Disease* Vol. 1 (eds Cohen, R.D., Lewis, B., Alberti, K.G.M.M. & Denman, A.M.), 550–570. With permission of the publisher W.B. Saunders.

8.3.3   The period of adapted starvation

From about three weeks of total starvation onwards, the body appears to be fully adapted to starvation and there is a kind of steady state, in which there is gradual depletion of the body's protein mass (minimised by the mechanisms discussed earlier), and steady depletion of the fat stores. Ketone body concentrations in the blood reach about 6–8 mmol/l, and ketone bodies provide about two-thirds of the metabolic requirement of the brain. Other tissues that require glucose (erythrocytes, renal medulla for instance) produce lactate, which is efficiently recycled, using energy derived from fatty acid oxidation. Thus, the rate of 'irreversible loss' of glucose is minimised. The major fuel flows in this state are summarised on Fig. 8.6.

We can see how the pattern of metabolism is governed by the physico-chemical features of fat and carbohydrate outlined in Chapter 1, so that fat – the most energy-dense fuel store – constitutes the major long-term fuel reserve and metabolism is geared to derive the maximum proportion of energy from fat oxidation. The changes that bring about this metabolic adaptation are mediated in a gradual way by changing concentrations of substrates in the blood, and

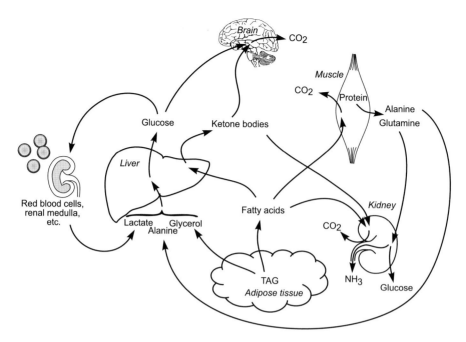

Fig. 8.6 Major fuel flows in prolonged starvation. Protein (especially that in muscle) and glycerol from triacylglycerol in adipose tissue are the only long-term sources of glucose. The complete oxidation of glucose is reduced by the production of ketone bodies which serve as an alternative fuel, e.g. for the brain. Those tissues that must use glucose (e.g. red blood cells, renal medulla) produce lactate, which is 'recycled' in gluconeogenesis. The major source of fuel for oxidation is thus adipose tissue triacylglycerol (TAG), providing fuel both in the form of non-esterified fatty acids and (via the liver) ketone bodies.

by the almost automatic responses of the endocrine system: insulin secretion decreases as the plasma glucose concentration falls, leptin secretion follows, while glucagon secretion increases. The central nervous system is involved in these responses, with mild activation of the adrenal medulla and sympathetic nervous system. However, the involvement of the central nervous system is very much less than in 'acute' situations such as exercise and trauma. A decrease in thyroid hormone secretion, via the hypothalamic-pituitary system, may in turn largely result from the 'peripheral' changes (via leptin).

The adapted state will, we hope, come to an end with refeeding. Otherwise it will continue, usually until weakness of the respiratory muscles leads to inability to clear the lungs properly, and pneumonia sets in and leads to death. There is some evidence that survival is determined by the size of the fat stores: when the fat stores are finally depleted as far as they can be, there is a sudden additional loss of protein and death follows quickly.

Nevertheless, it is worth pondering the ability of the metabolic pattern to adapt to such an extreme situation. We began our tour of metabolic regulation by looking at the changes that occur during normal daily life, with food coming in regularly three times a day. Many of us in the Western world are not used to missing a meal, let alone a day's food: the fact that the body could survive for around two months without any food intake is a clear illustration of the coordinated regulation of metabolism that not only underpins our daily lives, but also allows us to continue in some very extreme situations.

8.4   Exercise

Total starvation is a very extreme situation in one sense. On the other hand, as stressed in the earlier part of this chapter, it involves a relatively gradual adaptation. The flux through any particular metabolic pathway changes over a period of days or even weeks. Exercise represents a different type of extreme situation. In sprinting, for instance, it has been estimated that net flux through the glycolytic pathway in muscle increases at least a thousand-fold, and this must happen within a few seconds or even less. In strenuous endurance exercise, such as cross-country skiing or elite marathon running, the rate of whole-body energy expenditure increases by something like 18-fold over the resting level. This involves major changes in the transport of substrates through the blood, which could not be achieved without coordinated physiological changes, in the circulatory and respiratory systems, and metabolic changes.

8.4.1   Types of exercise

It is convenient to think of two extreme types of exercise, sometimes called *anaerobic* and *aerobic*.

Anaerobic exercise is typified by sprinting or weight-lifting; it is of short duration, but may involve great strength. It is dominated by the activity of the fast-twitch (Type II) muscle fibres (see Table 4.1).

For those with an understanding of physics, this can be confusing. Work is done when a force acts through a distance. Thus, apart from the initial snatch, it is not obvious that a weight lifter is doing any work in a physical sense when he or she holds a weight aloft for any length of time; and yet, we all know that this is tiring. The key to this lies in understanding that muscle contraction is only maintained by continued small contractions of individual muscles fibres; there has to be continued stimulation of the muscle by the somatic nerves and continued ATP production and utilisation within the muscle to maintain a contraction. A closely related term that may help to understand this is *isometric contraction* of the muscles (*isometric* meaning *equal length*): the muscle maintains a contraction without changing its length. In true 'isometric exercises' the muscles are tensed against a resistance. Again, no obvious outside work is done, but it certainly requires energy! The key feature of anaerobic exercise is rapid generation of energy over a short period. Energy is generated too rapidly for the diffusion into the muscle of substrates, including O_2, from the blood, and this is achieved by utilisation of the muscle's own energy stores, phosphocreatine and glycogen.

Aerobic exercise, on the other hand, involves prolonged exercise but at a lower intensity than can be achieved anaerobically. It is typified by long-distance running or swimming, or cross-country skiing. Here, the duration is such that it could not be maintained solely from the fuels stored within muscle: the fuel stores in the rest of the body (fat in adipose tissue, glycogen in the liver) must be used. Hence, these substrates must be brought to the muscle in the blood, and there are necessary adjustments to the circulatory system. The muscle fibres involved are predominantly the oxidative, Type I fibres. It is called *aerobic*, of course, because, to maximise efficiency, substrates (fatty acids and glucose) are completely oxidised.

8.4.2 Intensity of exercise

It will be useful to have an idea of the intensity of exercise in a quantitative sense. There are a number of terms and physical concepts that are related to this discussion. They are summarised in Table 8.3.

Force is defined as that which tends to cause a body to accelerate. It relates, for instance, to the strength of a muscle contraction. It is measured in newtons (N). Force may not *cause* a body to accelerate if it is opposed by an equal and opposite force. For instance, when we hold an object against the pull of gravity,

Table 8.3 Units related to energy and work.

Name	Brief definition	Units	Abbreviation	Notes
Force	That which tends to cause a body to accelerate	Newtons ($1\ N = 1\ kg\ m\ sec^{-2}$)	N	One newton is about the force needed to hold an apple against gravity
Work	Product of distance moved and the force exerted	Joules ($1\ J = 1\ kg\ m^2\ sec^{-2}$)	J	In dietary terms, it is useful to use kJ ($=10^3\ J$) and MJ ($=10^6\ J$)
Energy	Capacity to do work	Joules	J	Heat is one form of energy. When we speak of the 'energy' of food (e.g. dietary carbohydrate provides about 17 kJ/g) we refer to the heat liberated on complete oxidation
Power	Rate of doing work	Watts ($1\ W = 1$ joule/sec)	W	

Note that joules have replaced calories (1 cal = 4.18 J). Because calories are small (when dealing with nutrition) it was more common to use kilocalories (kcal, often abbreviated to Cal). Now kJ (1000 J) or MJ (1000 kJ) are convenient.

we exert a force on it. The force necessary to hold it steady will be equal to the mass of the object in kilograms multiplied by the acceleration due to gravity, about 9.8 m sec^{-2}.

Work is done on an object when a force acts on it over a distance. An example is lifting something through a height. The work done is the product of the distance moved (in metres) and the force exerted (which is, in turn, the mass of the object in kilograms multiplied by the acceleration due to gravity). This refers to the *external work* performed. It does not depend on the rate at which the object is moved: the amount of external work is the same when an object is moved through a given height, however quickly or slowly it is moved. This is because the object is being given *energy* (in this case, *potential energy*), and the gain in the object's potential energy is the same when it moves from the floor to the shelf (for instance) however fast it is moved. Another way of looking at energy is that it is the capacity to perform work: we could then lower the object down with a string over a pulley and make it do some work in return (turn a clock, for instance). Energy and work are measured in the same units, joules (J). One joule is the work done when a force of one newton acts over a distance of one metre.

It is not so obvious why external work is done when we move ourselves through a distance horizontally: if we only had frictionless roller skates (and no air resistance), we would need to expend no energy to keep going at a constant speed. In reality, we have to contend with friction against the air and loss of energy when our feet strike the ground. Running is not an efficient means of movement compared with wheels.

The *rate of doing work* is measured in energy units per unit of time (joules per second, called watts). This is called *power* or *power output*. Lifting an object against gravity is a convenient way of estimating power output. A useful practical exercise is to run as fast as possible up a flight of stairs, through a known height, and calculate the *external work* done against gravity (this is independent of the speed), and the *power output* (the work done divided by the time). An example calculation is given in Box 8.1.

However, the external work done is not the same as the energy expended by the person doing the work. The body is like any other machine that uses a fuel to produce external work. (The analogy with a petrol engine is obvious.) It is not fully efficient: some of the energy it uses from its store will be converted, not into external work, but into *heat*. As a rough approximation, the human body is about 25% efficient: of the energy it uses from its stores, about 25% is converted to external work, and 75% into heat. The rate of using our fuel stores is measured as *energy expenditure* by the whole body. We can assess this in two ways.

If we can measure the rate of heat production by the body, and add to this the rate of doing external work, then we can assess energy expenditure directly. This requires a form of *calorimeter*, or instrument for measuring heat. In this case it is known as a *direct calorimeter*, and in practice it is a room-sized cham-

Box 8.1   Measurement of power by climbing stairs

A volunteer runs up a flight of stairs and is timed with a stopwatch. The vertical height climbed is measured.

The results might be:

- the runner has a body weight (including clothing) of 70 kg
- the vertical height climbed is 2 m
- the time taken is 2.0 seconds

The potential energy gained = mass (kg) $\times$ g $\times$ height (m), where g is the acceleration due to gravity (9.8 m s^{-2})

$$= (70 \times 9.8 \times 2.0) \text{ J}$$

$$= 1715 \text{ J}$$

Then the rate of doing external work (power) = total work done/time taken

$$= 1715/2.0 \text{ J/s}$$

$$= 858 \text{ J/s, or } 858 \text{ W}$$

Notes

(1) A power output of 858 W would count as extremely heavy work on the scheme outlined in the text (where 200 W is regarded as 'heavy'); but the classification given in the text refers to *sustained* exercise, whereas much greater power output is feasible over a short time. In fact, power output measured over a very short time (a few seconds) is effectively a measure of the rate at which phosphocreatine can be used.

(2) A more accurate way of measuring short-term anaerobic power output is to time the subject over a shorter distance – for instance, to use electronic switch-pads under two stairs separated by 1 m vertically.

(3) You should realise that the calculation is an approximation. For instance, it ignores work done against friction of shoe on floor, etc. Nevertheless, in this situation it is true that by far the majority of work done will be the work against gravity, and it is a fairly good approximation.

(4) Another example is the annual race to run up 1860 steps to the top of the Empire State Building in New York (381 m in height). The time taken by an elite runner is about 11 min. Assuming a body mass of 70 kg gives an average power output of 400 W. This is less than the figure of 858 W above because that could only be sustained for a few seconds.

ber with temperature sensors of some sort in its walls to detect heat production. If the external work is done on an exercise bicycle by turning the pedals against friction, so that heat is produced, then there is no need to add separately the external work done: it will all be included in the total heat produced.

A direct calorimeter such as this is a sophisticated piece of equipment, and there are not many in the world. A simpler method for measuring the total energy expenditure is *indirect calorimetry*. Energy expenditure is assessed by the consumption of oxygen and, in more sophisticated systems, by the production of carbon dioxide. This is feasible because the body as a whole derives energy from the complete oxidation of substrates, excreting only water, CO_2 and urea. The principle of indirect calorimetry will be covered in detail in Chapter 11 (Box 11.2).

Thus, there are two ways of expressing the rate of working. We may measure it as external work done, usually referred to as *power* or *power output*, and measured in watts. Typical gradings of exercise are:

- 65 W: light
- 130 W: moderate
- 200 W: heavy exercise.

These refer to rates of doing *external work*.

Alternatively, we may measure the rate of whole-body energy expenditure, which will include both external work done and heat produced. This may also be measured in watts, although it is very convenient to relate it to the body's resting rate of energy expenditure. The unit *MET* (abbreviated from *metabolic rate*) has been coined for this measure. Some typical rates of energy expenditure expressed in this way are given in Table 8.4.

This enables us to answer a simple question that often comes up. We are about to walk up a mountain. We start by eating a confectionery bar to give us the energy. Is it enough energy – or might we even end up fatter than we started? The approximate calculation is given in Box 8.2.

8.4.3   Metabolic regulation during anaerobic exercise

Exercise begins in the brain. We decide to contract our muscles in that particular way which will move us forwards, upwards, backwards or whatever. The appropriate somatic nerves are activated, and electrical impulses travels towards the muscle(s) to be contracted. On arrival of the impulse at the nerve terminal, acetylcholine is liberated and attaches to the nicotinic receptors at the sole-plate (see Section 7.2.2.3 and Fig. 7.4). The binding of acetylcholine to these receptors sets a number of events in motion, described in Box 8.3.

ATP is hydrolysed as the muscle contracts. It must be replaced rapidly or the muscle would run out of energy; the amount of ATP present in skeletal muscle is sufficient for about 1 second of maximal effort. In fact measurements of the ATP concentration in contracting skeletal muscle show it to be remarkably

Table 8.4 Energy expenditure during various activities.

Activity	Energy expenditure (metabolic rate), MET
Resting (not asleep)	1.0
Sleeping	0.9
Light housework (e.g. sweeping floor)	2.5
Walking steadily (3 miles/h or 5 km/h)	3.5
Heavy housework (e.g. washing car, mopping floor)	4.5
Dancing	3–7
Swimming	6–11
Strenuous hill-walking (averaged over a whole walk including rests)	9
Jogging	10–12
Squash	12
Marathon running	18

One MET is defined as the normal resting metabolic rate (i.e. whole-body energy expenditure); it is about 4.8 kJ/min for a man of average size, and 3.8 kJ/min for a woman of average size. Note that 4.8 kJ/min is 4800/60 = 80 W (about the heat output of a light bulb). Remember that the figures given are for total energy expenditure by the body; the amount of *external work* done will be about one quarter of this (since the body as a machine has an efficiency of about 25%).

The figures in this table are, of course, approximations only. The data are taken from Newsholme & Leech (1983), Ainsworth *et al.* (1992) and Ainslie *et al.* (2002).

Box 8.2   Does a confectionery bar provide enough energy to climb a mountain?

Let's start with the pleasant bit – a 65 g confectionery bar provides 1230 kJ (294 kcal) of energy (if all oxidised).

Now for the climb: let's suppose:

- we are going to climb 1000 m (3000 ft)
- our body weight (with clothing, boots, rucksack containing a picnic for the top, etc.) is 75 kg.

The external work done (against gravity) in reaching the summit is:

force × height gained

= mass (kg) × g (m s^{-2}) × height gained (m),
where g is the acceleration due to gravity

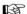

$$= (75 \times 9.8 \times 1000) \, J$$

$$= 735\,000 \, J, \text{ or } 735 \, kJ.$$

But the body is only about 25% efficient in converting chemical energy into external work. Therefore the total energy expenditure is about four times this, or:

$$4 \times 735 \, kJ, \times 3000 \, kJ, = 3 \, MJ.$$

Therefore we are permitted to stop halfway and eat another confectionery bar!

Note that the bar should not really be necessary; our fat stores (see Table 8.1) can provide typically about 540 MJ, enough for nearly 200 mountains without eating any more!

constant (Fig. 8.7). Mechanisms for resynthesising ATP must be turned on extremely rapidly. Initially the utilisation of ATP is 'buffered' by the phosphocreatine system (see Figs 4.10 and 8.7). But the amount of phosphocreatine is relatively small – it would sustain intense sprinting for about 4 seconds. The phosphagen store (phosphocreatine + ATP) must then be replenished, and this occurs initially by glycogen breakdown and glycolysis.

There is a rapid increase in the flux through the glycolytic pathway in muscle at the start of strenuous exercise. It may increase by something like 1000-fold. However, it is clear that the flux cannot increase unless there is substrate to sustain it, and in rapid, intense exercise this substrate is glucose 6-phosphate produced by glycogen breakdown, rather than glucose taken up from the plasma. Therefore, there must be a mechanism for coordinated stimulation of glycogenolysis and muscle contraction.

There are two aspects to this coordinated control. The first is that the elevation of sarcoplasmic Ca^{2+} concentration (Box 8.3) also activates glycogen phosphorylase (Fig. 8.8). The second is that glycogen phosphorylase cannot act unless the concentration of its co-substrate, inorganic phosphate (P_i), increases. This happens through the splitting of ATP in muscle contraction (Fig. 8.8). Since the ATP concentration is kept 'topped up' by phosphocreatine, this P_i really comes from phosphocreatine. Thus, glycogen breakdown and muscle contraction are intimately connected within the muscle: there is no need for rapid stimulation by hormones.

The increased flux through glycolysis, now that substrate is available, requires alterations in enzyme activity that are brought about by interconnected changes in the levels of metabolites within the cell, discussed in Box 8.4. Never-

Box 8.3   Events occurring in skeletal muscle on receipt of a somatic nerve impulse

The structure of the end of the nerve (the *end-plate*) and the receptive area (the *sole-plate*) on the muscle cell membrane (the *sarcolemma*) was shown in Fig. 7.4. On arrival of an impulse, acetylcholine is liberated into the synaptic cleft and binds to nicotinic receptors in the sole-plate. This causes opening of Na^+ channels and depolarisation of the sarcolemma (see Box 7.1 for a description of these processes). The depolarisation spreads across the sarcolemma as an *action potential*. It is relayed to invaginations of the sarcolemma which form tubes running into the muscle cell, the *T-tubules* (T for transverse). The arrival of the action potential causes the release into the muscle cell cytoplasm (the *sarcoplasm*) of Ca^{2+} ions from stores in the *sarcoplasmic reticulum*, a system of membranes within the cell. Thus, the sarcoplasmic Ca^{2+} concentration is rapidly elevated throughout the cell.

An increase in the concentration of Ca^{2+} causes contraction by binding to troponin C, a component of the *thin filaments* of muscle, and, via a conformation change, allowing the binding of the myosin heads (part of the *thick filaments*) to actin. Thin and thick filaments thus move ('slide') relative to one another to cause contraction. (See Section 4.3.1 for a brief description of muscle contraction, and Further Reading for Chapter 4 for more details.) The hydrolysis of ATP (to ADP and inorganic phosphate, P_i) by the myosin ATPase provides energy for this process. Thus, contraction and the hydrolysis of ATP are intimately linked.

☞

theless, the rate of change of glycolytic flux is so great that it seems unlikely that it can be accounted for solely by rapid changes in the concentrations of enzyme effectors. This has led to the idea that the sensitivity of metabolic regulation of this pathway may be increased by the existence of substrate cycles (see Box 8.4). Despite activation of the pathway of glycolysis in this way, studies of glycolytic flux made by magnetic resonance spectroscopy of muscle show that flux is only elevated when contraction occurs: flux falls almost to zero when contraction stops, although the concentrations of the metabolites that may activate phosphofructo-kinase remain high. This emphasises the important role of Ca^{2+} ions in coordinating contraction and metabolism, as shown in Fig. 8.8.

During intense exercise, energy is thus derived very rapidly from anaerobic glycolysis. There is no need for increased delivery of other substrates or oxygen in the plasma. Anaerobic glycolysis produces lactic acid which, at physiological pH, will be in the form of lactate ions and hydrogen ions. There is therefore an increase in the local hydrogen ion concentration in the muscle. This may be one cause of fatigue. A local fall in pH may have a number of effects that tend to cause lessening of the force of muscle contractions. These include effects on

These steps are shown diagrammatically below.

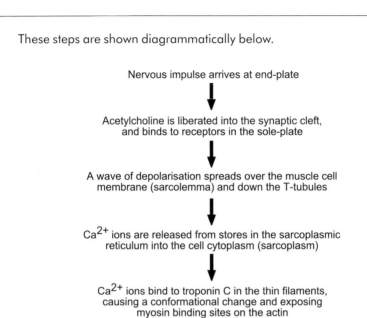

Nervous impulse arrives at end-plate

↓

Acetylcholine is liberated into the synaptic cleft,
and binds to receptors in the sole-plate

↓

A wave of depolarisation spreads over the muscle cell
membrane (sarcolemma) and down the T-tubules

↓

Ca^{2+} ions are released from stores in the sarcoplasmic
reticulum into the cell cytoplasm (sarcoplasm)

↓

Ca^{2+} ions bind to troponin C in the thin filaments,
causing a conformational change and exposing
myosin binding sites on the actin

↓

Myosin 'heads' in the thick filaments bind to actin; the filaments
'slide' relative to one another and thus the muscle contracts.
During this process ATP is hydrolysed to ADP + P_i

Fig. 8.3.1

In addition, the release of Ca^{2+} ions into the sarcoplasm leads to activation
of glycogen breakdown, as shown in Fig. 8.8.

the interaction between myosin and actin, on the binding of Ca^{2+} to troponin, and on the enzyme phosphofructokinase, an important regulatory enzyme in glycolysis that is inhibited at low pH (see Box 8.4).

The ability to perform this type of exercise depends largely upon the bulk of the glycolytic, Type II fibres, and this bulk can be increased through training (discussed in Section 8.4.9 below). Certain interventions may aid performance. Recently there has been considerable interest in dietary supplementation with creatine in amounts of 5 g/day. This has been shown to improve anaerobic performance, by increasing the amount of phosphocreatine in the muscles. Another intervention that has shown some success in experimental situations is to ingest large amounts of sodium bicarbonate ($NaHCO_3$), which acts as a buffer to minimise hydrogen ion accumulation and thus postpone fatigue.

8.4.4   Metabolic regulation during aerobic exercise

In Section 8.4.1, anaerobic and aerobic exercise were described as the two ex-

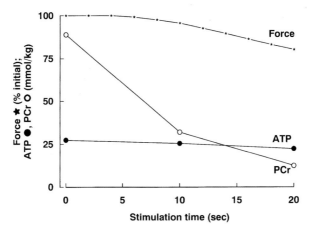

Fig. 8.7 Concentrations of ATP and of phosphocreatine (PCr) in Type II fibres in human muscle during contractions brought about by electrical stimulation. After 6 contractions (each 1.6 sec long; i.e. at ~10 sec) and after 12 contractions (~20 sec) a muscle biopsy was taken and rapidly frozen, and later the Type I and Type II fibres were separated for analysis. With repeated contractions, the force generated decreases slightly, the PCr concentration falls sharply, but the concentration of ATP remains almost constant. The implication is that ATP is being rapidly resynthesised at the expense of PCr. Adapted from Söderlund, K., Greenhaff, P.L. & Hultman, E. (1992) Energy metabolism in type I and type II human muscle fibres during short term electrical stimulation at different frequencies. *Acta Physiol Scand* 144: 15–22. With permission of the Scandinavian Physiological Society. Following Maughan *et al.* (1997).

treme forms of exercise. Many forms of exercise consist of a combination of the two. Games such as tennis and soccer require moments of intense power output (serving, kicking), accompanied by endurance performance (running about the court or pitch for 90 minutes or more). In running events, the 100 m sprint is virtually completely anaerobic: it is said that the elite sprinter has no need to draw breath during it. (Most of us would doubtless need several breaths!) The 400 m run is a combination of both anaerobic and aerobic exercise, and with increasing distance, the aerobic component becomes more dominant. The marathon run (42.2 km, 26.2 miles) is often taken as an example of almost pure aerobic exercise.

The characteristic of aerobic exercise is that it can be sustained for long periods. Of necessity, this means that stored fuels other than those in the muscles must be used, and must be completely oxidised so that partial breakdown products such as lactic acid do not build up. Complete oxidation of substrates also gives a much higher energy yield than partial breakdown: for instance, complete oxidation of 1 molecule of glucose gives rise to 31 molecules of ATP,[2] whereas anaerobic glycolysis to 2 molecules of lactate generates 3 molecules of ATP. Not surprisingly, then, the muscle fibres most involved in aerobic exercise are the more oxidative, slow-twitch Type I fibres (see Section 4.3.2). In order for these muscles to produce external work at a high rate over a long period, they must be supplied with substrates (including O_2), and the products of me-

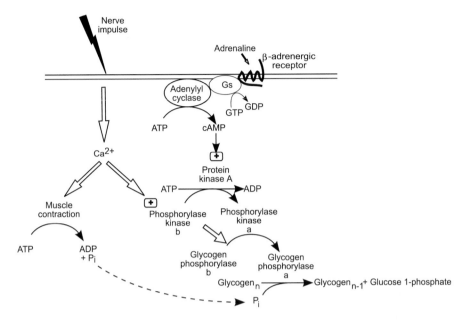

Fig. 8.8 Coordinated regulation of glycogenolysis and contraction by Ca²⁺ ions in skeletal muscle. Elevation of the concentration of Ca^{2+} ions in the sarcoplasm occurs in response to the arrival of a nerve impulse (see Box 8.3), and is responsible for the initiation of contraction. As discussed in Box 2.4, Fig. 2.4.2, Ca^{2+} ions can also activate phosphorylase kinase (independently of its phosphorylation state). Therefore glycogen breakdown is initiated by arrival of the nerve impulse. The figure also shows the activation of phosphorylase by adrenaline (as in liver). It has been suggested that the *anticipation* of exercise may 'prime' the system by an increase in adrenaline. Glycogen cannot be broken down until there is an increase in the concentration of inorganic phosphate (P_i), which is released as soon as contraction begins. The regulation of glycogen breakdown by Ca^{2+} ions is not confined to muscle; it can also occur in liver, and accounts for activation of glycogenolysis by catecholamines acting via α_1 adrenoceptors. However, the physiological significance is not known.

tabolism such as CO_2 must be removed, at a sufficiently high rate. This necessitates coordinated changes in the circulatory system.

It is illuminating to consider how much ATP is needed for endurance exercise – for instance, running a marathon. An approximate calculation is given in Box 8.5. A marathon runner will use almost his or her own body weight of ATP. Clearly this ATP was not all stored at the beginning of exercise! In fact the total amount of ATP is probably almost the same at the end of the race as at the beginning (see from Fig. 8.7 how the ATP content of muscle is maintained even during intense, anaerobic contractions). In other words, the ATP pool must be continuously resynthesised, to the extent that about 60–70 kg of ATP are synthesised during the race. The question now becomes: what are the metabolic fuels used for ATP resynthesis during aerobic exercise?

The major fuels used in aerobic exercise vary with the intensity of the exercise and with the duration. In relatively light exercise most of the energy required comes from non-esterified fatty acids delivered from adipose tissue.

Box 8.4   Activation of the pathway of glycolysis at the start of anaerobic exercise

At the start of intense anaerobic exercise, the net flux through the glycolytic pathway may increase about 1000-fold. In the text and Fig. 8.8 the link between contraction and glycogen breakdown is explained. Nevertheless, the enzymes of the pathway itself must be activated in order to allow this increase in flux. Regulation of the enzyme phosphofructokinase (PFK) is best understood and will be discussed here as an illustration.

Allosteric regulation
Regulation by fructose 2,6-bisphosphate, important in the liver, is probably not a major factor in exercising muscle. However, a number of intermediates act as allosteric effectors of PFK. These include:

Activators	Inhibitors
AMP	ATP
P_i	Citrate*
Fructose 1,6-bisphosphate	Phosphocreatine*
Fructose 6-phosphate	H^{+*}
NH_3	

*These potentiate the inhibitory effect of ATP.

During contraction, ATP is hydrolysed to ADP + P_i. It is partially replenished by phosphocreatine (see Fig. 8.7). The following associated reactions occur:

Reaction	Effect
ATP → ADP + P_i (associated with contraction)	ATP ↓, P_i ↑
2ADP → ATP + AMP (adenylate kinase)	AMP ↑
PCr + ADP → Cr + ATP (creatine kinase)	PCr ↓↓
AMP + H_2O → IMP + NH_3 (AMP deaminase)	NH_3 ↑

PCr, phosphocreatine; Cr, creatine; IMP, inosine monophosphate (a degradation product of AMP).

Thus, the changes in allosteric effectors all act to activate PFK.

Substrate cycling
However, it is difficult to envisage that an enzyme can alter its activity by a factor of 1000 in one second or so. For this reason, it has been proposed that the

sensitivity of control may be increased by the existence of a substrate cycle between fructose 6-phosphate (F 6-P) and fructose-1,6-bisphosphate (F 1,6-P_2). The reverse reaction is catalysed by fructose-1,6-bisphosphatase (FBPase).

The concept may be illustrated as shown in Fig. 8.4.1.

In the top scheme ('resting'), the flux through PFK is 55 (arbitrary units) and the reverse flux 5, giving a net flux along the pathway of 50 arbitrary units. On the starting blocks (middle scheme), anticipation (perhaps mediated via stress hormones) leads to a 36-fold activation of PFK and a 390-fold activation of FBPase (these are reasonable changes since they need not be instantaneous). The net flux (50 units) along the pathway remains unchanged. On the starting gun, an almost instantaneous change of 25.5-fold activation of PFK and halving of FBPase activity leads to a 1000-fold change in net flux through the pathway. The numbers illustrate the potential for increased sensitivity of metabolic control arising through substrate cycling, but are not based on physiological measurements.

This box and Fig. 8.4.1 are based largely on Newsholme & Leech (1983) with permission from John Wiley & Sons Ltd; quantitative estimates of the extent of substrate cycling *in vivo* are given by Newsholme & Challis (1992).

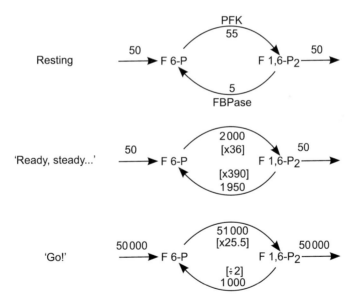

Fig. 8.4.1   Based on Newsholme, E.A. & Leech, A.R. *Biochemistry for the Medical Sciences.* 1983. © John Wiley & Sons Limited with permission.

Box 8.5   How much ATP is used in running a marathon?

There are several ways this problem might be approached. This is one.

Energy expenditure during marathon running ≈ 85 kJ/min

Oxidation of glucose liberates 17 kJ, so 85/17 ≈ 5 g glucose are used per min (Fat will also contribute, but this is only approximate)

5 g glucose/min = 5/180 mol glucose/min ≈ 0.028 mol glucose/min

Each mol glucose produces approximately 38 mol ATP on complete oxidation

Therefore ATP production ≈ 0.028 × 38 mol/min ≈ 1.06 mol ATP/min

If the race lasts 2 h 10 min (130 min) then total ATP production ≈ 130 × 1.06 mol ATP, ≈ 137 mol ATP

M_r for ATP ≈ 500

Therefore total ATP produced (and used) ≈ 500 × 137 g ≈ 69 kg ATP

(This is a very approximate calculation, but it is interesting that Buono & Kolkhorst (2001) approached it by an entirely different route and came to a similar figure.)

At higher intensities, carbohydrate tends to predominate early on, fat becoming more important later as glycogen stores are depleted. As we have seen several times, the amount of glucose present in the circulation and the extracellular fluid is small, and cannot be depleted without harmful effects. Therefore, the carbohydrate used during endurance exercise comes from glycogen stores, both in exercising skeletal muscle and in the liver. In principle, it might also come from gluconeogenesis: exercising muscles always produce some lactic acid, even in aerobic exercise, and this should be a good substrate for hepatic gluconeogenesis. In fact, gluconeogenesis seems to be restricted during exercise, perhaps because blood flow to the liver is restricted as blood is diverted to other organs and tissues (mainly, as discussed below, skeletal muscle). The use of different fuels at different intensities of exercise is illustrated in Fig. 8.9.

The contribution of fat to muscular work shows some odd characteristics. If we set out to design an 'exercise system' using our knowledge of metabolism gained so far, we might think that as large a proportion as possible of the energy

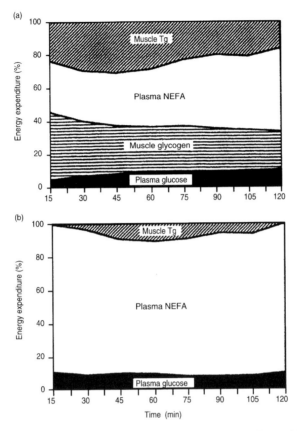

Fig. 8.9 Utilisation of different fuels during exercise at two intensities. The intensities of exercise are judged by oxygen consumption, in relation to the maximal rate of oxygen consumption for the individual ($\dot{V}O_2max$). Panel (a) shows exercise at 65% $\dot{V}O_2max$; 2 h at 65% $\dot{V}O_2max$ is relatively heavy exercise. (An elite marathon runner would maintain about 85% of $\dot{V}O_2max$ for 2 h 10 min.) Panel (b) shows exercise at 25% $\dot{V}O_2max$; 2 h at 25% $\dot{V}O_2max$ is relatively light. The figure shows the relative contribution to energy expenditure (total energy expenditure is taken in each case to be 100%, although it is 65/25 or 2.6 times greater in the top panel). The data were obtained by a combination of indirect calorimetry and use of isotopic tracers to measure the whole-body turnover of glucose, glycerol and fatty acids. Based on Romijn, J.A., Coyle, E.F., Sidossis, L.S. *et al.* (1993) Regulation of endogenous fat and carbohydrate metabolism in relation to exercise intensity and duration. *Am J Physiol* 265: E380–E391. With permission of the American Physiological Society.

for exercise should be generated by oxidation of fat. We have far more energy stored as fat than as carbohydrate, and there is not the same need to 'preserve' it for the functioning of organs such as the brain. In addition, fat is, as we have seen, a very 'light' way of storing a lot of energy. However, it appears from a number of studies that oxidation of fat can only support *around* 60% of the maximal aerobic power output. The evidence is briefly this. In ultra-endurance athletes (e.g. 24-hour runners), power output drops with time to about 50% of maximal aerobic power, at about the same time as the glycogen stores are depleted. In less well-trained subjects, it also appears that fat oxidation contributes a maximum of about 60% of muscle oxygen consumption.

Therefore, the maintenance of maximal aerobic power output requires that carbohydrate is oxidised as well as fat. Since this carbohydrate comes from the glycogen stores, the time for which maximal aerobic power can be sustained depends upon the amount of glycogen stored initially. Depletion of the glycogen stores leads to a sudden feeling of fatigue, described by marathon runners as 'hitting the wall'. The Swedish physician Jonas Bergström and a Swedish physiologist, Eric Hultman, showed this directly during the 1960s. They measured the content of glycogen in small samples (*biopsies*) of muscle, taken with a special needle, in a group of athletes who were each studied on two or three occasions, after consuming different diets. The different diets (mixed diet; low-carbohydrate diet; high-carbohydrate diet) produced different initial concentrations of muscle glycogen, and it was found that the 'time to exhaustion' when working at 75% of maximal aerobic power correlated with the initial muscle glycogen concentration (Fig. 8.10). This observation has led to the development of methods for boosting the muscle glycogen stores for endurance runners (*glycogen loading*).

Having looked at the overall pattern of fuel utilisation during aerobic exercise, we shall now consider in more detail the regulation of the utilisation of individual fuels, and how the delivery of energy is regulated by the hormonal and nervous systems.

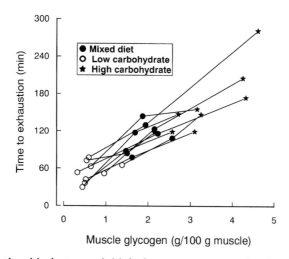

Fig. 8.10 Relationship between initial glycogen concentration in the quadriceps muscle and maximal work time (until exhaustion) in nine different subjects who followed different diets before each test. The greater the initial glycogen concentration, the longer the ability to sustain exercise. Redrawn from Bergström, J., Hermansen, E., Hultman, E. & Saltin, B. (1967) Diet, muscle glycogen and physical performance. *Acta Physiol Scand* 71: 140–150. With permission of the Scandinavian Physiological Society.

8.4.5   Nervous system and cardiovascular responses during aerobic exercise

Two components of the nervous system are intimately involved with metabolic regulation during aerobic exercise.

The somatic nervous system carries the stimuli for contraction of the appropriate muscles, and the arrival of a nervous impulse at the end-plate triggers both contraction and a coordinated activation of glycogen breakdown (Fig. 8.8). This is true just as much during aerobic exercise, and there appears to be 'obligatory' breakdown of muscle glycogen associated with muscle contraction, even if there are plentiful substrates in the blood (e.g. if the athlete has eaten well beforehand).

The sympathetic nervous system, accompanied by adrenaline secretion from the adrenal medulla, brings about the necessary changes in the cardiovascular system and the mobilisation of stored fuels, glycogen and triacylglycerol.

An important part of the physiological response during endurance exercise is an increase in cardiac output (both the rate and force of heart contraction increase), and an increased delivery of blood to skeletal muscle. The increase in cardiac output is mediated mainly by the sympathetic nervous system, acting on β-adrenergic receptors in the heart. An increase in cardiac output in itself might cause an increase in muscle blood flow, but there is an additional specific dilatation of the blood vessels in the muscle. Blood flow to the active muscle increases almost instantaneously at the onset of exercise. The mechanism that brings this about is not entirely clear. It used to be thought that this was mediated by cholinergic impulses from the sympathetic nerves (discussed in Chapter 7, Section 7.3.2 and Fig. 7.5). Skeletal muscle is unusual in that activation of the sympathetic nervous system causes vasodilatation; in other organs (e.g. skin, kidneys and abdominal organs) blood flow is restricted by sympathetic activation. However, the evidence that this occurs in humans is inconclusive and it is now thought to occur more through vasodilatory effects of substances released from the contracting muscle, including lactate ions and the accompanying hydrogen ions. Whatever the mechanism, the effect is that blood is diverted to the muscles, allowing greater delivery of substrates (including O_2), and also removal of the products of metabolism (lactic acid and CO_2 in particular) (Fig. 8.11).

Increased delivery of O_2 to the muscles and removal of CO_2 from the body also requires increased depth and rate of breathing. This is brought about mainly by the fall in blood pH (increase in H^+ ion concentration) which occurs as lactic acid and CO_2 are produced. The change in pH is sensed by receptors in the brainstem (see Section 7.2.1.2) which trigger changes in respiration.

8.4.6   Other hormonal responses during aerobic exercise

The sympathetic nervous system and adrenaline also bring about the mobilisation of stored fuels (discussed in detail below). Other hormones respond to aerobic exercise, and are involved in the regulation of fuel availability. Both growth

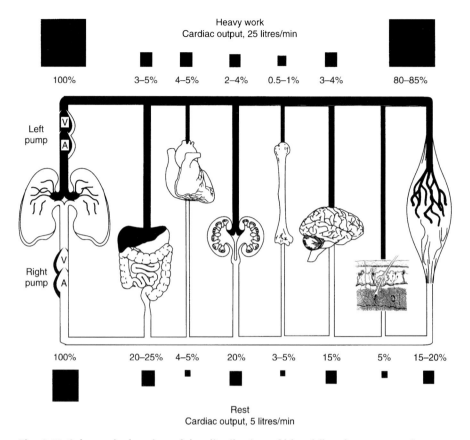

Fig. 8.11 Schematic drawing of the distribution of blood flow between various organs and tissues at rest (bottom) and during strenuous exercise (top) (distribution shown by the area of the black squares). Adipose tissue is not shown, but accounts for about 5–10% of cardiac output at rest, about 1% during exercise. Reproduced from Åstrand, P.-O. & Rodahl, K. (1977) *Textbook of Work Physiology*, 2nd edn. With permission of Mc-Graw-Hill Inc and the authors.

hormone and cortisol are secreted in response to exercise, rising in concentration in the plasma gradually over the first 30 minutes to 1 hour (Fig. 8.12) – i.e. these are relatively slow responses, and are likely to be involved particularly in the release of stored fuels during prolonged exercise. The plasma glucose concentration may rise or fall during exercise (discussed below), but the insulin concentration falls somewhat during endurance exercise (Fig. 8.13). This represents α-adrenergic inhibition of its secretion from the pancreas, brought about by the increased circulating adrenaline concentrations. Glucagon secretion may also increase, although this is not a major change except with very strenuous, prolonged exercise. The increase in adrenaline, glucagon, growth hormone and cortisol concentrations is a typical 'stress' response (see Fig. 7.6). Since the major effects of glucagon are on the liver, and liver metabolism may not be dominant during exercise because of restricted blood flow, there may be little role for glucagon in this situation.

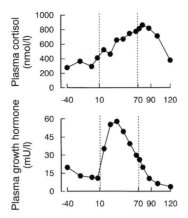

Fig. 8.12 Plasma concentrations of growth hormone (top panel) and cortisol (lower panel) during aerobic exercise at about 60% of maximal aerobic power. The exercise, on a bicycle, began with a 'warm-up' (shown as 0–10 minutes) and then carried on for 60 minutes (until 70 min on the X-axis). Based on Hodgetts, V., Coppack, S.W., Frayn, K.N. & Hockaday, T.D.R. (1991) Factors controlling fat mobilization from human subcutaneous adipose tissue during exercise. *J Appl Physiol* 71: 445–451. With permission of the American Physiological Society.

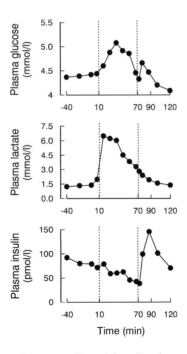

Fig. 8.13 Plasma glucose (top panel) and insulin (lower panel) concentrations during aerobic exercise at about 60% of maximal aerobic power. The protocol was the same as in Fig. 8.12. Note how the plasma insulin concentration falls during exercise, despite a rise in the plasma glucose concentration. The plasma lactate concentration is also shown (middle panel); it increases at the beginning of exercise and then subsides. Based on Hodgetts, V., Coppack, S.W., Frayn, K.N. & Hockaday, T.D.R. (1991) Factors controlling fat mobilization from human subcutaneous adipose tissue during exercise. *J Appl Physiol* 71: 445–451. With permission of the American Physiological Society.

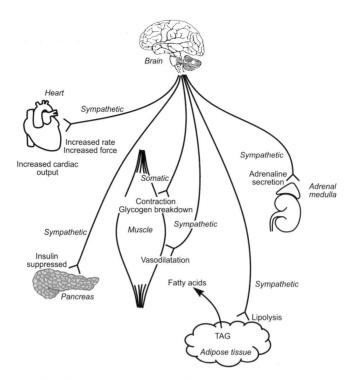

Fig. 8.14 Coordination of metabolism by the nervous system during endurance exercise. Adrenaline secreted from the adrenal medulla may be responsible, or may reinforce the effects of the sympathetic nerves, for increased lipolysis and for suppression of insulin secretion.

The way in which the somatic and sympathetic nervous systems coordinate physiological and metabolic changes during endurance exercise is illustrated in Fig. 8.14.

8.4.7   Carbohydrate metabolism during endurance exercise

Oxidation of glucose provides a major source of energy for the working muscles during aerobic exercise. During aerobic exercise at a high rate (e.g. 80–90% of maximal oxygen consumption, typical of an elite marathon runner) the rate of energy expenditure is around 80–90 kJ per minute. The proportion of this supplied by glucose oxidation varies according to the preceding diet and other factors, but 50% might be a reasonable estimate (i.e. 40–45 kJ/min from glucose). Oxidation of 1 g of glucose releases 17 kJ, so that 42.5/17 or about 2.5 g of glucose must be oxidised each minute.

The amount of glucose available in the blood and extracellular space is around 12 g (see Section 6.1). Therefore, even if it could all be used without adverse consequences, this could support high-intensity aerobic exercise for only a few minutes. The liver glycogen store is around 100 g (see Section 8.2.1). Therefore, this could support exercise for less than 1 hour. The total store of muscle glycogen may be around 300–400 g, giving rather longer. The utilisation of muscle glycogen is more extensive in those muscles being used for the exercise than in others, so not all the whole-body store of muscle glycogen may be used. Remember that these are all 'ball-park' figures. Note that the total store of glycogen store in liver and muscle could support glucose oxidation at a rate of 2.5 g/min for something over 2 h. It is probably not a coincidence that this is about the time taken for an elite runner to finish the marathon. When the glycogen store is depleted, the rate of energy expenditure will drop and performance will suffer. The marathon may be about the longest event that can be undertaken at such a high percentage of maximal oxygen consumption.

Hepatic gluconeogenesis has been ignored here; it probably does not make a large contribution, since hepatic blood flow may be decreased during exercise as the blood is diverted to working muscles. Moreover, much of the gluconeogenesis that occurs will be from lactate, released by the working muscles from their glycogen stores. Therefore, this is only part of the complete pathway for oxidation of those glycogen stores.

What are the factors responsible for mobilisation of the glycogen stores? In the working muscles, the effects of neural activation of contraction probably predominate, since the glycogen concentration in non-working muscles falls much less, if at all. This has been demonstrated in subjects performing one-legged exercise on a modified exercise bicycle; the glycogen content of the exercised leg falls whilst that of the other leg does not change (Fig. 8.15). As discussed earlier, the stimulation of contraction is intimately linked with the stimulation of glycogen breakdown (Fig. 8.8). An elevation in the concentra-

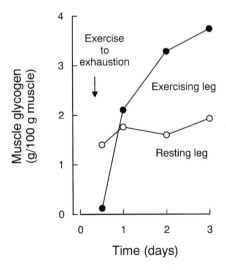

Fig. 8.15 Glycogen concentrations in leg muscle after one-legged exercise (bicycling on a specially adapted bicycle), in the exercised leg (solid points) and the non-exercised leg (open points). Average of two subjects. Based on Bergström & Hultman (1966).

tion of adrenaline may also contribute, potentiating the effect of somatic nerve stimulation; it is not a stimulus on its own, however, as evidenced by the one-legged exercise experiment, in which both legs are exposed to the same adrenaline concentration.

In the liver, the stimulus for glycogen breakdown is not entirely clear. Glucagon would be the obvious signal but, as noted earlier, its concentration is not always elevated during exercise. However, it should be remembered that when the concentration of glucagon is measured in 'peripheral blood' it may not reflect the concentration reaching the liver in the portal vein, so that there may be some increase in glucagon secretion. In addition, the concentration of glucose may rise or fall somewhat – largely depending on the nutritional state of the subject – but the plasma insulin concentration falls gently during sustained exercise (Fig. 8.13), probably representing the effects of increased α-adrenergic stimulation to the pancreas (via sympathetic nerves or plasma adrenaline). Therefore, the glucagon/insulin ratio reaching the liver will undoubtedly rise, favouring glycogen breakdown. In addition, there may be some direct effect of activation of the sympathetic innervation of the liver; this is very difficult to test in humans.

One other aspect of glycogen mobilisation is worthy of mention. Recall that glycogen, a hydrophilic molecule, is stored in hydrated form with about three times its own weight of water. When glycogen is mobilised, that water is released. Therefore, as well as providing the store of carbohydrate, glycogen also contributes to the water necessary for endurance exercise, helping to replace that lost as sweat, etc. If 300 g of glycogen are mobilised in all, this could mean almost one litre of water.

Note that the comment made above, that the plasma glucose concentration may not change much during endurance exercise, does not mean that there are no changes in glucose utilisation. The concentration of glucose in the plasma merely represents the balance between glucose production and glucose utilisation. The *turnover* of glucose in plasma increases several-fold during endurance exercise (see Romijn *et al.* 1993). The rate of glucose uptake by skeletal muscle must also increase several-fold. This is brought about by recruitment of GLUT4 transporters to the sarcolemma. But in this case, the recruitment is not driven by insulin. Muscle contraction itself can bring about this translocation. The stimulation of muscle glucose utilisation by the sympathetic nervous system (see Section 7.3.3.3) is also probably involved.

8.4.8   Fat metabolism during endurance exercise

The activity of muscle hexokinase is sufficient, in principle, for all the energy for sustained aerobic exercise to be derived from uptake of plasma glucose. In fact, as we have seen, this would reduce the length of time during which the exercise can be sustained at the highest rate. Simultaneous oxidation of glucose and fatty acids therefore produces the longest possible period of sustained high intensity exercise. The availability of fatty acids to the muscles also reduces the rate of glucose oxidation, by operation of the glucose–fatty acid cycle (see Section 6.4.1.2). There is experimental evidence that increasing the availability of fatty acids leads to sparing of glycogen, thus at least in principle allowing high-intensity exercise to be continued for longer.[3]

The fatty acids oxidised during endurance exercise come from two main sources: triacylglycerol stored in adipose tissue, and triacylglycerol stored in the muscles themselves. The latter is difficult to study and the factors controlling muscle triacylglycerol utilisation are not clear. Nevertheless, the muscle triacylglycerol concentration falls during intense, long-lasting exercise. The regulation of fat mobilisation from adipose tissue is better understood. The main stimulus for this to increase during exercise is adrenergic. Blockade of β-adrenergic receptors in adipose tissue with the drug propranolol prevents the increase in lipolysis during exercise (see Fig. 7.7). The main stimulus may be circulating adrenaline or activation of the sympathetic nerves. Studies of exercise in people who have had spinal cord injuries, so that some of their adipose tissue is innervated whilst some is not, suggest that circulating adrenaline is more important than the sympathetic innervation. The adrenergic stimulation of lipolysis may be reinforced by the slight fall in insulin concentration (thus relieving the normal suppression of lipolysis by insulin). In sustained exercise (longer than, say, 30–60 min) then the increases in plasma growth hormone and cortisol concentrations (Fig. 8.12) may potentiate the adrenergic stimulation of lipolysis, perhaps by an increase in the amount of enzyme (hormone-sensitive lipase) present.

The fatty acids liberated in adipose tissue must be transported through the plasma bound to albumin to the muscles for uptake and oxidation. It may be a step in this pathway which limits the rate at which fatty acids can be oxidised, leading to the restriction of the contribution of fatty acid oxidation to about 60% of the maximal sustainable rate of energy expenditure. The evidence, from experiments in which the availability of fatty acids in the plasma is increased by the means described earlier, suggests the following. In moderate-intensity exercise, up to about 65% of the maximal aerobic power, increased availability of fatty acids increases the rate of fat oxidation, implying that the normal limitation on their oxidation is at the level of release from adipose tissue. However, in higher intensity exercise (an elite marathon runner maintains 80–85% of maximal aerobic power) then increased availability of fatty acids leads to very little increase in fat oxidation: it appears that the rate of fatty acid utilisation by muscle is limited.

There is some information as to why these steps may be limiting. The release of non-esterified fatty acids into the plasma depends upon the availability of albumin. If the blood flow through adipose tissue is restricted, there may be insufficient albumin available to carry away all the fatty acids formed in lipolysis. Non-esterified fatty acids may then accumulate in the tissue, as described in the case of physical trauma (Section 7.3.3.2 and Table 7.1). To some extent this may cause an increase in their re-esterification to form triacylglycerol, but it also appears that they accumulate as such. When exercise stops, there is often a sudden release of fatty acids into the general circulation not accompanied by the expected one mole of glycerol for each three moles of fatty acids. It is not, perhaps, surprising that blood flow through adipose tissue should be restricted. We have already seen that a high sympathetic activity or circulating adrenaline concentration can restrict blood flow through many tissues by α-adrenergic effects on the blood vessels, and during exercise this occurs as part of the re-distribution of blood to the working muscles. Adipose tissue is affected in just this way.

At higher intensities of exercise, the muscles appear unable to oxidise more fatty acids even if they are available in the plasma. The reason may be this. Glucose metabolism in muscle proceeds at a high rate during intense aerobic exercise. Acetyl-CoA is produced, via the action of pyruvate dehydrogenase, but will primarily be oxidised in the tricarboxylic acid cycle. However, the high concentration may cause some increase in flux through the first part of the pathway of *de novo* lipogenesis, thus increasing the concentration of the next intermediate in that pathway, malonyl-CoA (see Box 4.3). (Fatty acid synthase is not expressed in muscle.) As was discussed in Section 4.1.2.2, malonyl-CoA inhibits the entry of fatty acids into the mitochondrion for oxidation. Thus, glucose oxidation proceeding at a high rate may limit the muscles' ability to oxidise fat.

Thus, fat metabolism during high-intensity endurance exercise does not follow the rules we might expect on the basis of everything we know about human metabolism. The contribution of fatty acids is limited and the avail-ability of glycogen limits the time for which high-intensity exercise can be maintained. We may speculate that perhaps the ability to run at high intensity for long periods was not important in terms of the evolution of *Homo sapiens*. Maybe the ability to sprint, to escape from a predator, was more important.

8.4.9   The effects of training

Exercise training has a number of effects, which cannot be discussed at length in this book. They occur over various time-spans. A single bout of exercise will bring about some metabolic changes that are relevant to the theme of this book.

Expression of muscle lipoprotein lipase increases after exercise, and this increase lasts around 24–48 hours. We can imagine that this is an adaptation allowing the muscle to use more circulating triacylglycerol-fatty acids. It has a clear consequence. The ability of the body to handle incoming, dietary fat is improved within 24 h of a single bout of exercise (Fig. 8.16). Since impaired ability to handle a fat load is a marker of risk of cardiovascular disease, this may be one mechanism by which exercise protects against such disease (discussed in more detail in Chapter 9, see Section 9.4.3). Note, however, that since the in-crease in lipoprotein lipase activity is fairly short-lived, exercise must be regular to sustain this benefit.

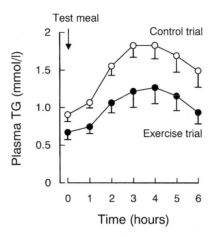

Fig. 8.16 Plasma triacylglycerol (TG) concentrations after a high-fat test meal on two occasions. In one trial, participants had exercised for 2 h at 70% maximal aerobic power 24 h previously ('Exercise trial'); on the other occasion, they had rested the day before ('Control trial'). Both the fasting TG concentration and the rise in concentration after the test meal are significantly reduced in the exercise trial. Data are from eight normal subjects and are shown as mean ± standard error. Data from Malkova *et al.* (2000).

Similarly, if tested 24 h after exercise, there is improvement in glucose utilisation in response to insulin (tested, for instance, by infusing both glucose and insulin intravenously). Resistance to the effects of insulin, common in sedentary people (discussed in more detail in Chapter 10, Box 10.2), is a marker of increased risk both of developing diabetes and of developing cardiovascular disease. Again, therefore, this may be a mechanism by which regular exercise helps to protect against these conditions.

Beyond these rather early changes, prolonged training will bring about longer-lasting structural changes in muscle. In the case of *anaerobic exercise* (such as weight-lifting or sprinting) the changes brought about by training are largely increased muscle bulk and strength. The increase in muscle bulk is mainly the result of muscle *hypertrophy* rather than *hyperplasia*: that is, muscle cells become bigger rather than increasing in number. A weight lifter, sprinter or high-jumper will have a higher proportion of Type II fibres than a long distance runner (see Fig. 3.7), but this is not primarily a result of training; it appears to be genetically determined. Rather, he or she is a weight lifter or sprinter *because* he or she has a high proportion of Type II fibres.

The changes occurring with endurance training are rather more varied. They are listed in Table 8.5. They concern increased ability to deliver O_2 and other substrates to the working muscle, and increased ability within the muscle to utilise substrates. Note that the activity of glycogen synthase is usually found to be increased whilst that of glycogen phosphorylase is not; presumably the activity of glycogen phosphorylase is not usually limiting for generation of power in endurance exercise.

Table 8.5 Changes occurring with endurance training.

Cardiovascular and whole-body
Increased cardiac output, and ability to increase this during exercise
Improved respiratory function
Increased lean body mass (mainly muscle bulk)
Decreased body fat
Increased bone strength
Structural changes in muscle
Increased density of capillaries
Increased number of mitochondria
Increased size of mitochondria
Increased myoglobin concentration
Metabolic changes in muscle
Increased expression of GLUT4
Increased sensitivity to insulin (discussed in text)
Increased activity of lipoprotein lipase (discussed in text)
Increased activity of oxidative enzymes in mitochondria
   (tricarboxylic acid cycle and β-oxidation)
Increased glycogen synthase activity

Based in part on Åstrand & Rodahl (1977) and on Holloszy & Booth (1976).

8.5   Further reading

Starvation
Cahill, G.F., Herrerra, M.G., Morgan, A.P. *et al.* (1966) Hormone-fuel inter-
    relationships during fasting. *J Clin Invest* 45: 1751–1769.
Cahill, G.F.J. (1976) Starvation in man. *Clin Endocr Metab* 5: 397–415. *These
    two papers by Cahill and colleagues review the classic studies of human
    starvation (mostly in initially obese subjects) upon which much of our
    present knowledge is based.*
Henry, C.J.K. (1990) Body mass index and the limits of human survival. *Eur J
    Clin Nutr* 44: 329–335.
Collins, S. (1995) The limit of human adaptation to starvation. *Nature Med* 1:
    810–814.
Dulloo, A.G. & Jacquet, J. (1999) The control of partitioning between protein
    and fat during human starvation: its internal determinants and biological
    significance. *Br J Nutr* 82: 339–356.
Elia, M., Stubbs, R.J. & Henry, C.J. (1999) Differences in fat, carbohydrate,
    and protein metabolism between lean and obese subjects undergoing total
    starvation. *Obes Res* 7: 597–604. *The authors caution that most of our
    understanding of the responses to starvation is based upon studies in ini-*

tially obese subjects. Here they review differences between lean and obese subjects in their responses to starvation.

Elia, M. (2000) Hunger disease. *Clin Nutr* 19: 379–386.

Flier, J.S., Harris, M. & Hollenberg, A.N. (2000) Leptin, nutrition, and the thyroid: the why, the wherefore, and the wiring. *J Clin Invest* 105: 859–861.

Prentice, A.M. (2001) Fires of life: the struggles of an ancient metabolism in a modern world. *British Nutrition Foundation Nutrition Bulletin* 26: 13–27. *In an extraordinarily illuminating article, the author reviews evidence that famine has imposed an evolutionary pressure throughout human evolution.*

Exercise

Bergström, J. & Hultman, E. (1972) Nutrition for maximal sports performance. JAMA 221: 999–1006. *This old paper reviews much of the classical data on muscle glycogen and exercise.*

Spurway, N.C. (1992) Aerobic exercise, anaerobic exercise and the lactate threshold. *Br Med Bull* 48: 569–591.

Coyle, E.F. (1995) Substrate utilization during exercise in active people. *Am J Clin Nutr* 61(suppl): 968S–979S.

Jones, N.L. & Heigenhauser, G.J. (1996) Getting rid of carbon dioxide during exercise. *Clin Sci* 90: 323–335.

Maughan, R., Gleeson, M. & Greenhaff, P.L. (1997) *Biochemistry of Exercise and Training.* Oxford: Oxford University Press. *A compact textbook on exercise biochemistry.*

Joyner, M.J. & Halliwill, J.R. (2000) Sympathetic vasodilatation in human limbs. *J Physiol* 526: 471–480.

Wyss, M. & Kaddurah-Daouk, R. (2000) Creatine and creatinine metabolism. *Physiol Rev* 80: 1107–1213.

Schnermann, J. (2002) Exercise. *Am J Physiol Regulatory Integrative Comp Physiol* 283: R2–R6.

Sakamoto, K. & Goodyear, L.J. (2002) Intracellular signaling in contracting skeletal muscle. *J Appl Physiol* 93: 369–383.

Wojtaszewski, J.F.P., Nielsen, J.N. & Richter, E.A. (2002) Effect of acute exercise on insulin signaling and action in humans. *J Appl Physiol* 93: 384–392.

Notes

1   This is very variable, and can be expanded considerably under certain conditions, such as high carbohydrate intake after exercise.

2   Biochemistry textbooks may say 38 ATP per glucose, but modern values are lower. This is discussed in Chapter 6 of Salway (1999).

3   The availability of fatty acids may be increased experimentally as follows.
    The subject or animal is either fed a high-fat meal or given a triacylglycerol
    emulsion into a vein. Then the substance *heparin* (an anticoagulant) is
    given. This displaces the enzyme lipoprotein lipase, bound to capillary en-
    dothelial cells, into the bloodstream where it acts rapidly on the circulating
    triacylglycerol to release fatty acids into the plasma. Examples of such stud-
    ies in exercise are given by Costill *et al.* (1977) and Dyck *et al.* (1993).

9

Lipoprotein Metabolism

9.1 Introduction to lipoprotein metabolism

The major energy store of the body is a hydrophobic compound, triacylglycerol, for reasons discussed in earlier chapters. Other hydrophobic molecules play important roles in cellular function, particularly the sterol cholesterol and its esters (*cholesteryl esters*). Mechanisms for transporting these non-water soluble lipid species in the blood have therefore evolved.

Non-esterified fatty acids are carried in the plasma bound to albumin. Some fat-soluble micronutrients and regulators of metabolism – e.g. fat-soluble vitamins and steroid hormones – are transported in the plasma by specific carrier proteins such as the *cortisol-binding globulin*, which carries cortisol. The transport of both triacylglycerol and cholesterol occurs in specialised macromolecular structures known as *lipoproteins*. Because triacylglycerol and cholesterol are carried by the same system, the metabolism of these two types of lipid in the plasma is closely interrelated.

The lipoproteins are particles with a lipid, highly hydrophobic core and a relatively hydrophilic outer surface. A typical lipoprotein particle (Fig. 9.1) consists of a *core* of triacylglycerol and cholesteryl ester, with an outer *surface monolayer* of phospholipid and free cholesterol. (As discussed in Section 1.2.1.1, cholesteryl esters are highly hydrophobic. By comparison, free cholesterol – i.e. unesterified cholesterol – has amphipathic properties because of its hydroxyl group.) The amphipathic phospholipids and cholesterol stabilise the particle in the aqueous environment of the plasma: their hydrophobic (polar) heads face outwards, and their hydrophilic tails protrude into the particle. The term 'particle' is a technical one: these are not solid particles, but more like small lipid droplets. In fact they are emulsion particles. They enable fat to be stably incorporated into plasma in the same way as the phospholipids

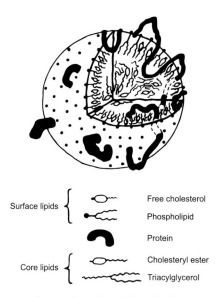

Surface lipids { Free cholesterol
                 Phospholipid

                 Protein

Core lipids { Cholesteryl ester
              Triacylglycerol

Fig. 9.1 A typical lipoprotein particle. From *Hyperlipidaemia: diagnosis and management*, 2nd edition, by P.N. Durrington (1995). Reprinted by permission of Elsevier Science Ltd.

present in egg yolk (mainly phosphatidylcholine) stabilise olive oil in vinegar when making mayonnaise, and in the same way that droplets of triacylglycerol are stabilised by phospholipids in milk.

Each lipoprotein particle has associated with it one or more protein molecules, the *apolipoproteins*. These proteins have hydrophobic domains, which 'dip into' the core and anchor the protein to the particle, and also hydrophilic domains that are exposed at the surface.

The lipoproteins consist of a heterogeneous group of particles with different lipid and protein compositions, and different sizes. They have traditionally been separated into groups, or fractions, based on either electrophoretic mobility or flotation in an ultracentrifuge. The latter technique has given rise to a much-used classification system, which will be used here. It could almost be viewed as a coincidence that the fractions isolated in the ultracentrifuge also have some functional distinction. However, the distinctions are not absolute, and each ultracentrifugal fraction may consist of a range of particles with somewhat different metabolic functions.

The characteristics of the major lipoprotein fractions are listed in Table 9.1. The chylomicron and VLDL particles are relatively rich in triacylglycerol and are often referred to together as the triacylglycerol-rich lipoproteins; they are mainly concerned with delivery of triacylglycerol to tissues. The smaller LDL and HDL particles, on the other hand, are more involved with transport of cholesterol to and from cells. The major apolipoproteins involved in lipoprotein metabolism are listed in Box 9.1, and some important enzymes involved with the lipoproteins in the plasma are listed in Box 9.2.

Table 9.1 Characteristics of the major lipoprotein classes.

Fraction	Density range, g/ml	Diameter, nm	Major lipids	Major apolipoproteins	Composition (percentage by weight)			
					Protein	TG	Cholesterol	PL
Chylomicrons	< 0.950	80–1000	Dietary TG	B48, AI, AII, C, E	1	90	5	4
Very low density lipoproteins (VLDL)	0.950–1.006	30–80	Endogenous TG (from liver)	B100, C, E	10	65	13	13
Low density lipoproteins (LDL)	1.019–1.063	20–25	Cholesterol and cholesteryl ester	B100	20	10	45	23
High density lipoproteins (HDL)	1.063–1.210	9–15	Cholesteryl ester and PL	AI, AII, C, E	50	2	18	30

TG, triacylglycerol; PL, phospholipid.

Notes:

1 There are other fractions and sub-fractions not distinguished here. For instance, between VLDL and LDL there is an intermediate density lipoprotein (IDL) fraction; its half-life is short and its concentration normally low.

2 The proportions shown are approximate only and vary within each major class.

3 Apolipoprotein C refers to the presence of apolipoproteins CI, CII and CIII (see Box 9.1); these are usually found together.

Box 9.1   The major apolipoproteins involved in lipoprotein metabolism

The complete amino acid sequences of the nine major human apolipoproteins are now known (AI, AII, AIV, B (48 and 100), CI, CII, CIII, D and E). The apolipoproteins other than apoB are often referred to as soluble apolipoproteins. They may exist in lipid-free form in the plasma and they may exchange between lipoprotein particles. Apolipoproteins of the groups A, C and E have similar gene structures and some homologous stretches of sequence, and are believed to have evolved from a common ancestral gene, whereas the genes for apoB and apoD have distinct structures.

Apolipoproteins AI, AII

These apolipoproteins are not closely related except in that they often occur together in lipoprotein fractions. AI is the better characterised. It has a relative molecular mass (M_r) of 28 000 (243 amino acids) and it has two major functions in lipoprotein metabolism. It is an activator of the enzyme lecithin-cholesterol acyl transferase (LCAT – see below). In addition, its amino acid sequence contains six repeated 22-amino acid sequences, which fold into alpha-helices with strong polar and non-polar faces. Thus, it has amphipathic properties that enable it to bind very strongly to various lipid classes including phospholipids and cholesterol. This property may give it a special role in interacting with cell membranes and 'collecting' cholesterol from the cells. It is produced in the cells of the small intestine and the liver.

Apolipoprotein B

This is a large protein found in chylomicrons, VLDL and LDL. There are two isoforms, called apolipoprotein B100 and apolipoprotein B48. The former contains 4536 amino acids (M_r 513 000). Apolipoprotein B48 is the N-terminal 2152 amino acids of this (M_r 241 000); in other words it represents about 48% of the apolipoprotein B100 molecule (and hence their names). It is produced from the same gene, by editing of the messenger RNA (in the cytoplasm) to introduce a stop codon. Apolipoprotein B48 is produced in intestinal cells and incorporated into chylomicrons, whereas B100 is produced in the liver and incorporated into VLDL. Since LDL are mostly produced from VLDL (see the text), LDL particles also contain B100. There is just one molecule of apolipoprotein B (B100 or B48) per particle: it wraps around the particle, its hydrophobic regions 'dipping down' into the core to anchor it. It functions as a receptor ligand.

Apolipoproteins CI, CII and CIII

Like the apolipoproteins A, these are not closely structurally related, but are often found together. Apolipoprotein CII is the best understood. It is a protein of M_r 8900 with 78 amino acids. It is an essential activator of the enzyme lipoprotein lipase (discussed earlier, in Sections 4.5.3.1 and 6.2.4.2); without it, lipoprotein lipase is not active. Thus, lipoprotein lipase can only act on the triacylglycerol in particles that contain apolipoprotein CII. It is produced in the liver. Apolipoprotein CIII may inhibit lipoprotein lipase, so that the ratio of CII to CIII in a particle seems to determine its susceptibility to lipolysis by lipoprotein lipase.

Apolipoprotein E
Apolipoprotein E is a protein of M_r 34 000 (299 amino acids), which exists in three major isoforms (known as E2, E3 and E4). Each person carries two alleles: thus, an individual may be E2/E3, E3/E3, etc. Apolipoprotein E functions as a receptor ligand. The different isoforms have different affinities for the receptor, and contribute to the variation in lipoprotein concentrations found within any population. Apolipoprotein E is found in association with the triacylglycerol-rich particles, chylomicrons and VLDL, and also in HDL. It is synthesised in many tissues, but the major source of apolipoprotein E in the plasma is probably the liver.

9.2   Outline of the pathways of lipoprotein metabolism

9.2.1   Chylomicron metabolism – the exogenous pathway

The metabolism of chylomicrons is often called the *exogenous pathway* of lipoprotein metabolism. *Exogenous* means 'from outside the body', since this is the pathway for transporting fat from outside the body – in fact, fat which has been eaten. The pathway is summarised in Fig. 9.2. We have already seen how triacylglycerol and cholesterol are absorbed and re-esterified in the cells of the intestinal wall, and secreted as chylomicron particles, via the lymphatics, into the circulation (Section 3.3.3). The newly secreted chylomicron particles consist of a core of cholesteryl ester and triacylglycerol, with a surface of unesterified cholesterol and phospholipid, and the apolipoproteins B48 and AI. There is just one molecule of apolipoprotein B48 per particle: the particle is synthesised in the enterocyte around this protein, which will stay with the particle throughout its lifetime. The particles also carry some apolipoprotein AIV, described in Section 3.2.3.2.

In the circulation, they interact with other particles, and some of the smaller apolipoproteins are passed from one particle to another, probably passively by diffusion down concentration gradients. In particular, chylomicrons rapidly acquire apolipoprotein CII, which makes them substrates for the action of lipoprotein lipase as they pass through capillaries of tissues expressing this enzyme

Box 9.2   Some important enzymes involved in lipoprotein metabolism

Lipoprotein lipase (LPL)
This enzyme is found in a number of tissues outside the liver, particularly adipose tissue, skeletal muscle and heart muscle. Its role in lipid metabolism has already been discussed (Sections 4.5.3.1 and 6.2.4.2). It is synthesised within the cells of the tissue (e.g. the adipocytes or the muscle fibres) and exported to the capillaries, where it is attached to the endothelial cells. Here it is bound (non-covalently) to highly negatively charged glycosaminoglycan chains such as heparan sulphate. LPL acts on lipoprotein particles passing through the capillaries, hydrolysing triacylglycerol molecules to release non-esterified fatty acids which may be taken up into the tissue for esterification (and hence storage – mainly in adipose tissue) or oxidation (in muscle). It can only do this if the particles contain apolipoprotein CII (see Box 9.1). LPL activity in adipose tissue is stimulated by insulin, over a relatively long time-course (a few hours). In muscle it is slightly suppressed by insulin but its activity is increased by exercise (both acutely and by training).

Hepatic lipase (HL)
This enzyme is structurally related to LPL, but has a number of different characteristics. It does not require apolipoprotein CII for activity, and it is present in the liver. It has an affinity for smaller particles than does LPL: the significance of this will be discussed below. In addition, it will hydrolyse both triacylglycerol and cholesteryl esters. HL and LPL are members of the same family as pancreatic lipase, the principal enzyme of intestinal fat digestion (Section 3.2.3.3).

Lecithin-cholesterol acyl transferase (LCAT)
This enzyme comes from the liver and is found in the plasma. It associates with particles containing apolipoprotein AI (which activates it). It transfers a fatty acid from position 2 of phosphatidylcholine (present in HDL particles) to unesterified cholesterol, forming a cholesteryl ester (see Fig. 1.6 for the structures of these species). The remaining lysophosphatidylcholine is transferred to plasma albumin from which it is rapidly removed from blood and reacylated.

Acyl-coenzyme A:cholesterol acyltransferase (ACAT)
There are two isoforms, ACAT1 and ACAT2. These are intracellular enzymes responsible for the synthesis of cholesteryl esters from cholesterol and acyl-CoA. They are responsible for esterification of dietary cholesterol within the enterocyte (for package into the chylomicron), formation of cholesteryl ester droplets for storage within cells, and providing cholesteryl esters for VLDL

secretion from the liver. ACAT1 is widely expressed, whereas ACAT2 is mainly expressed in the enterocytes of the small intestine and in the liver. There has been considerable interest in the possibility of inhibition of ACAT2 by drugs to reduce cholesterol absorption.

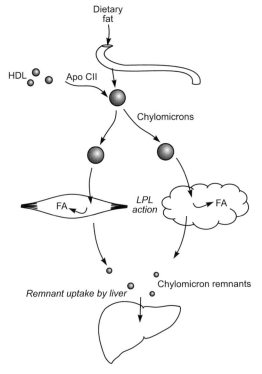

Fig. 9.2 The exogenous pathway of lipoprotein metabolism. Apo, apolipoprotein; FA, fatty acids; LPL, lipoprotein lipase.

such as adipose tissue and muscle. Their triacylglycerol is thus hydrolysed, and the particles shrink. At the same time, they must lose some surface coat, which they do by dissociating some unesterified cholesterol and phospholipid, and some apolipoproteins, which are taken up by other particles such as HDL.

These 'slimmed down' chylomicron particles are known as *chylomicron remnants*. They are relatively enriched in cholesteryl ester, since they have lost their triacylglycerol. As we will see later (Section 9.4.3), these remnants are potentially harmful if they persist in the circulation. The apolipoproteins on their surface must adopt a different conformation in the smaller particle compared with the original chylomicron, and this makes them ligands for a receptor in the liver. This is the receptor known as LRP, the LDL-receptor related protein (also known as the α2-macroglobulin receptor). Other receptors may also be involved: this is currently an area of intense research. Thus, dietary triacylglycerol is delivered to the tissues, some unesterified cholesterol enters the HDL fraction, and some triacylglycerol and cholesteryl ester is delivered, in the remnant particles, to the liver.

9.2.2   VLDL and LDL metabolism

9.2.2.1   VLDL metabolism – the endogenous pathway

In contrast to the metabolism of chylomicrons, there is an *endogenous pathway* of lipoprotein metabolism in which triacylglycerol is distributed from the liver to other tissues. It is summarised in Fig. 9.3. VLDL particles are secreted by the liver. When secreted, they contain triacylglycerol, cholesteryl ester, apolipoprotein B100 and small amounts of apolipoproteins E and C. (See Box 9.1 for further description of these apolipoproteins. Apolipoprotein C refers to a group

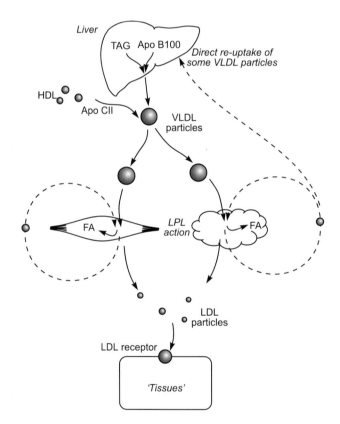

Fig. 9.3 The endogenous pathway of lipoprotein metabolism. Particles may undergo several cycles of hydrolysis by lipoprotein lipase (LPL) in capillary beds (dashed lines), forming smaller particles which may be taken up directly by receptors in the liver; others remain in the circulation as low-density-lipoprotein (LDL) particles. These are eventually removed by uptake into tissues via the LDL receptor (Box 9.3).

of related small proteins.) Like the chylomicron particle and apolipoprotein B48, each VLDL particle contains just one molecule of apolipoprotein B100, which will stay with the particle throughout its lifetime. VLDL particles have a surface coat, like all lipoprotein particles, of phospholipids and unesterified cholesterol. The content of apolipoproteins E and C rapidly increases in the plasma, by transfer from other lipoproteins, mainly HDL.

VLDL particles are also substrates for lipoprotein lipase in capillary beds, and so deliver triacylglycerol from the liver to other tissues. This is a means of distributing lipid energy to the tissues. The particles may undergo several cycles of lipolysis by lipoprotein lipase as they pass again and again through tissues. As with chylomicrons, hydrolysis of the triacylglycerol core by lipoprotein lipase leads to redundant surface material that is passed to other particles, again mainly those of the HDL fraction. The relatively cholesteryl ester-enriched particles which result have two possible fates. They may be taken up directly by a receptor in the liver and other tissues, which binds a homologous region in apolipoprotein B100 and in apolipoprotein E: it is called the *LDL receptor* or sometimes the *B/E receptor.* Thus, they deliver cholesteryl ester to tissues. Alternatively, they may remain in the circulation, having shrunk through the action of lipoprotein lipase and hepatic lipase (which becomes more important as the particles become smaller – see Box 9.2) until they have lost all surface components except apolipoprotein B100 and a shell of phospholipid and free cholesterol, and they have a core enriched in cholesteryl ester – in fact, they have become LDL particles.

9.2.2.2 LDL metabolism and regulation of cellular cholesterol content
LDL particles have a relatively long half-life in the circulation – about 3 days. During this time they are relatively stable metabolically. They leave the circulation mainly through uptake into various tissues by the LDL receptor (Box 9.3), and thus deliver cholesterol to tissues. LDL particles vary in size, a feature that will be discussed again later (Box 9.6).

As tissues take up LDL particles, the cellular cholesterol content is regulated through the SCAP-SREBP2 system (see Fig. 2.6 and Box 9.3). This means that the increase in cellular cholesterol content potentially caused by uptake of LDL-cholesterol by the LDL receptor is self-limiting.

There is an important variation on this theme. Some cells, particularly macrophages, express different receptors which will take up LDL particles. One of these alternative receptors is known as the *scavenger receptor.* These receptors are not subject to down-regulation like the LDL receptor, and therefore, especially in people with a high plasma LDL-cholesterol concentration, the macrophages may become excessively cholesterol-laden.

These scavenger receptors do not have a high affinity for normal LDL particles, but they bind avidly to LDL particles that have been chemically modified in various ways. In the body, this modification is probably oxidative damage to the lipids and the apolipoprotein-B100 that the particle contains. This oxida-

Box 9.3   The LDL receptor and regulation of cellular cholesterol content

The LDL receptor is a protein of M_r 120 000. It has a short intracellular domain and a long extracellular domain, terminating in the ligand-binding N-terminus. It is expressed in most nucleated cells, but LDL uptake is particularly active in the liver and in some tissues that need cholesterol for particular biosynthetic purposes – e.g. the adrenals and ovaries, where it serves as a precursor for steroid hormone synthesis.

LDL particles bind to the receptor, which is then internalised by endocytosis. The cholesteryl ester contained in the LDL particle is hydrolysed in the lysosomes, liberating cholesterol, which forms part of the cellular cholesterol pool. This is used for incorporation into membranes (see Fig. 1.5), for synthesis of steroid hormones, and – in the liver – for synthesis of bile acids and formation of VLDL. The sterol content of intracellular membranes is sensed by the SCAP-SREBP2 system (Fig. 2.6), which regulates gene expression. The synthesis of new LDL receptors and of the enzymes for cholesterol synthesis, including the major regulatory enzyme, 3-hydroxy-3-methylglutaryl-CoA (HMG-CoA) reductase (Box 4.3), is suppressed when cellular cholesterol content is high, but stimulated by SREBP2 when cellular cholesterol is low.

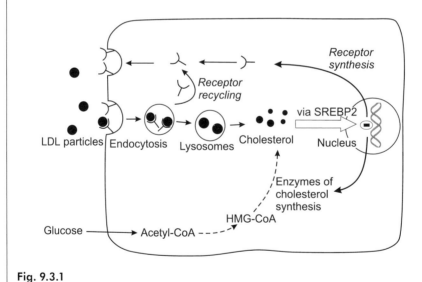

Fig. 9.3.1

tion may occur once LDL particles have left the plasma and entered the sub-endothelial space, or the *intima*, where there are several cell types that can cause oxidative damage. The process of uptake by scavenger receptors is presumably intended to remove the occasional 'damaged' particle, but when the number of such particles increases beyond a certain level the process becomes pathological. This is discussed in a little more detail below (Section 9.4.3 and Box 9.6).

This uptake of cholesterol-rich particles by macrophages in the arterial wall may be the beginning of the process of *atherosclerosis*, deposition of fatty material in the arterial wall, leading to an inflammatory process and the formation of an atherosclerotic plaque (see Section 9.4.1 for more detail).

9.2.3   HDL metabolism

Whilst LDL particles regulate the cholesterol content of cells by delivering cholesterol, HDL particles bring about the opposite process – the removal of cholesterol, which is transported to the liver for ultimate excretion.

9.2.3.1   HDL and reverse cholesterol transport

HDL particles begin their life as apolipoprotein AI molecules secreted from the liver and intestine, associated with some phospholipid. These nascent particles are called *pre-β HDL* from their migration pattern on electrophoresis. As they acquire phopholipids and cholesterol, they form disc-shaped molecular aggregates, so-called *discoidal HDL*. Nascent HDL acquire cholesterol in two ways. First, they interact with cells and collect excess cellular cholesterol. Secondly, they acquire the excess surface material released during the lipolysis of the triacylglycerol-rich lipoproteins by lipoprotein lipase (Sections 9.2.1, 9.2.2). The unesterified cholesterol that is acquired by these routes is esterified to a long-chain fatty acid by the action of the enzyme LCAT associated with HDL particles (Box 9.2), which is activated by apolipoprotein AI. Thus, the particles acquire a core of hydrophobic cholesteryl esters, and 'mature' into spherical, cholesterol-rich particles. These larger, cholesterol-rich particles can be sub-fractionated by ultracentrifugation into HDL_2 (larger particles) and HDL_3 (smaller). The larger particles give up their cholesterol to the liver, both by interaction with specific receptors, and indirectly by transferring cholesteryl ester to the triacylglycerol-rich lipoproteins for return to the liver (this mechanism is discussed further below in Section 9.2.3.2). The smaller HDL particles and relatively lipid-poor apolipoprotein AI resulting are then ready to accept further cholesterol from peripheral tissues. Thus, there is a constant recycling of HDL particles between smaller, cholesterol-depleted and larger, cholesterol-rich forms (Fig. 9.4).

The interaction of HDL particles with cells has recently been understood in molecular detail. HDL particles acquire cellular cholesterol by interacting with a membrane-associated protein that is a member of a large family of proteins with the ability to bind ATP on their cytoplasmic domain. This particular ATP-binding motif gives them the name of ATP-binding cassette or ABC proteins. The one involved with transfer of cholesterol to HDL is known as ABC-A1. It transfers cholesterol from cell membranes to HDL. Note that the action of LCAT associated with HDL is essential to this process: by esterifying cholesterol, it maintains the concentration gradient so that more cholesterol can be taken up by the particle. At the hepatocyte, mature HDL particles interact with

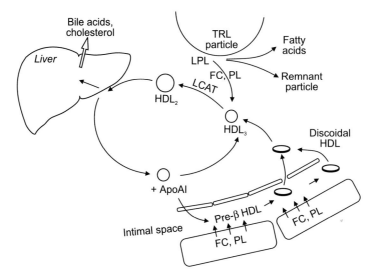

Fig. 9.4 HDL metabolism. Pre-β HDL is apolipoprotein AI (apoAI) associated with some phospholipid. It acquires free cholesterol (FC) and further phospholipid (PL) by interaction with cells and forms discoidal HDL particles, which acquire further FC and PL that is shed from triacylglycerol-rich lipoprotein (TRL) particles as lipoprotein lipase (LPL) acts upon them. Lecithin-cholesterol acyltransferase (LCAT) esterifies the FC the HDL particles have acquired and by this means they mature into spherical, cholesterol-rich HDL$_2$ particles. These may give up their cholesterol and some phospholipid to the liver from where the cholesterol can be excreted in the bile. The lipid-poor apolipoprotein AI is thereby regenerated and begins the cycle again. Based on Fielding, P.E. & Fielding, C.J. (1996) Dynamics of lipoprotein transport in the human circulatory system. In: *Biochemistry of Lipids, Lipoproteins and Membranes* (eds Vance, D.E. & Vance, J.E.), 495–516. With permission of Elsevier Science.

a receptor that is a member of a large family of receptors known as scavenger receptors, because their role is generally to remove 'debris' by phagocytosis (especially in macrophages). This particular receptor is known as scavenger receptor (SR)-BI and is expressed in the liver and also in steroidogenic tissues (e.g. adrenal gland and ovary). 'Docking' of HDL particles with SR-BI is followed by off-loading of their cholesteryl ester content. The cholesteryl esters enter the cellular pool and may be hydrolysed by lysosomal hydrolases as shown for LDL-receptor mediated uptake (Box 9.3). This process is fundamentally different from the uptake of LDL particles by the LDL-receptor, however, and has been called 'selective lipid uptake'. The difference is that the particle itself is not internalised and the cholesterol-depleted particle leaves the receptor to re-enter the cycle of the HDL pathway.

By these means, excess cholesterol is transferred from peripheral tissues to the liver, from where it can be excreted as cholesterol and as bile salts in the bile (see Boxes 3.1 and 9.4). This process of removal of cholesterol from the tissues, transport to the liver and ultimate excretion from the body is the opposite of the delivery of cholesterol by LDL: it is known as *reverse cholesterol transport* (Fig. 9.5).

Box 9.4   Cholesterol homeostasis in the body

The body pool of cholesterol is about 140 g. Of this, about 8 g is present in the plasma, mainly in LDL.

About 1 g of cholesterol enters the body pool each day, 400 mg from intestinal absorption and 600 mg from biosynthesis; i.e. there is < 1% turnover per day of the body cholesterol pool. Note that this does not conflict with the figure of 1 g per day of cholesterol in the diet given in Table 3.1 since cholesterol absorption is incomplete.

There is a turnover of about 5 g plasma cholesterol/day, cholesterol entering the plasma in chylomicrons and VLDL particles, and from tissues into HDL, and leaving in the form of chylomicron-remnants, VLDL particles, LDL particles and by removal from HDL.

There is also turnover of cholesterol in the *enterohepatic circulation* (see Box 3.1). Bile salts, formed from cholesterol in the liver, are secreted in the bile and largely reabsorbed in the ileum. The total pool of 2.5–4 g of bile acids is recycled about twice with each meal, i.e. the turnover is rapid: about 18 g/day leaves in the bile and most of this (approximately 17.5 g) is reabsorbed. Cholesterol is also secreted in the bile, about 1 g/day; of this, about half is reabsorbed and the remainder lost in the faeces. The net loss of cholesterol and bile acids is around 1 g/day, matching input from diet and synthesis.

The enterohepatic circulation may be interrupted by a resin such as *cholestyramine* or *cholestipol* which binds the bile acids, prevents their re-absorption and leads to their excretion in faeces. More cholesterol is converted to bile acids to keep the total amount constant. If completely efficient, this treatment could lead to the loss of about 18 g of cholesterol each day – many times the normal turnover rate of the body cholesterol pool. It can thus help to lower the plasma cholesterol concentration. However, the powerful feedback control of cellular cholesterol content on HMG-CoA reductase will minimise its effect.

Data for this box taken from Newsholme & Leech (1983), Hunt & Groff (1990) and Lewis (1990).

9.2.3.2   Cholesteryl ester transfer protein

A circulating protein known as *cholesteryl ester transfer protein* (CETP) catalyses the exchange of hydrophobic lipids – cholesteryl esters and triacylglycerol – between lipoprotein particles (Fig. 9.5). They exchange by facilitated diffusion along concentration gradients. When the plasma concentration of triacylglycerol is high – for instance, after a meal when triacylglycerol-laden chylomicrons are present – CETP will catalyse the exchange of cholesteryl ester from HDL to triacylglycerol-rich lipoproteins, whilst triacylglycerol moves in the opposite direction. The cholesteryl esters remain with the triacylglycerol-rich lipoprotein particle until it is taken up by the liver as a remnant. The HDL

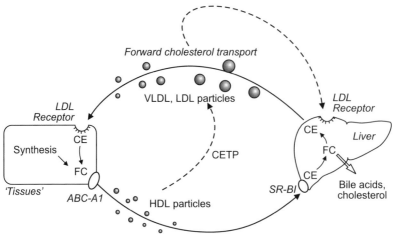

Fig. 9.5 Forward and reverse cholesterol transport. Cholesterol is secreted by the liver in VLDL particles; these become LDL particles after hydrolysis of their triacylglycerol by lipoprotein lipase and hepatic lipase (see Fig. 9.3) and are taken up by tissues via the LDL receptor. A proportion of the particles will be taken up again by the liver. Cholesterol is removed from peripheral tissues by HDL particles via interaction with the receptor ABC-A1 (more details of HDL metabolism are in Fig. 9.4). This cholesterol is transferred to the liver by interaction with the receptor SR-BI and may be excreted in the bile. An alternative fate for the cholesterol in HDL particles is transfer via the action of cholesteryl ester transfer protein (CETP) to triacylglycerol-rich particles whose remnants thus become cholesterol-enriched. This is an alternative route for transfer of cholesterol to the liver. CE, cholesteryl ester; FC, free cholesterol.

has now become enriched with triacylglycerol. This HDL-triacylglycerol can be hydrolysed by hepatic lipase, leaving smaller, cholesteryl ester-depleted HDL_3 particles which can then pick up further cholesterol from cells as outlined in the previous section.

   In terms of defence against coronary heart disease this may sound a beneficial process. Unfortunately, things are not so simple. Some species – such as the rat – do not have CETP activity, and they do not suffer from atherosclerosis. Some families have been described in whom CETP is lacking; they have high HDL-cholesterol concentrations and appear to be protected against atherosclerosis. Probably the culprit is the cholesteryl ester-enriched remnant particle that results from CETP action. This will be considered again below (Section 9.4.3).

9.3   Regulation of lipoprotein metabolism

The pathways of lipoprotein metabolism are regulated at many stages. It will come as no surprise that insulin plays a major role.

9.3.1   Insulin and triacylglycerol metabolism

The enzyme lipoprotein lipase is activated in adipose tissue by insulin, as noted in previous chapters (see Section 4.5.3.1). Thus, in the postprandial period, clearance of the triacylglycerol-rich lipoproteins is increased, and this increase in clearance occurs at the time of the peak triacylglycerol concentration in plasma, a few hours after a fatty meal. The removal of chylomicron-triacylglycerol is a saturable process, reflecting limited activity of lipoprotein lipase. After a fat-rich meal this pathway may become saturated. Both chylomicrons and VLDL compete for hydrolysis by lipoprotein lipase, a process that has been termed the *common saturable removal mechanism*. For reasons that are not entirely clear, lipoprotein lipase acts preferentially on larger particles, so chylomicrons tend to 'win'. One corollary of this competition is that the rapidity of clearance of excess triacylglycerol from the plasma in the postprandial period (i.e. after a meal) is dependent upon the subject's VLDL-triacylglycerol concentration: in someone with a low VLDL-triacylglycerol concentration, clearance of triacylglycerol after a meal tends to be more rapid. Because of the competition between chylomicron- and VLDL-triacylglycerol for hydrolysis by lipoprotein lipase, the VLDL-triacylglycerol concentration usually rises after a fatty meal (because its clearance is decreased).

It is beneficial to the individual to be able to clear excess triacylglycerol rapidly from the plasma after a meal (see Section 9.4.3, later). Thus, it makes sense for the body not to add extra VLDL-triacylglycerol to the plasma in this period. A number of studies of hepatocytes *in vitro* show that insulin suppresses VLDL output in the short term. These studies are difficult to perform *in vivo*, but in studies in which insulin has been infused into a vein, production especially of the larger, more triacylglycerol-rich VLDL particles is suppressed. In addition, the rate of VLDL-triacylglycerol secretion depends strongly on the delivery of non-esterified fatty acids from the plasma as a substrate for triacylglycerol synthesis. These are taken up by hepatocytes and esterified for secretion as VLDL-triacylglycerol. As we saw in Chapter 6 (Fig. 6.9), the concentration of non-esterified fatty acids in plasma falls after a meal due to suppression of adipose tissue lipolysis by insulin. On balance of the evidence, therefore, it seems likely that VLDL-triacylglycerol secretion is inhibited in the postprandial period.

There is an interesting parallel here with glucose metabolism following a meal. In both cases it seems that the body is 'buffering' the entry of substrates into the circulation. In the case of glucose, the entry of endogenous glucose (from hepatocytes) is suppressed after a meal, and the rate of clearance of glucose from the circulation is increased (mainly in skeletal muscle). Therefore the rise in blood glucose concentration is minimised. In the case of fat ingestion (at least when this occurs as part of a mixed meal, so that insulin release is stimulated) there is probably also a suppression of the entry of endogenous triacylglycerol into the circulation, and an increase in triacylglycerol clearance (mainly by adipose tissue). When this beautiful coordination breaks down, adverse consequences follow. In the case of glucose metabolism, failure of coordination leads to diabetes mellitus (Chapter 10). In the case of fat metabolism, it may lead to atherosclerosis (see Section 9.4.3).

9.3.2   Relationship between plasma triacylglycerol and HDL-cholesterol concentrations

In studies of large numbers of individuals, an inverse relationship is usually observed between plasma triacylglycerol and HDL-cholesterol concentrations: the higher the subject's plasma triacylglycerol concentration, the lower tends to be the HDL-cholesterol concentration. We can now see how this inverse relationship is brought about.

Because the hydrolysis of the triacylglycerol-rich lipoproteins by lipoprotein lipase is accompanied by the transfer of cholesterol and other surface components into HDL, the HDL concentration can be increased by a rapid lipoprotein lipase action in the postprandial period. A rapid action of lipoprotein lipase may reflect a high activity of the enzyme (this might reflect physical fitness, for example, when its activity in skeletal muscle will be high) and/or it may reflect low competition from VLDL-triacylglycerol. In both cases this is likely to be reflected in a low fasting triacylglycerol concentration. At the other extreme, if removal of triacylglycerol is slow, then there will be increased opportunity for lipid exchange via the action of CETP. Thus, HDL will become depleted of cholesteryl esters, and the triacylglycerol-rich lipoprotein remnants will become enriched with them. Again, the inverse relationship between plasma triacylglycerol and HDL-cholesterol concentrations will result.

9.3.3   Cholesterol homeostasis

There is continuous turnover of the body's pool of about 140 g of cholesterol (free and esterified). This is discussed in Box 9.4.

Insulin may regulate cholesterol turnover at a number of points. Insulin activates the enzyme HMG-CoA reductase by reversible dephosphorylation. Thus, insulin increases cholesterol synthesis. However, this effect is probably less important than the control by cellular cholesterol content discussed above (Box 9.3). Insulin also seems to stimulate expression of the LDL receptor: during insulin infusion, in an experimental situation, removal of LDL-cholesterol is increased, and the effect has been demonstrated in hepatocyte cultures *in vitro*. It is not known whether this occurs in all tissues or just in the liver. However, again, hormonal effects on cholesterol homeostasis do not seem to be of major importance compared with the regulation by cellular cholesterol content.

9.4   Disturbances of lipoprotein metabolism

9.4.1   Cholesterol and atherosclerosis

Lipoprotein metabolism has come to prominence because of its link with coronary heart disease. Coronary heart disease means a blockage – partial or complete – of one or more of the *coronary arteries* which supply blood to the muscular walls of the heart (the *myocardium*) (see Section 4.5). It arises initially because of the development of fatty deposits in the arterial walls – the process known as *atherosclerosis*. Atherosclerosis may affect arteries anywhere in the body, and can lead to impaired blood supply to the limbs, for instance – a particular problem in heavy smokers. But when it affects the blood supply to the heart, then the results can be fatal. At first, the restriction on blood supply to the myocardium may appear as chest pains (*angina*) during exercise, when the demand on the myocardium increases. Later, complete blockage may occur as the result of a blood clot at the site of the atherosclerotic lesion – this is a *coronary thrombosis*, or heart attack, also called a *myocardial infarction*. The region of myocardium supplied by the artery may necrose (die). More importantly in the short term, local disturbances in contraction of the heart can lead to disturbances in the electrical coordination of contraction, and the heart may go into uncoordinated fluttering (*ventricular fibrillation*) or stop completely (*asystole* or *cardiac arrest*). This is a serious situation with a high mortality.

The fatty deposit is known as an *atherosclerotic plaque*. It is a complex structure, involving inflammation and proliferation of the smooth muscle cells of the arterial wall and connective tissue (collagen fibrils) as well as a pool of cholesterol-rich lipid. It is thought to begin as a smaller lesion called the *fatty streak*; this fatty deposit is one of the earliest visible signs during the development of atherosclerosis. The fatty streak stems from the accumulation of so-called *foam cells*. These are cells that, under light microscopy, appear to be laden with foam. In fact they are macrophages, and the foamy appearance reflects an accumulation of lipid, mainly cholesterol. Hence, cholesterol accumulation is one of the first events in the development of atherosclerosis.

The link between cholesterol in the blood and coronary heart disease was recognised in part because the incidence of coronary heart disease varies widely from one country to another: in Finland, for instance, the incidence is almost ten times the incidence in Japan, although this differential is changing as the diets and lifestyles of countries change. The average concentration of cholesterol in the blood also varies widely from country to country, and it varies almost exactly in parallel with the incidence of coronary heart disease (Fig. 9.6). Within any one country, the incidence of coronary heart disease also varies with the plasma cholesterol concentration. These are *epidemiological* findings and not proof of cause and effect. In recent years, however, several long-term studies in people at high risk of coronary heart disease have shown that lowering of the plasma cholesterol concentration significantly reduces mortality from coronary heart disease.

9.4.2   Conditions leading to elevation of the blood cholesterol concentration

The average concentration of cholesterol in the blood of people in the United

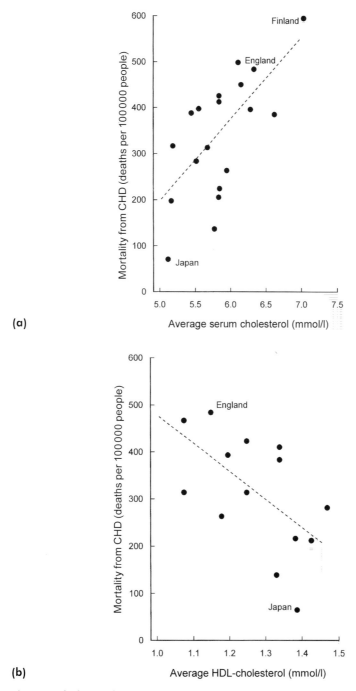

(a)

(b)

Fig. 9.6 Cholesterol and heart disease. The top panel shows the relationship between average serum cholesterol concentration and mortality from coronary heart disease in males in different countries. The lower panel shows the inverse relationship between average serum HDL-cholesterol concentration and mortality from coronary heart disease in males in different countries. The dashed lines are the regression lines. Redrawn, based on Simons L.A. (1986) Interrelations of lipids and lipoproteins with coronary artery disease mortality in 19 countries. *Am J. Cardiol* 57: 5G–10G, with permission from Excerpta Medica Inc.

Kingdom is about 6 mmol/l, of which the major portion – around 4 mmol/l – is carried in the LDL fraction. The average concentration of triacylglycerol in the blood after an overnight fast is about 1–2 mmol/l. An elevated concentration of lipids in the blood is referred to as *hyperlipidaemia*. When it is necessary to distinguish the contribution of different lipids, then elevation of the cholesterol concentration is known as *hypercholesterolaemia*, elevation of the triacylglycerol concentration as *hypertriglyceridaemia*. (The correct chemical term used in this book is triacylglycerol rather than triglyceride, but physicians are not quite ready to battle with hypertriacylglycerolaemia.)

The blood lipid concentration may be elevated because the subject has a genetic disposition to a raised concentration (*primary hyperlipidaemia*), or because of factors in the individual's environment – diet, lifestyle, other diseases, etc. (*secondary hyperlipidaemia*). There is an alternative classification, completely based on the phenotype without consideration of the underlying cause (the Fredrickson classification), although sometimes the underlying cause may be inferred from the phenotype (Table 9.2).

Table 9.2 The classification of hyperlipidaemias according to phenotype.

Type	Plasma cholesterol	Plasma triacylglycerol	Particles accumulating	Usual underlying defect
I	+	+++	Chylomicrons	Lipoprotein lipase deficiency, apolipoprotein CII deficiency
IIa	++	N	LDL	LDL receptor defect or LDL overproduction
IIb	++	++	VLDL, LDL	VLDL or LDL overproduction or impaired clearance
III	++	++	Chylomicron- and VLDL-remnants	Impaired remnant removal; may be due to particular isoform of apolipoprotein E, or apo-E deficiency
IV	N or +	++	VLDL	VLDL overproduction or clearance defect
V	+	+++	Chylomicrons, VLDL and remnants	Lipoprotein lipase defect (not complete absence) or apolipoprotein CII deficiency

This is known as the Fredrickson classification after the American clinician and biochemist, Donald Fredrickson. N, normal; +, mildly raised; ++, moderately raised; +++, severely raised.

9.4.2.1   Primary hyperlipoproteinaemias

The most dramatic primary hyperlipidaemias are those known as *familial hypercholesterolaemia* (FH) and *Type I hyperlipoproteinaemia* (Table 9.2), also known as *chylomicronaemia syndrome*.

The first of these, FH, is manifest by a consistently raised blood cholesterol concentration, typically 8–10 mmol/l in people heterozygous for the disease (about 1 in 500 people in the UK), but more like 15–20 mmol/l in people who are homozygous (i.e. who have two copies of the gene which causes it). The incidence of coronary heart disease in such people is very high unless they are adequately treated to lower the cholesterol concentration. This is another reason for believing that there is a direct cause-and-effect link between elevated blood cholesterol concentration and atherosclerosis. The defect in FH is in the amino acid sequence of the LDL receptor. Many genetic defects have been described: some lead to LDL receptors that cannot bind LDL particles normally, others prevent expression of the receptor on the cell surface. The net result is that LDL particles remain in the circulation. Recently, it has been realised that defects in the sequence of apolipoprotein B may produce a very similar syndrome. Because lipoprotein cholesterol is not being taken up into cells, the pathway of cholesterol synthesis is not repressed, and this adds to the problem.

Treatment of FH may involve a low-cholesterol diet, and substances (resins) which bind cholesterol and bile salts in the intestine, preventing their reabsorption (see Box 9.4). However, the preferred form of treatment now is the use of drugs (the *statins*) which inhibit the pathway of cholesterol synthesis at the enzyme HMG-CoA reductase. The effect of this is not just to reduce cholesterol synthesis. Because cellular cholesterol content is reduced, the synthesis of LDL receptors is up-regulated by the SCAP-SREBP2 system (see Fig. 2.6 and Box 9.3). Increased expression of LDL receptors, especially in the liver, means that LDL particles are removed from the blood and so the blood cholesterol concentration falls.

Type I hyperlipoproteinaemia is a very rare condition, also inherited, in which chylomicrons accumulate in the plasma, giving it a creamy appearance. The major abnormality, unlike FH, is therefore accumulation of triacylglycerol rather than cholesterol. The plasma triacylglycerol concentration may reach 50 or even 100 mmol/l. Interestingly, people with this condition seem not to be at increased risk of coronary heart disease. (This is disputed by some, but the risk is certainly not as high as in FH.) They are at risk of inflammation of the pancreas (*pancreatitis*). This can be very serious: if the pancreatic juices, with their potent digestive enzymes, leak into the abdominal cavity, the results can be life-threatening. So the disease must be treated, but this can be done very effectively by means of a low-fat diet. Without dietary fat, chylomicrons do not accumulate. The defect in Type I hyperlipoproteinaemia is usually in the enzyme lipoprotein lipase: sufferers are deficient in this enzyme. The condition is only noticed in people who are homozygous for the defect: heterozygotes have sufficient lipoprotein lipase activity to remove chylomicrons relatively normally. In a few cases, the lipoprotein lipase is normal, but the sufferers lack apolipoprotein CII, the essential co-factor for lipoprotein lipase activity.

Type III hyperlipoproteinaemia is another condition with a genetic basis. The particles that accumulate are remnants of VLDL and chylomicrons. We all carry two copies of the gene for apolipoprotein E (apoE) (as we do of all genes except for those on the sex chromosomes). There are two common genetic variations in the apoE gene, leading to either a cysteine or an arginine at position 112, and the same at position 158. This leads to three common forms of apoE: cysteine at both positions (known as apoE2), cystine at 122, arginine at 158 (apoE3) and arginine at both positions (apoE4). (ApoE1 was identified at one time but then recognised to represent the presence of a carbohydrate group, sialic acid: thus it is not a sequence variant. There are also other mutations in apoE at different positions that give similar electrophoretic mobilities to the variants described above.) ApoE is involved in the binding of remnant particles to the LDL receptor. ApoE2 binds much less well than the other forms, and people who have two copies of apoE2 therefore have a defect in removal of remnant particles from their plasma. About 1 in 10 000 people have Type III hyperlipoproteinaemia, although about 1 in 100 people are homozygous for apoE2. The disease becomes manifest when some other condition is present, such as obesity, diabetes or hypothyroidism, or when other genetic variations are present that in themselves might not result in disease. Accordingly, type III hyperlipoproteinaemia is inherited in a polygenic fashion, rather than the monogenic inheritance pattern of Type I hyperlipoproteinaemia or familial hypercholesterolaemia.

9.4.2.2 Secondary hyperlipoproteinaemias

Secondary hyperlipidaemias arise because of diet, bodily factors (e.g. obesity) or other diseases (e.g. diabetes). Here, we will look briefly only at the first of these. The effects of obesity and diabetes will be covered in the next two chapters.

The average blood cholesterol concentration varies widely, as we saw earlier, from country to country. This might reflect racial genetic differences, but it does not seem to. Japanese people who have moved to the USA have cholesterol concentrations and rates of coronary heart disease which are as high as, or even higher than, other Americans. Something in the Japanese lifestyle keeps the cholesterol concentration low, and evidence suggests that this is a dietary factor. Dietary factors and the serum cholesterol concentration are discussed in Box 9.5.

As Box 9.5 makes clear, dietary fatty acids play a much more important role in determining the serum cholesterol concentration than does dietary cholesterol. The means by which individual fatty acids affect the plasma cholesterol concentration are not entirely clear, although one mechanism has been elucidated. It appears that saturated fatty acids in the liver affect the distribution of hepatic cholesterol between unesterified and esterified forms. In the presence

Box 9.5 Dietary influences on the serum cholesterol concentration

Dietary cholesterol
Perhaps surprisingly, the amount of cholesterol in the diet is not a major factor affecting the blood cholesterol concentration. The amount of cholesterol we eat is not large in comparison with the body pool: we eat less than 1 g per day whereas the amount of cholesterol in the body is more like 140 g, of which about 8 g is present in the plasma (Box 9.4). Contrast this with glucose, where we eat several 'plasma's-worth' in a single meal (see Section 6.1). And cholesterol is not rapidly absorbed like glucose: it enters the plasma slowly, even more so than triacylglycerol. Further, cholesterol intake leads to cholesterol entering cells, which effectively suppresses cholesterol synthesis. The blood cholesterol concentration is related far more closely to the dietary intake of particular fatty acids, especially the ratio of saturated to polyunsaturated fatty acids.

Dietary fatty acids
The initial evidence for the role of saturated fatty acids in raising serum cholesterol concentrations was epidemiological: the wide differences in average plasma cholesterol concentration between different countries were found to relate to the average consumption of saturated fatty acids. More detailed studies since have shown that this is an over-generalisation. Particular saturated fatty acids are worse 'culprits' than others: stearic acid (18:0) seems to be relatively inert whereas palmitic acid (16:0) and myristic acid (14:0) raise the cholesterol concentration. In contrast, polyunsaturated fatty acids (e.g. linoleic acid, 18:2 *n*-6) have a cholesterol-lowering effect. There has been debate about the effect of monounsaturated fatty acids (oleic acid, 18:1, found in olive oil, is the most common example in the diet). These were until recently thought to be relatively neutral in terms of cholesterol concentrations, but recent evidence suggests that they also lower blood cholesterol. (The experiments to test this are difficult to design: if an experimenter wants to increase the proportion of monounsaturated fatty acid in the diet, something else has to be left out, and the answer may well depend on what is omitted.)

A change in the fatty acid content of the diet will produce a fairly predictable change in serum cholesterol concentration, and formulae have been derived to predict this, such as:

$$\Delta \text{Serum cholesterol} = 0.026 \times (2.16\Delta S - 1.65\Delta P + 6.66\Delta C - 0.53)$$

where ΔSerum cholesterol represents the change in serum cholesterol concentration in mmol/l, ΔS the change in dietary saturated fatty acids (expressed as percentage of energy derived from them), ΔP the change in dietary polyunsaturated fatty acids, and ΔC the change in dietary cholesterol expressed in 100 mg per day. The factor 0.026 converts from mg/dl to mmol/l. Source: Hegsted *et al.* (1965).

The important point is that dietary saturated fatty acids have a larger detrimental effect than the beneficial effect of polyunsaturated fatty acids (the factor for ΔS in the equation is greater than that for ΔP): hence the advice for many people to change from dairy products such as butter, which contain a high proportion of saturated fatty acids, to spreads based on vegetable oils containing more unsaturated fats.

A few points should be stressed. Firstly, such a change alone may make an insignificant difference to coronary heart disease risk in any one individual, and other lifestyle factors (e.g. smoking, physical activity, body weight) may need to be modified as well to influence risk of coronary heart disease. Secondly, many people are misled into thinking that spreads containing unsaturated fatty acids are less *fattening* than dairy products: this is, of course, not so.

Margarines are made by hardening unsaturated vegetable oils by the process of *hydrogenation* – reduction of some of the double bonds. (Remember from Chapter 1 that the more saturated fatty acids have higher melting points.) In this process, some of the double bonds are converted to the *trans*-configuration rather than the usual *cis*-. *Trans*-unsaturated fatty acids seem to behave similarly to saturated fatty acids with respect to cholesterol-raising. Most spread manufacturers, at least in the UK, have now recognised this and largely removed *trans*-unsaturated fatty acids from their products.

This box concerns effects on the serum cholesterol concentration. The polyunsaturated fatty acids referred to above are predominantly those of the *n*-6 family. The *n*-3 polyunsaturated fatty acids, as found in fish oils, have different effects. They are relatively neutral in terms of serum cholesterol, but they are quite potent in lowering serum triacylglycerol concentrations. They also have other beneficial effects in relation to coronary heart disease, such as reducing the tendency of platelets to aggregate.

of saturated fatty acids, there is less conversion of unesterified cholesterol to cholesteryl esters. Since it is the tissue unesterified cholesterol content which down-regulates LDL-receptor expression, this change will lead to decreased expression of hepatic LDL-receptors, and thus an elevation of the plasma LDL concentration.

9.4.3   HDL-cholesterol, plasma triacylglycerol and coronary heart disease

Although an elevated LDL-cholesterol concentration is certainly an important marker for risk of coronary heart disease, it is also true that if people who suffer a heart attack, especially those who do so at a relatively early age, are studied, a large proportion will not have elevated cholesterol concentrations. In terms of total risk in the population, factors other than LDL-cholesterol are more important. One important marker of risk is the combination of reduced HDL-cholesterol and elevated triacylglycerol concentrations.

Unlike LDL-cholesterol, elevated HDL-cholesterol concentrations are associated with *decreased* risk of coronary heart disease (Fig. 9.6). The converse is that a low HDL-cholesterol concentration is a marker of increased risk.

It was mentioned earlier that, in studies of large numbers of people, an inverse relationship is observed between plasma triacylglycerol and HDL-cholesterol concentrations. We have seen already (Section 9.3.2) how the inverse relationship between HDL-cholesterol and plasma triacylglycerol concentrations may be brought about. There are two lines of thought about their relationships with coronary heart disease risk. Firstly, HDL-cholesterol may in itself be associated with protection against coronary heart disease. This may reflect the fact that it is a marker of the efficiency of reverse cholesterol transport, the removal of cholesterol from tissues.

Alternatively, low HDL-cholesterol concentrations (and thus increased risk) may be a marker for some defect in the metabolism of the triacylglycerol-rich lipoproteins. One implication of defective metabolism of the triacylglycerol-rich lipoproteins is that their remnant particles remain for longer in the circulation whilst they are reduced to a sufficiently small size for receptor-mediated uptake. They also become cholesterol-enriched through the action of CETP. These cholesterol-rich remnants themselves may be taken up to initiate the formation of atherosclerotic lesions.

The idea that remnant particles have atherogenic potential explains neatly why people with lipoprotein lipase deficiency and enormously elevated plasma triacylglycerol concentrations are not at risk of coronary heart disease; if their particles are not metabolised at all, no smaller remnants will be produced. In this view, a 'sluggish' metabolism of the triacylglycerol-rich lipoproteins is worse than none at all. Such a condition may result from a genetic change in the lipoprotein lipase sequence, such that the enzyme is not completely ineffective but is less effective than normal. Alternatively it may reflect an increased concentration of VLDL-triacylglycerol which will prevent efficient clearance of chylomicron-triacylglycerol because of competition for lipoprotein lipase. This may result, in turn, from increased hepatic VLDL synthesis or impaired clearance. These are very much areas of current research.

An alternative view of why the combination of low HDL-cholesterol and elevated triacylglycerol concentrations leads to atherosclerosis is that these changes are also associated with alterations in the nature of LDL particles, in a combination of lipoprotein alterations called the *atherogenic lipoprotein phenotype*. This is discussed in Box 9.6.

A common theme relevant to the low HDL-cholesterol/elevated triacylglycerol combination is that of impaired postprandial lipid metabolism. Giv-

Box 9.6   The atherogenic lipoprotein phenotype

In the text the combination of a low HDL-cholesterol concentration with an elevated triacylglycerol concentration is described. These two are closely related with another change in lipoproteins: the LDL particles in the circulation are smaller and more dense than normal. This combination is often called the atherogenic lipoprotein phenotype. It is more common than simple elevation of the plasma cholesterol concentration, and may therefore be a bigger risk factor in population terms for coronary heart disease.

LDL particles are not all of the same size. In any one individual there is a population of particles with different sizes. As for all lipoprotein particles, the larger particles are less dense. In the atherogenic lipoprotein phenotype, the population of particles is skewed towards the smaller, denser end of the spectrum. The mechanism by which this occurs is outlined in Fig. 9.6.1.

Why does this shift in the density of LDL particles matter? It is proposed that small LDL particles may be particularly likely to leave the circulation by penetrating the endothelial lining, and enter the sub-endothelial space. Here they may be exposed to oxidative stress, and small, dense lipid-depleted particles may be particularly at risk of oxidative damage because in losing their core lipid, they may have lost fat-soluble antioxidant vitamins. These oxidatively damaged particles may then be taken up by macrophage scavenger receptors (see Section 9.2.2.2) to begin the process of foam-cell formation and eventually atherosclerosis.

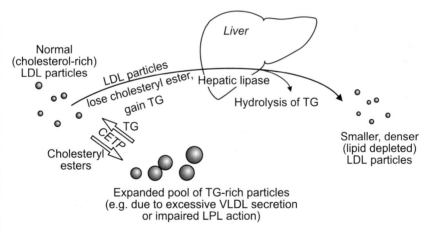

Fig. 9.6.1   CETP, cholesteryl ester transfer protein (see Section 9.2.3.2); TG, triacylglycerol.

ing a fatty meal 'stresses' the fat metabolism system and may unmask defects (Fig. 9.7), just as giving oral glucose can be used to test for adequate glucose metabolism (discussed in Chapter 10; see Box 10.2). But eating meals that contain fat is also part of everyday life. Suppose someone has a reduced ability to clear triacylglycerol from the circulation in the period following a meal. This may reflect low activity of lipoprotein lipase, increased competition for clearance from VLDL particles, or many other factors (see Section 9.3.1). The consequence will be a reduced transfer of cholesterol (from the action of lipoprotein lipase on triacylglycerol-rich particles) into HDL particles, and also, through the action of CETP, loss of cholesterol from the HDL pool (these mechanisms were explained in more detail in Section 9.3.2). In addition, the walls of blood vessels will be exposed for longer to the potentially atherogenic remnants of the triacylglycerol-rich lipoproteins. Impaired postprandial lipid metabolism may be more than just a diagnostic test: it may reflect a situation that occurs several times a day, day after day, leading to atherosclerosis. It is, incidentally, a common feature of conditions in which insulin is not as effective as usual (*insulin resistance*: see Box 10.1), for reasons which are relatively obvious if we think about the normal roles of insulin in coordinating lipid metabolism. These conditions include physical inactivity, obesity and Type II diabetes mellitus, in all of which there is a predisposition to atherosclerosis.

Treatment of this condition may involve modification of the factors that predispose to it, e.g. increasing physical activity and losing of weight. But there is one group of drugs that is particularly effective in reducing elevated triacyl-

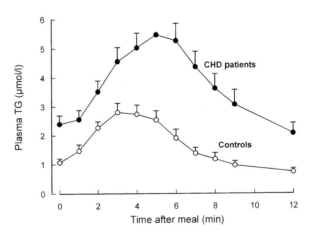

Fig. 9.7 Impaired postprandial triacylglycerol metabolism in patients with coronary heart disease. A meal containing a relatively large amount of fat (50 g per m² body surface area; around 100 g for most people) was given at time 0. Open points show healthy controls (*n* = 10); solid point show patients who have had a myocardial infarction (at least 5 years before the test) (*n* = 34). The patients show elevated triacylglycerol (TG) concentrations in the fasting state (time 0) and an exaggerated rise in plasma triacylglycerol concentration after the fat load, showing an impairment of the normal rapid metabolism of dietary triacylglycerol. From Karpe *et al.* (1992) with permission.

glycerol concentrations and raising HDL-cholesterol. These are the fibric acid derivatives or *fibrates*. The fibrates are agonists for the liver nuclear receptor PPARα (see Section 2.1.3.2). By activating this receptor, they increase fatty acid oxidation and reduce triacylglycerol synthesis. Activation of PPARα also affects apolipoprotein synthesis in the liver. Expression of apo-AI and apo-AII increases. Since these are important components of HDL, more HDL particles may be formed and the HDL-cholesterol concentration increases. Expression of apo-CIII is reduced. Since this apolipoprotein may be an inhibitor of lipo-protein lipase (Box 9.1) this will enhance triacylglycerol clearance from the circulation. Activation of PPARα can in addition induce lipoprotein lipase ex-pression. The significance of this is not immediately clear since this would be a hepatic effect (PPARα is expressed mainly in the liver) but the adult liver does not normally express lipoprotein lipase. In animal experiments, it seems that the fibrates do indeed reactivate lipoprotein lipase expression in the liver (it is normally switched off early in life) but the situation is not clear in humans.

9.5   Further reading

General on lipid metabolism
Gurr, M.I., Harwood, J.L. & Frayn, K.N. (2002) *Lipid Biochemistry: An Introduction*, 5th edn. Oxford: Blackwell Science.

Lipoprotein lipase and triacylglycerol-rich lipoprotein metabolism
(See also Further Reading in Chapters 4 and 6 for additional reviews on lipo-protein lipase)
Braun, J.E.A. & Severson, D.L. (1992) Regulation of the synthesis, processing and translocation of lipoprotein lipase. *Biochem J* 287: 337–347.
Havel, R.J. (1997) Postprandial lipid metabolism: an overview. *Proc Nutr Soc* 56: 659–666.
White, D.A., Bennett, A.J., Billett, M.A. & Salter, A.M. (1998) The assembly of triacylglycerol-rich lipoproteins: an essential role for the microsomal triacylglycerol transfer protein. *Br J Nutr* 80: 219–229.
Karpe, F. (1999) Postprandial lipoprotein metabolism and atherosclerosis. *J Intern Med* 246: 341–355.

Cholesterol metabolism
Rye, K.A., Clay, M.A. & Barter, P.J. (1999) Remodelling of high density lipoproteins by plasma factors. *Atherosclerosis* 145: 227–238.
Tall, A.R., Jiang, X.-C., Luo, Y. & Silver, D. (2000) 1999 George Lyman Duff memorial lecture: lipid transfer proteins, HDL metabolism, and atherogenesis. *Arterioscler Thromb Vasc Biol* 20: 1185–1188.

Chang, T.-Y., Chang, C.C.Y., Lin, S., Yu, C., Li, B.-L.& Miyazaki, A. (2001) Roles of acyl-coenzyme A:cholesterol acyltransferase-1 and -2. *Curr Opin Lipidol* 12: 289–296.

Groenendijk, M., Cantor, R.M., de Bruin, T.W., Dalling, A. & Thie, G.M. (2001) The apoAI-CIII-AIV gene cluster. *Atherosclerosis* 157: 1–11.

Oram, J.F. & Lawn, R.M. (2001) ABCA1. The gatekeeper for eliminating excess tissue cholesterol. *J Lipid Res* 42: 1173–1179.

Lin, G. (2002) Insights of high-density lipoprotein apolipoprotein-mediated lipid efflux from cells. *Biochem Biophys Res Commun* 291: 727–731.

(See also Further Reading in Chapter 2 for additional reviews on ABC family transporters)

Nutrition, exercise and lipoproteins

Hardman, A.E. (1999) Physical activity, obesity and blood lipids. *Int J Obes* 23 Suppl 3:S64–S71.

Schaefer, E.J. (2002) Lipoproteins, nutrition, and heart disease. *Am J Clin Nutr* 75: 191–212.

Disorders of lipoprotein metabolism, atherosclerosis and treatment

Durrington, P.N. (1995) *Hyperlipidaemia: Diagnosis and Management*, 2nd edn. Oxford: Butterworth-Heinemann Ltd.

Havel, R.J, & Rapaport, E. (1995) Management of primary hyperlipidemia. *New Engl J Med* 332: 1491–1498.

Brewer, H.B., Jr. (2000) The lipid-laden foam cell: an elusive target for therapeutic intervention. *J Clin Invest* 105: 703–705.

Barbier, O., Pineda Torra, I., Duguay, Y. *et al.* (2002) Pleiotropic actions of peroxisome proliferator-activated receptors in lipid metabolism and atherosclerosis. *Arterioscler Thromb Vasc Biol* 22: 717–726.

10

Diabetes Mellitus

10.1 Different types of diabetes

The disease *diabetes mellitus*, if untreated, is characterised by intense thirst and frequent urination. Hence its name *diabetes*, from the Greek for syphon. The term *mellitus* means to do with honey – i.e. sweet. It refers to the fact that the urine is sticky and sweet with glucose. There is a completely different, and much rarer, disease also called diabetes: this is *diabetes insipidus*. Diabetes insipidus is also characterised by thirst and urination, but the urine is *insipid* or watery, and not sweet. Diabetes insipidus is caused by a failure of the *antidiuretic hormone* (also called *vasopressin* – see Section 5.3.2) to act, either because of a lack of the hormone, or because of a defect in the receptors for antidiuretic hormone in the kidney. Diabetes insipidus will not be considered further here.

Diabetes mellitus (which will be referred to simply as diabetes in this chapter) can itself be divided into two main types (Table 10.1). In one, the disease usually develops during childhood or adolescence. People with this type of diabetes tend to be on the thin side. In this type of diabetes, lack of treatment leads to severe illness; and the only effective treatment is injection of the hormone insulin. This is known as *Type 1 diabetes mellitus* or in older literature as *insulin-dependent diabetes mellitus* (IDDM). In the other, more common form, the disease usually starts later in life – from the mid-thirties onwards. Those who develop this form of the disease are very often overweight. This form of the disease is not life-threatening in the short term even if not treated, and adequate treatment does not require the use of insulin in the early stages. But it is a mistake to think of this as a milder form of diabetes, as we shall see: the longer-term consequences of lack of treatment are just as severe as in Type 1 diabetes. This form of diabetes is known as *Type 2 diabetes mellitus* or, in older literature, *non-insulin dependent diabetes mellitus* (NIDDM).

Table 10.1 Different forms of diabetes mellitus.

	Type 1 diabetes	Type 2 diabetes
Other names	Juvenile-onset diabetes; insulin-dependent diabetes mellitus (IDDM)	Maturity-onset diabetes; non-insulin-dependent diabetes mellitus (NIDDM)
Defect	Auto-immune destruction of β-cells	Defective insulin secretion *and* insulin resistance
Age of onset (typical)	1–25	> 40*
Bodily physique (typical)	Lean (weight loss at diagnosis)	Obese
Prevalence (whole population)	0.5%	2%
Inheritance	ca. 50%	ca. 70–80%
Treatment	Insulin injections	Diet, drugs, later insulin injections

*But there is an alarming trend to the development of Type 2 diabetes at earlier ages, even in childhood, as children in affluent societies become fatter and less physically active.

10.2   History of the study of diabetes, and its clinical features

10.2.1   History of diabetes

The disease of diabetes mellitus has been described since antiquity. The earliest known record is in an Egyptian papyrus dating from around 1500 BC. The Greek physician Aretaeus of Cappadocia named the disease 'diabetes' in the first century AD and described the short and painful life of sufferers: 'it consists in the flesh and bones running together into urine; the patients are tortured with an unquenchable thirst; the whole body wastes away...'. It is often claimed that the English physician, Thomas Willis, was the first to notice the sweet taste of the urine in 1679, but this fact is actually recorded in much earlier writings from the East. Indian medical writings, for instance, noted that ants find a particular interest in the urine of sufferers. The same writings also distinguished the two types of sufferer: young and thin, or older and overweight.

Important milestones in understanding the disease occurred in the nineteenth century. These were the discovery of the islets of Langerhans in the pancreas in 1869 (see Section 5.2.1), and the observation by Oskar Minkowski and Joseph von Mering in Strasbourg in 1889 that removal of a dog's pancreas led to diabetes. This was a chance observation, made whilst they investigated the role of the pancreas in fat absorption. Minkowski and von Mering also noted that if they attached a small piece of pancreas to the inside of the abdominal cavity, the dog did not develop diabetes; and this led to the idea that the pancreas produced a substance that was essential for normal metabolism. The name *insulin* was given to this hypothetical substance by the English physiologist Edward Sharpey-Schafer, from *insula*, the Latin for island. By that time, a link between the diabetes and destruction of the pancreatic islets was suspected. This was based partly on the observations of an American pathologist, Eugene Opie, at the turn of the century, that the islets were destroyed in the pancreas of patients who had died of diabetes – which was then, of course, a fatal disease. In 1921 in Toronto Dr Frederick Banting and Charles Best, a medical student assisting him, made an extract of pancreas which, when injected into a dog (called Marjorie) made diabetic by removal of her pancreas, restored her to health. Production of this extract from the pancreases of cows and pigs was increased as rapidly as possible and it was soon made available (at first in small quantities) for treatment of human sufferers. The first person to be treated was a 14-year-old boy, Leonard Thompson. For such people it was a life-saving treatment (Fig. 10.1).

10.2.2 Type 1 diabetes mellitus

Type 1 diabetes results from destruction of the insulin-secreting cells of the islets of Langerhans. This destruction is auto-immune in nature – i.e. it is brought about by the body's own natural defences, but directed against one of its own tissues. The liability to develop Type 1 diabetes is to some extent inherited, but

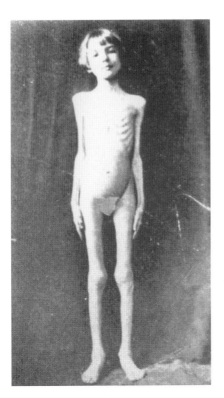 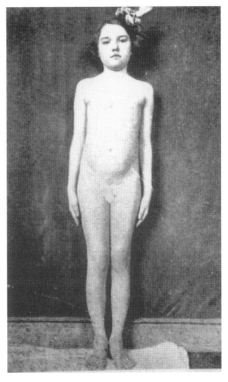

Fig. 10.1 A sufferer from Type 1 diabetes mellitus in the early days of insulin therapy, before (left) and after (right) treatment with insulin. Reproduced from Bliss (1983).

amongst identical twins (who have the same genetic complement), if one has Type 1 diabetes, only around 40% of their twins will have the disease.[1] Thus, something in the environment must set the disease process in motion. There are a number of theories about what this trigger might be, including a belief that the trigger is a viral infection. Some people also believe that a traumatic episode can trigger off diabetes. However, none of these theories is proven. What is clear is that the metabolic changes in Type 1 diabetes essentially represent a deficiency of insulin, and can largely be treated by injection of insulin. Type 1 diabetes is not a very common disease; it is present in about 0.5% of the population in the United Kingdom, and rather less in warmer parts of the world. However, the incidence of Type 1 diabetes is increasing in some parts of the world, including the United Kingdom and particularly Scandinavia.

10.2.3 Type 2 diabetes mellitus

Type 2 diabetes mellitus does not result so clearly from insulin deficiency. Defects in insulin secretion in people with Type 2 diabetes can be unmasked by laboratory tests: in particular, the initial phase of insulin secretion in re-sponse to a glucose load appears to be defective at an early stage in the disease. However, the prominent defect in Type 2 diabetes is not so much a deficiency of insulin, as a failure of insulin, at relatively normal concentrations, to exert its normal effects: this is the condition known as *insulin resistance* (Fig. 10.2). Insulin resistance may have widespread effects (Box 10.1).

   Insulin resistance is also a prominent feature of obesity (see Section 11.4.4). One very plausible hypothesis for the development of Type 2 diabetes is the fol-lowing. When people become obese, their tissues become resistant to the ac-

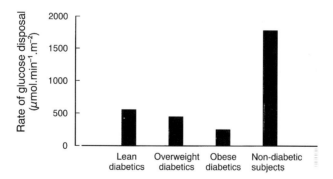

Fig. 10.2 Rates of insulin-stimulated glucose disposal in non-diabetic controls, and in lean, overweight and obese people with Type 2 diabetes. Insulin was infused intravenously to produce the same plasma insulin concentration in all subjects. None of the diabetic subjects responds to the same extent as the controls – this is the phenomenon of *insulin resistance* (Box 10.1). Amongst the diabetics, the more overweight are more severely affected. Based on Alberti, K.G.M.M., Boucher, B.J., Hitman, G.A. & Taylor, R. (1990) Diabetes mellitus. In: *The Metabolic and Molecular Basis of Acquired Disease* Vol. 1 (eds Cohen, R.D., Lewis, B., Alberti, K.G.M.M. & Denman, A.M.), 765–840. With permission of the publisher W.B. Saunders.

tions of insulin. Therefore, the concentration of glucose in the blood increases, initially only a little, and insulin is released in greater quantities from the pancreas. In obese subjects, concentrations of insulin in the plasma, and their response to a glucose load, are thus actually greater than normal. Some people can maintain this increased insulin secretion throughout their life, and carry on as obese but non-diabetic individuals. In others, however, who are predisposed genetically, the ability of the islets to sustain high rates of insulin production begins to fail. At first insulin levels may fall to a little less than necessary, so the glucose concentration rises somewhat, but insulin levels may still be greater than in insulin-sensitive people. Then they may fall further, to typical 'normal' levels, but with an elevated glucose concentration; and in the later stages of the disease to less than normal. Insulin resistance will still be prominent. The result is clinically evident diabetes. However, because some pancreatic insulin secretion remains, these people do not usually need insulin for treatment in the early stages. In those who manage to lose considerable amounts of weight (especially early in the disease) the diabetes may revert almost to normal, and some patients are managed on strict diet alone.

Type 2 diabetes is a more common disease than Type 1 diabetes. It is present in about 2% of the population in the Western world, but its incidence increases steeply with age: in the over-70 year age group, for instance, the prevalence approaches 10%. It is more strongly inherited than is Type 1 diabetes: amongst identical twins, if one twin has Type 2 diabetes, the chances are more than 90% that the other twin will have the disease. But again environment must play an important part. For instance, the incidence of Type 2 diabetes in people living in rural areas in the Indian subcontinent is low, but in Indians living in Britain the incidence is very high, and increasing: it is thought that some feature of the lifestyle here, probably related to diet and lack of exercise, leads to the development of the disease in a group who are genetically predisposed.

10.3   Alterations in metabolism in diabetes mellitus

It is important to draw a distinction here between the metabolic alterations that occur in untreated diabetes mellitus, and those which occur in people with the disease nowadays, who usually receive treatment. The former may be studied in animal models of the disease in which drugs which are selectively toxic to the pancreatic islets are given to abolish or severely restrict insulin secretion.

It is a mistake to think, however, that people with treated diabetes are free from metabolic problems. It is now rare, at least in the developed world, for them to die from acute lack of insulin. But their life expectancy is reduced, and their quality of life may be reduced by progressive onset of so-called *diabetic complications*. These will be considered further below, together with the reasons why treatment does not always produce a totally healthy individual.

10.3.1 Untreated Type 1 diabetes

The metabolic picture in untreated Type 1 diabetes, outlined in Fig. 10.3, is very much what we might predict from knowledge of the normal role of insulin. It is a *catabolic state*, i.e. there is breakdown of fuel stores and tissues. Lack of insulin leads to a net mobilisation of glycogen. Glucagon secretion is increased in this condition, perhaps because the general 'stress' state leads to increased sympatho-adrenal activity. This, together with lack of insulin, leads to increased gluconeogenesis. Thus, hepatic glucose production is increased. In addition, the supply of amino acid substrate for gluconeogenesis is increased because there is net breakdown of tissue protein, especially of the large amount in skeletal muscle. Glucose utilisation in tissues in which it is normally activated by insulin, particularly skeletal muscle, is impaired or abolished. This is reinforced by increased availability of fatty acids (see below) for oxidation; these will displace glucose as the oxidative fuel by the *glucose–fatty acid cycle* mechanism described in Section 6.4.1.2. Thus, the concentration of glucose

---

Box 10.1   Insulin resistance

The term insulin resistance was originally used to describe the condition of people with Type 1 diabetes who were treated with early, relatively impure preparations of animal insulins and who developed antibodies against the injected (foreign) proteins. Then these people required larger and larger doses of insulin for blood glucose control. However, it had also long been recognised that non-diabetic people differ widely in the sensitivity of their metabolic processes to insulin. There is a spectrum from the very insulin-sensitive to the very insulin-resistant. Sensitivity to insulin can be measured, for instance, by injecting a small dose of insulin intravenously and measuring the rate of fall of the blood glucose concentration. It is now recognised that the condition of insulin resistance is associated with a number of adverse metabolic changes that increase the risk of developing Type 2 diabetes, coronary heart disease and hypertension.

The mechanism by which insulin resistance develops is not clear. At one time it was thought that there was a deficit of cell-surface insulin receptors, but this is not now thought to be a general explanation. There seem to be alterations in a number of the steps of the signal chain that links insulin receptor-binding to metabolic processes (see Box 2.4). A metabolic explanation is that increased flux of fatty acids from adipose tissue impairs glucose utilisation through the action of the glucose–fatty acid cycle (see Section 6.4.1.2).

Insulin resistance is a prominent feature of both Type 2 diabetes (see Fig. 10.2) and obesity (see Section 10.2.3 for how these are linked) and appears to be more prominent in 'central' (or abdominal) obesity (Section 11.4.4).

Table 10.1.1 Features associated with insulin resistance.

Feature	Linked to	Mechanism	See Section
Glucose intolerance	Increased risk of developing Type 2 diabetes	Impairment of insulin action on glucose metabolism (definition of insulin resistance)	10.2.3
Elevated fasting and (especially) postprandial plasma triacylglycerol concentration	Increased risk of developing coronary heart disease	Failure of insulin action on lipid metabolism	9.4.3
Reduced plasma HDL-cholesterol concentration	Increased risk of developing coronary heart disease	Failure of insulin action on lipid metabolism	9.4.3
Presence of small, dense (lipid-depleted) LDL particles	Increased risk of developing coronary heart disease	Linked to impairment of triacylglycerol metabolism	Box 9.6
Impairment of endothelial function	Increased risk of developing both diabetes and coronary heart disease	Impaired insulin action on nitric oxide production, and probably other mechanisms	4.7.1; 10.5.5
High blood pressure	Increased risk of vascular disease	In part impairment of endothelial function	
Increased tendency to blood coagulation	Increased risk of vascular disease	Insulin-stimulated production of factors that tend to increase clotting	
Increased blood uric acid concentration	Increased risk of gout; uric acid is also linked to coronary heart disease risk (maybe through its association with insulin resistance)	Insulin increases renal tubular reabsorption of uric acid: high insulin concentrations therefore retain more uric acid	

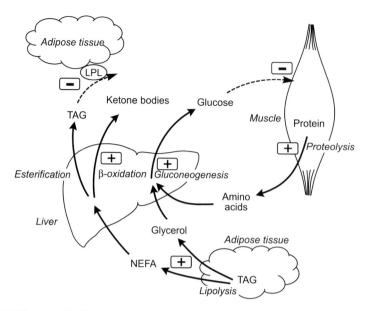

Fig. 10.3 The metabolic pattern in untreated Type 1 diabetes. Pathways accelerated by insulin deficiency are marked '+', pathways inhibited (particularly glucose uptake by insulin-sensitive tissues such as muscle, and triacylglycerol removal by lipoprotein lipase), are marked '–'. LPL, lipoprotein lipase; NEFA, non-esterified fatty acids; TAG, triacylglycerol.

in the blood rises dramatically. The normal 'resting' concentration of around 5 mmol/l may increase to 10, 20 or even 50 mmol/l as the disease progresses. In addition, the change in blood glucose concentration when glucose or carbohydrate is ingested becomes exaggerated – the person is said to display poor *glucose tolerance*. This feature is commonly used for diagnosis of diabetes mellitus (Box 10.2).

The increased glucose concentration of the blood, known as *hyperglycaemia*, leads to loss of glucose in the urine. At normal blood glucose concentrations, glucose is not lost by the kidney; it is filtered at the glomerulus and reabsorbed in the proximal tubules. But when the blood concentration rises above about 12 mmol/l, the level known as the *renal threshold*, reabsorption becomes saturated and glucose 'spills over' into the urine. This would lead to a hyperosmolar urine, so more water is lost through the process known as *osmotic diuresis*. Hence we see the classic sign of increased production of sugary urine. Loss of this extra water leads, of course, to thirst, the other classic sign of diabetes mellitus. People who develop Type 1 diabetes are usually first driven to their doctor by a combination of weight loss, thirst and frequent urination; treatment with insulin rapidly reverses these changes and restores their feeling of health.

The changes in glucose metabolism are usually regarded as the 'hallmark' of diabetes mellitus, and treatment is always monitored by the level of glucose in the blood. However, it has been said that if it were as easy to measure fatty

Box 10.2   Diagnosis of diabetes mellitus

Diabetes mellitus is defined as an elevation of the plasma (or blood) glucose concentration. It may be diagnosed by a measurement of the plasma glucose concentration after an overnight fast, but usually the disease is more clearly unmasked by observing the response of the plasma glucose concentration after drinking a solution of 75 g glucose, the *oral glucose tolerance test*. The World Health Organization has specified limits for definition of diabetes and of less severe changes known as *impaired fasting glucose* and *impaired glucose tolerance*: the last two categories are not recognised as diseases themselves but they show people at risk of developing diabetes.

	Typical control values	Impaired fasting glucose	Impaired glucose tolerance	Diabetes mellitus
Fasting	4.5–5.0	6.1–6.9	—	≥ 7.0
2 h after 75 g glucose	4.5–6.0	—	7.8–11.0	≥ 11.1

Venous plasma glucose concentrations in mmol/l: typical non-diabetic control values are shown for comparison. Taken from Alberti & Zimmet (1998).

The figure shows typical results from an oral glucose tolerance test in non-diabetic people, and people with Type 2 diabetes.

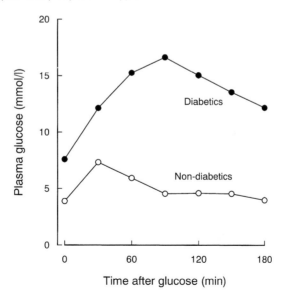

Fig. 10.2.1   Redrawn from Felber *et al.* (1993).

acids in blood as it is to measure glucose, we would think of diabetes mellitus mainly as a disorder of fat metabolism. Lack of insulin leads to unrestrained release of non-esterified fatty acids from adipose tissue, and also to lack of activation of adipose tissue lipoprotein lipase. Thus, adipocytes fail to take up triacylglycerol from the blood, and there is a dramatic net loss of fat from adipose depots. This, together with the breakdown of protein, leads to the catabolic state and rapidly developing wasted appearance of sufferers who do not receive treatment (see Fig. 10.1).

The concentration of non-esterified fatty acids in the plasma in untreated diabetes mellitus (normally in the range 0.2–1.0 mmol/l in healthy subjects) may reach 3–4 mmol/l. These high concentrations of non-esterified fatty acids, together with the lack of insulin (and possibly increase in glucagon) lead to increased fatty acid oxidation and ketone body production in the liver (see Fig. 10.3). The combined concentration of the ketone bodies 3-hydroxy-butyrate and acetoacetate in the blood is normally less than 0.2 mmol/l. In untreated diabetes, their combined concentration may reach 10–20 mmol/l. Remember that the ketone bodies are produced as the corresponding acids, 3-hydroxybutyric acid and acetoacetic acid. Thus, the level of acidity of the blood also increases – i.e. the pH falls, from the normal value of about 7.4 to perhaps around 7.1. This is a dangerous situation, known as *diabetic ketoacidosis*.

In addition, excess non-esterified fatty acids may be diverted into esterification in the liver despite the lack of insulin, and increased VLDL-triacylglycerol secretion may result. Triacylglycerol clearance from the plasma is much reduced because of lack of activation of adipose tissue lipoprotein lipase (Fig. 10.3). Thus, hypertriglyceridaemia is another feature of untreated diabetes mellitus.

The accumulation of substances such as ketone bodies and glucose in the blood, together with dehydration, leads to an increase in the osmolality of the blood. This, in combination with the increased acidity in the blood, causes changes in brain function which may lead eventually to unconsciousness – *diabetic coma*, or *hyperglycaemic coma*. This will progress to death if not treated. This was the fate of sufferers from Type 1 diabetes before the introduction of insulin treatment. Treatment of diabetic ketoacidosis consists of insulin together with fluid. Deaths from diabetic ketoacidosis are now, fortunately, rare.

The tendency to develop ketoacidosis is one feature that distinguishes Type 1 from Type 2 diabetes clinically. Those with Type 2 diabetes are generally more resistant to development of ketosis, presumably because the small amount of insulin secretion that remains is sufficient to prevent excessive ketone body formation. However, ketosis may occur when there is an additional metabolic stress such as infection.

10.3.2 Metabolic alterations in Type 2 diabetes

The plasma glucose concentration in Type 2 diabetes varies according to the severity of the condition, but if a patient neglects his or her treatment and then attends a diabetic clinic, it would not be uncommon to find a plasma glucose concentration of 20 mmol/l. The plasma glucose concentration is consistently raised throughout the day (Fig. 10.4), with an exaggerated response to meals. This highlights the important role of insulin in minimising the postprandial 'excursions' in plasma glucose concentration, which is impaired in Type 2 diabetes. In addition, plasma non-esterified fatty acid concentrations may be elevated throughout the day (Fig. 10.5). This elevation of plasma non-esterified fatty acid concentration may aggravate a number of features of the condition, reducing further the ability of insulin to stimulate glucose uptake by skeletal muscle and promoting hepatic VLDL-triacylglycerol secretion.

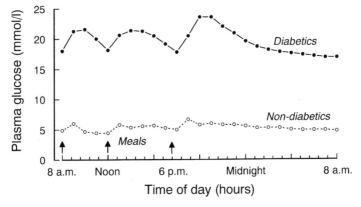

Fig. 10.4 Twenty-four-hour profiles of plasma glucose concentration in non-diabetic subjects and subjects with severe Type 2 diabetes. The non-diabetic subjects were also shown in Fig. 6.1. Redrawn from data in Reaven *et al.* (1988), Copyright © 1988 American Diabetes Association. From *Diabetes*, Vol. 37, 1988; 1020–1024. With permission of the American Diabetes Association.

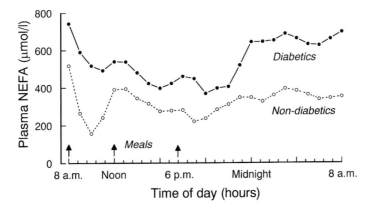

Fig. 10.5 Twenty-four-hour profiles of plasma non-esterified fatty acid (NEFA) concentration in non-diabetic subjects and subjects with severe Type 2 diabetes. Plasma glucose concentrations in these subjects are shown in Fig. 10.4. Redrawn from data in Reaven *et al.* (1988), Copyright © 1988 American Diabetes Association. From *Diabetes*, Vol. 37, 1988; 1020–1024. With permission of the American Diabetes Association.

10.4   Treatment of diabetes mellitus

10.4.1   Type 1 diabetes

In Type 1 diabetes, the only satisfactory treatment is to replace the missing insulin. However, this simple statement is not easy to put into practice. First, we must find some insulin. Until the last two decades, all insulin used by people with diabetes was extracted from the pancreas of cows and pigs. This had two disadvantages. The supply was finite and there were worries that it would never be sufficient to meet the needs of diabetic patients worldwide. In addition, both bovine and porcine insulin differ slightly from human insulin in amino acid sequence, and also the extracts were not completely pure; and these two factors together led to the development of *insulin antibodies* in people treated with these preparations – i.e. antibodies made against what the body sees as a foreign protein. In people who reacted particularly strongly in this way, the concentration of insulin antibodies became so high (binding the insulin that was given) that enormous doses of insulin had to be used; in fact, this was the original condition known as insulin resistance. Now, a protein identical with human insulin is produced by bacteria in culture, using recombinant DNA techniques; the supply is effectively infinite, the preparations are pure and the protein does not cause antibodies.

Even with a suitable insulin preparation, however, it has to be given to the subject. It cannot be swallowed because, like any other protein, it is broken down into its constituent amino acids before absorption from the intestine. Therefore it has to be injected. Nobody actually likes having an injection, and the number of injections given per day should ideally be as few as possible. But a major theme of this book has been the way in which metabolism is regulated by constantly changing, subtle alterations in the secretion of insulin. How can this possibly be mimicked by two or three injections each day? In addition, the anatomical relationship of the liver and the pancreas have been stressed in this book: insulin is secreted into the portal vein and exerts its initial effects on the liver. We cannot inject into the portal vein, and insulin is usually given into the subcutaneous adipose tissue (Fig. 10.6). How different will metabolic regulation be if insulin reaches the peripheral circulation in concentrations which can only change slowly, and which do not respond directly to changes in the concentration of glucose in the blood? The answer is that, with a suitable combination of injections three times a day, surprisingly normal glucose concentrations can be maintained in the blood: but never completely normal.

One important reason for the lack of complete normalisation is the balancing act which a person with Type 1 diabetes must perform between too little and too much insulin. Too little and the blood glucose concentration rises unduly and ketoacidosis begins; too much and the blood glucose concentration will fall below normal levels. This can happen very quickly, particularly if, for instance, the subject unexpectedly has to miss a meal or to take some exercise, having injected his or her normal amount of insulin. If the blood glucose con-

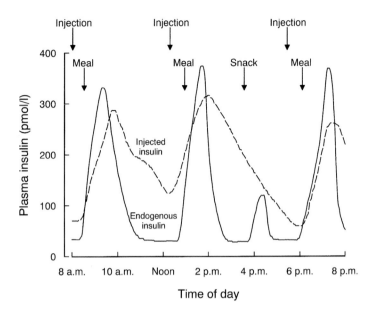

Fig. 10.6 Plasma insulin concentrations in non-diabetic subjects and people with Type 1 diabetes having three injections of insulin during the day. Based on Alberti, K.G.M.M., Boucher, B.J., Hitman, G.A. & Taylor, R. (1990) Diabetes mellitus. In: *The Metabolic and Molecular Basis of Acquired Disease* Vol. 1 (eds Cohen, R.D., Lewis, B., Alberti, K.G.M.M. & Denman, A.M.), 765–840. With permission of the publisher W.B. Saunders.

centration falls below about 2 mmol/l, then (as discussed in Section 4.2) the brain will suffer from a lack of substrate and changes in mood – e.g. irritability, slurred speech – will follow; if the glucose falls further, unconsciousness may occur. This is the condition of *hypoglycaemia*, or, if it leads to unconsciousness, *hypoglycaemic coma*. Because this condition can develop so rapidly, and because its consequences can be so severe, many people with diabetes tend to keep their plasma glucose concentration on the higher side of normal rather than the lower side. For many people nowadays, the process of checking their treatment has been made enormously simpler by the availability of portable devices to measure the glucose concentration in a drop of blood from a finger-prick.

10.4.2 Type 2 diabetes

For those with Type 2 diabetes, the balancing act is somewhat easier. Many can control their blood glucose concentration reasonably well either by strict adherence to a diet, or by use of drugs. However, people with Type 2 diabetes may also need treatment with insulin to achieve satisfactory control of blood glucose concentrations, especially when they have the condition for some years.

Dietary measures are largely based on what we know about the processes of digestion, absorption and postprandial metabolism (Chapters 3 and 6). The content of simple sugars (mono- and disaccharides) in the food should be low since these lead to a rapid rise in the concentration of glucose in the blood; a high content of fibre in the diet helps to slow down the rate of absorption of carbohydrate and thus minimise the postprandial excursions in blood glucose concentration. In addition, of course, energy intake must be controlled in order to maintain as low a body weight as possible, since excess weight is associated with insulin resistance.

Several classes of drug are available for treatment of Type 2 diabetes. Acarbose is an inhibitor of α-amylase, the pancreatic enzyme that digests starch (Section 3.2.3.3). It is given with meals and slows carbohydrate digestion, and therefore reduces postprandial excursions in blood glucose concentration. The *sulphonylureas* act directly upon the pancreatic β-cells to promote insulin release by closing the ATP-sensitive K^+ channels in the cell membrane (see Fig. 5.4). In the longer term, the sulphonylureas also lead also to improved sensitivity to insulin. The *biguanide* drug, metformin, acts in a way which is not entirely clear, mainly to improve the sensitivity of the tissues to insulin, i.e. to reduce insulin resistance. In the last decade a new class of drugs has become available, the *thiazolidinediones* or *glitazones*. These drugs are activators of the transcription factor PPARγ in adipose tissue. Their action was described in Section 2.4.2.2. Their overall effect is to improve sensitivity to insulin in all tissues, including skeletal muscle and the liver.

10.5   The longer-term complications of diabetes

10.5.1   Macrovascular and microvascular disease and their relationship to glucose concentrations

People with diabetes may lead very active, normal long lives. For some, however, their life is marred by the development of diabetic complications. These complications are so-called because they seem to be secondary, long-term effects of the disease rather than direct, short-term effects of lack of insulin. However, the distinction is not absolute and it could be argued that they are just as much a feature of the disease as, for instance, ketoacidosis.

There has been a long-standing debate about whether the progression of complications is related to the degree of *glycaemic control* – i.e. if a normal blood glucose concentration could be maintained, would complications not occur? This simple question has been extraordinarily difficult to answer. Recently two long-term prospective studies have produced clear results. In the Diabetes Control and Complications Trial (DCCT) conducted in the USA, people with Type 1 diabetes were randomly allocated to receive either normal insulin treatment or special, intensive insulin treatment which maintained their glucose concentrations closer to normal over a period of 6–7 years. In the group with intensified treatment, the progression of complications was significantly less. In the United Kingdom Prospective Diabetes Study, people with Type 2 diabetes were randomised to various types of control and, over a 10-year period, the development of complications was again related to average blood glucose concentrations. Therefore, it is now firmly believed that complications develop because of prolonged elevation of the glucose concentration. However, the downside in both DCCT and UKPDS was that people in the intensive treatment groups suffered more episodes of hypoglycaemia.

The complications include vascular disease – in turn divided into *microvascular disease* (affecting the capillaries) and *macrovascular disease* (affecting large vessels), kidney problems (*nephropathy*), nerve problems (*neuropathy*) and eye problems (*retinopathy* and cataract). The development of high blood pressure (*hypertension*) is also a complication of diabetes, related to both nephropathy and insulin resistance. Microvascular disease and diseases of the nerves and kidneys may be interrelated through changes in the *basement membrane*, a membranous structure which surrounds the capillaries in many tissues. In diabetes, this becomes thickened and may restrict permeability.

Macrovascular disease means disease of the large vessels, or essentially, atherosclerosis, the process outlined in Section 9.4.1. In diabetes, this typically affects arteries in the limbs as well as the coronary arteries. It can then lead to impaired blood supply to a leg, for instance, to the extent that the viability of the leg is threatened. Blood supply to damaged tissues is also reduced, so that healing of wounds in the leg, for instance, can be slow and ulcers may form that are difficult to treat. In addition, coronary atherosclerosis is a common finding; in people with diabetes, cardiovascular disease is the commonest cause of death.

In untreated or poorly controlled diabetes, there are alterations in lipid metabolism which may give rise to the abnormalities usually associated with atherosclerosis. For instance, lack of insulin leads to failure to activate adipose tissue lipoprotein lipase normally after meals, with the consequences outlined in Section 9.4.3. But in those with apparently well-controlled diabetes, the concentrations of lipoprotein constituents in plasma may be relatively normal. It is probable that more subtle alterations in lipoprotein composition occur, which are not fully understood. One mechanism may be non-enzymatic glycation (see Section 10.5.2, below) of the apolipoproteins, which could affect their ability to interact normally with receptors. In addition, a number of adverse changes have been attributed to chronic (long-standing) elevation of insulin concentrations. This will be the situation in many people with diabetes who are treated either with insulin or with insulin-releasing drugs (sulphonylureas), in the presence of some degree of insulin resistance. This chronic *hyperinsulinaemia* is thought to bring about changes in the arterial wall, particularly promotion of the proliferation of smooth muscle cells. As we saw in Section 9.4.1, this is an important component of atherosclerosis. It may also lead to 'inflexibility' of the blood vessels which control the resistance of the peripheral circulation, and thus to inability to regulate blood pressure normally: hypertension (high blood pressure) may therefore result.

A number of biochemical mechanisms have been proposed to underlie these apparently diverse changes.

10.5.2 Non-enzymatic glycation of proteins

The mechanism is illustrated in Fig. 10.7. This changes the function of proteins – for instance, changes in collagen structure may result. Since glycation is a non-enzymatic process, its progression is dependent mainly upon the prevailing glucose concentration. It probably occurs in everybody over the years, and it is easy to see how it could be a mechanism which relates an increased 'average' glucose concentration over a number of years to the premature development of tissue damage. There are drugs available to inhibit the generation of AGEs (advanced glycation end-products), which have shown promising results in experimental trials. The AGEs may bind to specific receptors, one of which is known as the receptor for AGEs (RAGE). If the RAGE receptor is blocked, in experimental models of diabetes, some of the complications of diabetes are lessened.

10.5.3 The polyol pathway

Another biochemical mechanism which may relate to the average glucose concentration is the formation of the polyhydric alcohol, sorbitol. The pathway by which this occurs (Fig. 10.8) is a normal, physiological one; for instance, it is responsible for the production of fructose, which is a normal constituent of seminal fluid. But, again, it occurs at an increased rate when the glucose concentration is elevated. It may be particularly responsible for the development of diabetic cataract (opacity of the lens); sorbitol accumulates in the lens, and this may lead to osmotic tissue swelling and damage. Alternatively, it has been suggested that utilisation of NADPH by this pathway leaves the cell open to oxidative damage, since NADPH is normally involved in regenerating the

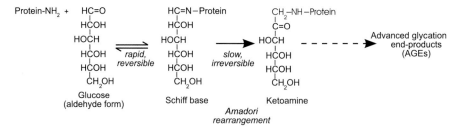

Fig. 10.7 Non-enzymatic glycation of proteins. A sugar molecule in its straight-chain, aldehyde form reacts non-enzymatically with a lysine-NH_2 group in a protein. The resultant Schiff's base is converted with time to an irreversible, ketoamine linkage which may disrupt the functioning of the protein. With further time (perhaps over a matter of years) further changes occur, leading to the so-called *advanced glycation end-products* (AGEs), usually brown-coloured. The rate of the first reaction is proportional to the concentration of sugar molecules.

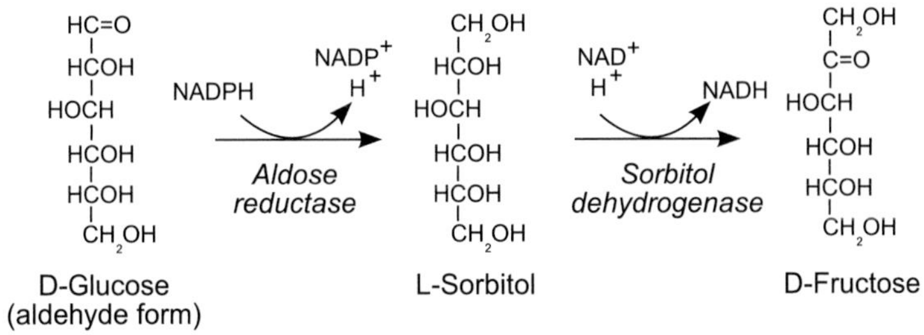

Fig. 10.8 The polyol pathway for production and further metabolism of sorbitol. The enzyme *aldose reductase* is present in a number of tissues including nerve cells and the eye lens. It has a high K_m for glucose: thus, the higher the glucose concentration, the greater the rate of conversion to sorbitol.

antioxidant compound glutathione. Drugs are available that inhibit aldose reductase. Results from clinical trials have been mixed.

10.5.4   The hexosamine pathway

Glucose can also follow the pathway that leads proteoglycan synthesis (e.g. the formation of compounds such as heparan sulphate; see Section 4.5.3.1). In this pathway, the amide group of glutamine is transferred to sugars to form hexosamines. It has been suggested that hexosamines are involved both in insulin resistance and in altering gene expression in a way that might accentuate the complications of diabetes.

10.5.5   Protein kinase C activation

The family of isoforms of protein kinase C (PKC) was described in Box 2.3. PKC-α and PKC-β are activated by diacylglycerol. It has been suggested that activation of these particular isoforms is brought about by synthesis of diacylglycerol from acyl-CoA and glycerol 3-phosphate formed from glycolysis (see Fig. 4.3) in response to high intracellular glucose concentrations. Activation of PKC may alter gene expression in such a way as to increase diabetic complications. In particular, this may happen in endothelial cells, where consequences may include decreased expression of the endothelial nitric oxide synthase (Section 4.7.1) and hence impaired endothelial function, and increased expression of the adhesion molecules that lead to leukocyte entry into the sub-endothelial space.

10.5.6   A common pathway?

Recently it has been suggested that all these pathways interrelate through one common mechanism: exposure of cells to increased oxidative stress. The proposal is that elevated glucose concentrations lead to increased flux of reducing equivalents through the electron transport chain (see Fig. 4.13) and that this, in turn, leads to generation of reactive oxygen species, oxygen-derived radicals that may cause cellular damage. There is support for this from animal models of diabetes, in which overexpression of either the enzyme superoxide dismutase, that breaks down reactive oxygen radicals, or of UCP-1 (Fig. 4.13), which discharges the mitochondrial proton gradient, will reduce the progression of complications.

10.6   Further reading

Articles marked * all come from a Nature Insight section on Diabetes in which there are also other good reviews: *Nature* 2001; 414: 781–827.

General diabetes, insulin resistance
Reaven, G.M. (1988) Role of insulin resistance in human disease. Diabetes 37: 1595–1607. *This is a 'classic' article in which Gerald Reaven set out the now well-accepted idea that insulin resistance was an underlying feature of several conditions associated with increased risk of developing Type 2 diabetes and coronary heart disease.*
*Zimmet, P., Alberti, K.G. & Shaw, J. (2001) Global and societal implications of the diabetes epidemic. *Nature* 414: 782–787.

Genetics of diabetes
McCarthy, M. & Menzel, S. (2001) The genetics of type 2 diabetes. *Br J Clin Pharmacol* 51: 195–199.
Redondo, M.J. & Eisenbarth, G.S. (2002) Genetic control of autoimmunity in Type 1 diabetes and associated disorders. *Diabetologia* 45: 605–622.

Metabolism and insulin secretion in diabetes mellitus and its treatment
*Bell, G.I. & Polonsky, K.S. (2001) Diabetes mellitus and genetically pro-grammed defects in β-cell function. *Nature* 414: 788–791.
Langin, D. (2001) Diabetes, insulin secretion, and the pancreatic beta-cell mi-tochondrion. *N Engl J Med* 345: 1772–1774.
*Moller, D.E. (2001) New drug targets for type 2 diabetes and the metabolic syndrome. *Nature* 414: 821–827.
*Saltiel, A.R. & Kahn, C.R. (2001) Insulin signalling and the regulation of glucose and lipid metabolism. *Nature* 414: 799–806.

Diabetes complications
Tomlinson, D.R. (1999) Mitogen-activated protein kinases as glucose trans-ducers for diabetic complications. *Diabetologia* 42: 1271–1281.
*Brownlee, M. (2001) Biochemistry and molecular cell biology of diabetic complications. *Nature* 414: 813–820.
Singh, R., Barden, A., Mori, T. & Beilin, L. (2001) Advanced glycation end-products: a review. *Diabetologia* 44: 129–146.

Gutterman, D.D. (2002) Vascular dysfunction in hyperglycemia: is protein kinase C the culprit? *Circ Res* 90: 5–7.

Note

1   Figures vary from 36% to 54%: this is a difficult estimate to make because of bias in the selection of twins (if both have diabetes, they are more likely to register themselves for such a study). See Leslie *et al.* (1989) and Hitman & Niven (1989).

11

Energy Balance and Body Weight Regulation

11.1   Energy balance

The first law of thermodynamics states that energy can neither be created nor destroyed, although it may be interconverted between different forms. The human body is, as we have seen, a device for taking in chemical energy and converting that chemical energy, by controlled oxidation of fuels, into other forms of chemical energy (e.g. by the synthesis of storage compounds), into mechanical work and into heat. The first law of thermodynamics applies to the human body as to any other isolated system. Therefore, the amount of chemical energy taken in, after correction for any lost as waste products, must equal the total output of heat and mechanical work plus the chemical energy used in biosynthetic reactions; any chemical energy remaining will be stored. This may be written simply as:

Energy intake (food) = Energy expended (heat, work) + Energy stored

'Energy stored' may include a change in the heat stored – i.e. a change in body temperature, but over any reasonably long period this will be relatively constant.

On an hour-to-hour basis, the energy intake and energy expenditure may not match each other at all (see Fig. 1.2 in Chapter 1). This is why it is necessary to have short-term storage compounds such as glycogen and triacylglycerol, which can 'buffer' these mismatches between intake and expenditure of energy. In the longer term – over a period of months or years – then the glycogen stores, which have a finite and fairly small capacity (see Table 8.1), cannot buffer mismatches between intake and expenditure. The stores of triacylglycerol in adipose tissue are our long-term buffer for mismatches between energy intake and energy expenditure. In other words, if energy intake exceeds energy expenditure consistently, then triacylglycerol accumulates in adipose tissue, which accords with common observation.

It is interesting to ask how precisely energy intake and energy expenditure usually match each other over the long term. Many people maintain a *relatively* constant body weight throughout their adult lives. Suppose that from the age of 25 to the age of 75 a particular individual changes body weight by 10 kg. That's quite a big change, and many people will change much less. We can translate that into a change in energy stores in adipose tissue. Adipose tissue is not all lipid, and its energy density is about 30 MJ per kg. This means that over the person's adult lifetime there has been an imbalance between energy intake and energy expenditure of 300 MJ over 50 years, which, by simple arithmetic, is about 16 kJ (4 kcal) per day. Therefore, many people balance their energy intake and energy expenditure over their adult life to the extent of about 5 kJ (about 1kcal) *per meal*, and indeed many people even more precisely than that. We can look at the precision involved in this example in another way. Most people take in about 10 MJ of food energy each day, or $50 \times 365 \times 10$ MJ (182 500 MJ) over adult life (about 20 tonnes of food!). The imbalance with expenditure might amount, as we have seen, to around 300 MJ. This represents an imbalance between intake and expenditure of about 0.2% of the throughput, a pretty impressive figure.

Clearly, there is no way in which we can judge the energy content of individual meals to this degree of precision, and this sort of reasoning has led many people to believe that there are biological control mechanisms that regulate either energy intake (via changes in appetite) or energy expenditure. One such mechanism is leptin (see Fig. 5.11). It is important also to remember that, for humans, there are external cues, such as the tightness of one's belt or the reading on the bathroom scales, which can, perhaps subconsciously, affect one's eating or exercise pattern, especially over reasonably long time periods.

The aim of this chapter is to fill in some of the background to what is known about the regulation of energy intake and expenditure, and also to show how an understanding of metabolic regulation in the way it has been discussed in the book enables you to take a fairly commonsense look at ideas about body weight regulation.

11.2   Energy intake

Evidence that there is regulation of energy intake has long been available from studies of laboratory animals. For instance, rats or mice have been underfed from an early age. Then, when their weight is significantly less than control animals allowed *ad libitum* feeding (feeding as much as they want), the underfed animals are returned to *ad libitum* feeding. The result is always that their weight rapidly increases until it reaches the same value as control animals of a similar age. This led many years ago to the concept of a 'set-point' for body weight (as there is a set-point for temperature in a system with a thermostat: see Fig. 6.2). What determines this set-point? Some people argued for a 'ponderostat', a system that responds according to ponderal index or the degree of overweight. The British physiologist G.C. Kennedy, in the 1950s, argued for a 'lipostat', a system that responds according to the size of the body's fat stores. The discovery of leptin (see Section 5.6 and Fig. 5.11) proved this conjecture to be basically correct. Leptin, as described in Section 5.6, is a signal from adipose tissue. Its plasma concentration reflects the size of the fat stores, and signals to the hypothalamus to restrict energy intake (and also, in small animals, to increase energy expenditure).

The discovery of leptin in 1994 led to an explosion of work in the field of energy intake regulation. It is now recognised that there are several pathways within the central nervous system that regulate food intake in both positive and negative directions. Some of these are summarised in Box 11.1.

Box 11.1   Regulation of energy intake

Most of the detail of appetite regulation has been worked out in laboratory animals, but the discovery of some relatively rare single-gene mutations causing obesity in humans gives support to the idea that the pathways are basically similar.

There are short-term and long-term regulatory pathways. These converge within the central nervous system.

Long-term signals feed information on the 'energy status' of the organism to the brain. Those clearly identified are leptin and insulin: leptin signals the state of the fat stores, insulin the state of 'carbohydrate repleteness'. These act through complex pathways in the hypothalamus that involve a variety of neurotransmitters and neuropeptides. They inhibit hunger pathways and stimulate satiety pathways. Conversely, if leptin and insulin concentrations are low, signalling a need for energy, hunger pathways are stimulated and satiety is suppressed. Some key peptides involved in these hypothalamic pathways are:

- Neuropeptide Y (NPY): this is a powerful hunger signal; injection of neuropeptide Y into the brains of rats brings about eating.
- Peptides related to pro-opiomelanocortin (POMC) (see Section 5.3.1): POMC is a large peptide that is cleaved to generate a number of biologically active peptides including ACTH and melanocyte-stimulating hormone (MSH) (one of a family of peptides known as melanocortins). MSH was, as its name suggests, first identified as a stimulator of pigment (melanin) production in the skin, but also acts on a variety of receptors in the hypothalamus to suppress appetite. One of these receptors in particular is

the melanocortin-4 receptor (Mc4 receptor). Mice lacking the Mc4 receptor overeat and become obese, and recently some children with early-onset obesity have been found to have mutations in the Mc4 receptor.

Short-term signals arise from the intestinal tract, the hepatic portal vein and the liver. Generally they serve to produce satiety, bringing about the end of a meal. These signals are transmitted partly in afferent fibres of the vagus nerve (see Section 7.2.2.2) and partly through the blood. There are many candidate 'satiety' hormones including glucagon-like peptide-1 (Section 5.7) and cholecystokinin (CCK, Section 3.2.3.2), and also apolipoprotein-AIV secreted from the small intestine as a component of chylomicrons. Ghrelin is a peptide released from the stomach (ghrelin gets its name from its first-recognised action of stimulating growth hormone *release*) that stimulates appetite: its secretion rises during fasting and is suppressed following feeding.

These pathways and their interaction are summarised in Fig. 11.1.1. Note that this is very over-simplified; see Further Reading for more detailed accounts.

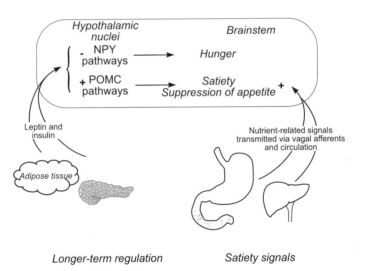

Fig. 11.1.1   Summary of central pathways regulating appetite.

There has been some scepticism over whether these systems, mostly discovered in small animals, operate in humans. Plasma leptin concentrations in obese humans are almost always elevated compared with lean people: there is a positive relationship, as expected, with fat mass (Fig. 11.1). Therefore the majority of human obesity is not explained by a defect in leptin secretion (as is seen in the *ob/ob* mouse); in fact, people remain obese despite high levels of leptin.

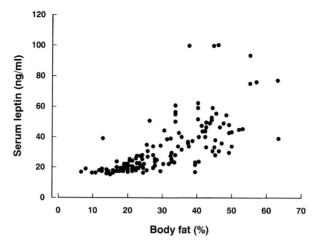

Fig. 11.1 Relationship between serum leptin concentration and percentage body fat in 179 subjects with a wide range of fatness. There is generally a positive relationship: the more fat one has, the higher the leptin concentration. However, for any particular value of body fat (40%, for instance), there is a wide range of leptin concentrations, so generalisations are dangerous. Adapted from Considine, R.V., Sinha, M.K. & Heiman, M.L. *et al.* (1996) Serum immunoreactive-leptin concentrations in normal-weight and obese humans. *N Engl J Med* 334: 292–295. With permission. Copyright © 1996 Massachusetts Medical Society. All rights reserved.

However, recent developments have shown that this system is, indeed, of fundamental importance to human energy balance. The group of Professor Stephen O'Rahilly in Cambridge, UK, have specialised in studying cases of severe childhood obesity. In 1997 they reported two young cousins who had shown phenomenal growth, and compulsive eating behaviour, since birth. When they attempted to measure the plasma leptin concentrations in these children, they could find none. Sequencing of their leptin genes showed that both are homozygous for a frameshift mutation[1] in the leptin gene. They cannot produce functional leptin, and the impact for them is almost as severe as if they could not produce insulin (although quite different in nature). The cousins have now been treated with human leptin (produced by recombinant DNA techniques as discussed in Section 5.6). Data have been published for one of them. She has shown progressive weight loss, and remarkable normalisation of her eating behaviour, for the first time in her life (Fig. 11.2). Since that time, there have been reports of several further families with mutations either in the leptin gene or in the gene for the leptin receptor (although this is still an extraordinarily rare cause of obesity). The phenotype is similar, and, in older people, includes sexual immaturity, emphasising that leptin is an important signal to the reproductive system as well as to the systems regulating energy intake (see Section 5.6). We can no longer believe that human energy intake is not regulated by internal mechanisms, although clearly these mechanisms, when they are working normally, can easily be overridden.

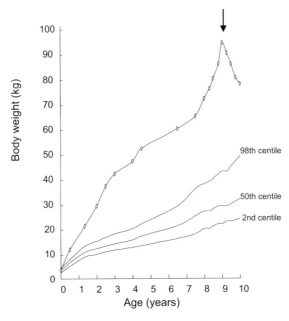

Fig. 11.2 Growth of a child with leptin deficiency due to a mutation in the leptin gene. The lower lines show normal growth curves. The data for the child are marked with diamonds. The point at which treatment with recombinant leptin was started is shown by the arrow. From Farooqi, I.S., Jebb, S.A. & Langmack, G. *et al.* (1999) Effects of recombinant leptin therapy in a child with congenital leptin deficiency. *N Engl J Med* 341: 879–884. With permission. Copyright © 1996 Massachusetts Medical Society. All rights reserved.

There are two schools of thought as to why many people can remain obese despite high plasma leptin concentrations. One holds that there is a condition of 'leptin resistance', akin to insulin resistance (Box 10.1), which may have a molecular basis, and which may therefore be amenable at some time in the future to alteration by drugs. The other believes that the leptin system is primarily a 'starvation' signal: in starvation, leptin levels fall, and this causes an intense drive to eat (as seen also when the system is defective). But in normal life, when food is readily available, the signal may be very weak in comparison with the effect of all that readily available, highly palatable and energy-rich food that surrounds us in modern societies.

Work from Professor O'Rahilly's group, and others, has also identified children with obesity due to mutations in other components of the system shown in Box 11.1. The commonest is a mutation in the melanocortin-4 receptor. This defect accounts for about 5% of severe childhood obesity. Therefore we can also be certain that other components of the system shown in Box 11.1 also act in humans, and pharmaceutical companies are busy trying to manipulate these systems in order to treat obesity. However, it would be a mistake to draw the conclusion that most obesity is due to such single-gene mutations: they remain relatively rare as causes of obesity. Although human obesity has quite a strong genetic component (estimates vary, but around 30–50% of the variation of human body mass index (BMI) may be explained by genetics), it is mostly polygenic and very few of the genes involved have been identified.

11.3   Energy expenditure

11.3.1   Measurement of energy expenditure

The measurement of metabolic rate has a long history. Probably Antoine Lavoisier (1743–1794), the French chemist and physiologist, was the first to study the metabolic rate of a human, his assistant Séguin.

There are two basic approaches. First, we may measure directly the heat liberated by the body. This can be done by constructing a special insulated chamber whose walls contain devices for measurement of heat liberated. Either they may contain pipes through which water is circulated; the small difference in temperature between water entering and water leaving the system must be accurately measured. Alternatively, the walls may contain a large number of thermocouples that respond electrically according to the temperature. This technique gives a direct measurement of heat liberation, and is known as *direct calorimetry*.

Direct calorimetry requires sophisticated equipment, and can only be applied in conditions which somewhat restrict the subject. The alternative approach – used by Lavoisier – is that of *indirect calorimetry*. In this, energy expenditure is assessed from measurement of the oxidation of fuels, assessed in turn from the whole-body consumption of O_2 and production of CO_2. The basic principles are outlined in Box 11.2. In its simplest form, the subject breathes into a bag, whose contents are later analysed for O_2 and CO_2 concentrations. More commonly nowadays, a clear plastic 'hood' or 'canopy' is placed over the subject's head, and air is drawn through this by a pump, so that all the expired air is collected and its contents of O_2 and CO_2 are measured by onstream analysers. An indirect calorimeter can also be constructed in the form of a room in which a subject may live a relatively normal, although somewhat constrained, life for several days.

Indirect calorimetry is usually performed over a period which ranges from minutes, breathing into a bag, to a few days in a chamber. Even this is not entirely satisfactory for assessing energy expenditure in people living their normal daily lives. For this, another technique is normally used, the *double-labelled water* technique (outlined in Box 11.3). This is a technique for estimating CO_2 production over a period of 2–3 weeks. Energy expenditure can be assessed from CO_2 production alone with reasonable accuracy, although some estimate of the ratio of CO_2 production to O_2 consumption makes the calculation more reliable. This may be done by the subject keeping a diary of food intake, and using this to assess the ratio of CO_2 production to O_2 consumption if all this food were combusted (the *food quotient* or FQ); it is reasonable to assume that the same ratio for the body (the *respiratory quotient*, RQ or *respiratory exchange ratio*, RER) will approximate the FQ over a period of time. The advantage of the double-labelled water technique is that it allows the measurement of energy expenditure in subjects living their normal lives outside the laboratory: a subject reports to the laboratory to receive a glass of labelled water, and then simply has to report back at intervals – say once each week – to provide a sample of urine or saliva.

11.3.2   The components of energy expenditure

We expend energy continuously over each 24-hour period. Some of this energy expenditure represents the basic requirements for staying alive: at the cellular level, pumping of ions across membranes to maintain normal gradients, turnover of proteins and other cellular constituents; at the organ level, pumping of blood around the body, respiration, etc. This 'basal' level of metabolic activity is known as the *basal metabolic rate*. Basal metabolic rate is measured after an overnight fast, in a room at a comfortable temperature, with the subject awake but resting; these conditions have been found to give very reproducible answers. When we sleep, the metabolic rate (rate of energy expenditure) is lower than the basal metabolic rate, but at all other times during normal daily life it is higher. Energy expenditure is increased by physical activity. It is also increased after meals. The increase in the rate of energy expenditure after meals used to be called the *specific dynamic action* of food; more usually now it is referred to as *diet-induced thermogenesis* or DIT, thermogenesis meaning the generation of heat. DIT represents the energy cost of gastrointestinal tract activity, digestion, absorption and the metabolic cost of storing the fuels (e.g. the formation of glycogen by the direct pathway from glucose involves the hydrolysis of two high-energy phosphates, one ATP and one UTP, per molecule of glucose).

The total expenditure of energy over a 24-hour period can be broken down into the basal metabolic rate, the energy cost of physical activity and diet-induced thermogenesis (Fig. 11.3). Physical activity varies considerably from person to person. However, the largest component of the 24-hour energy expenditure is, for most people, the basal component. The basal metabolic rate is very closely related to the amount of non-fat tissue in the body, the *fat-free mass* or *lean body mass*.[2] The larger someone's fat free mass, the larger (in general) their basal metabolic rate (this will be illustrated later, in Fig. 11.5). The basal metabolic rate is also regulated by hormones, primarily by the thyroid hormone, triiodothyronine. During starvation or food deprivation thyroid hormone concentrations fall and basal metabolic rate decreases (see Section 7.3.2.1). The significance of this for weight reduction programmes will be discussed again later. Leptin does not seem directly to regulate energy expenditure significantly in humans as it does in rodents; this is based on evidence from measurements of energy expenditure in the children with leptin deficiency (Fig. 11.2).

Box 11.2   The principles of indirect calorimetry

The human body takes in the macronutrients carbohydrate, fat and protein. They eventually leave the body as CO_2, H_2O and urea. There is almost no loss of other products (e.g. partial oxidation products such as pyruvic acid or ketone bodies); in other words, the macronutrients are virtually completely oxidised (with the exception of urea formation from protein). The body produces heat and external work from the oxidation of these substances. It is irrelevant that the process of oxidation within the body may not be direct – e.g. glucose may form glycogen, then lactate, then be recycled as glucose before oxidation; or even that glucose may be converted to fat before oxidation. The net heat production will be the same as if the oxidation occurred directly.

The equations for oxidation of the individual fuels are given below:

Glucose
(the quantities are shown for one mole of glucose):

$$C_6H_{12}O_6 + 6\,O_2 \rightarrow 6\,CO_2 + 6\,H_2O - \Delta H$$

180 g   6 × 22.4 litres   6 × 22.4 litres   6 × 18 g   2.80 MJ

(ΔH is the enthalpy change – i.e. heat produced; the negative sign is the convention when heat is liberated.)

Note that oxidation of 1 g of glucose liberates 2.80/180 MJ or 15.6 kJ.

The ratio of CO_2 production to O_2 consumption, the *respiratory quotient* (RQ) for this reaction, is 6/6 or 1.00.

Fat
(the quantities are shown for one mole of a typical triacylglycerol, palmitoyl, stearoyl, oleoyl-glycerol, $C_{55}H_{106}O_6$):

$$2C_{55}H_{106}O_6 + 157\,O_2 \rightarrow 110\,CO_2 + 106\,H_2O - \Delta H$$

2 × 862 g   157 × 22.4 litres   110 × 22.4 litres   106 × 18 g   68.0 MJ

Note that oxidation of 1 g of triacylglycerol liberates 68.0/1724 MJ or 39.4 kJ.

The RQ for this reaction is 110/157, or 0.70.

☞

Protein
(the quantities are shown for one mole of a standard protein):

$$C_{100}H_{159}N_{32}O_{32}S_{0.7} + 104\ O_2 \rightarrow$$

2257 g 104×22.4 litres

86.6 CO_2 + 50.6 H_2O + other products   – ΔH

86.6×22.4 litres 50.6×18 g   45.4 MJ

The other products are assumed to be urea (11.7 mol), ammonia (1.3 mol), creatinine (0.43 mol) and sulphuric acid (0.7 mol).

Note that oxidation of 1 g of standard protein liberates 45.4/2257 MJ or 20.1 kJ.

The RQ for this reaction is 86.6/104, or 0.83.

We may look at this another way, by calculating the heat liberated for each litre of O_2 used:

	Energy equivalent of 1 litre O_2	Respiratory quotient
Glucose*	20.8 kJ	1.00
Fat	19.6 kJ	0.71
Protein (forming urea)	19.4 kJ	0.83

*Slightly different values will be obtained depending upon whether the substrate is assumed to be pure glucose, or a glucose polymer such as glycogen. The same also applies to fat and protein: different fats and proteins give slightly different values.

Note that the heat produced per litre of O_2 consumed is almost constant. Thus, measurement of O_2 consumption alone allows the calculation of energy expenditure (heat production) to a reasonable accuracy. However, the estimate can be improved by also measuring CO_2 production and urinary urea (or total nitrogen) excretion, to allow the appropriate energy values to be used.

These figures may be combined into a formula such as:

$$\text{Energy expenditure (kJ)} = 15.9\ VO_2 + 5.2\ VCO_2 - 4.65\ N$$

where VO_2 represents the volume of O_2 consumed (litres), VCO_2 the volume of CO_2 produced (litres) and N the amount of urinary nitrogen excretion (g), over whatever measurement period is used.

Data taken, in part, from Elia & Livesey (1992).

Box 11.3 Measurement of energy expenditure using double-labelled water

The subject is given water ($^2H_2{}^{18}O$) in which both the oxygen and hydrogen atoms are isotopically labelled with a *stable isotope* (i.e. it is not radioactive), so that these atoms can be 'traced'. The oxygen atoms equilibrate with CO_2 through the action of the enzyme carbonic anhydrase in blood. Then the loss of ^{18}O atoms from the body is related to the rate of expiration of CO_2. However, ^{18}O is also lost in water (in sweat, breath, urine, etc.). This is allowed for by following the loss of ^2H. Thus, ^{18}O is lost somewhat faster than ^2H, and the difference (averaged over 2–3 weeks) gives a measure of the rate of CO_2 production. As described in the text, this can be used to derive an estimate of energy expenditure. A typical experimental result is shown below.

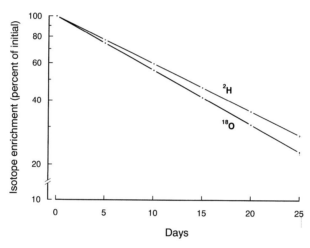

Fig. 11.3.1 Data for the example are reproduced from Garrow, J.S. (1988) *Obesity and related diseases*. With permission of Churchill Livingstone.

Some recent work has suggested that people may vary considerably in a component of energy expenditure that reflects involuntary physical activity or 'fidgeting'. This has been called non-exercise activity thermogenesis (NEAT). People with a low degree of fidgeting have been shown to have an increased risk of weight gain.

11.4 Obesity

11.4.1 Definition of obesity
Clearly obesity cannot be defined simply from the body weight since a tall thin

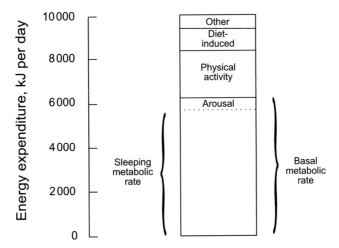

Fig. 11.3 Components of energy expenditure. A typical 24-hour energy expenditure of 10 000 kJ is shown with its components.

person may have the same body weight as a short, plump one. The Belgian astronomer Quetelet observed in 1869 that, amongst a large group of individuals, the weight varied roughly in proportion to the square of the height. Thus, for people of identical build, the figure given by weight/height² will be roughly constant. This ratio is known as the *body mass index* (universally denoted BMI) or *Quetelet's index*, or sometimes the *ponderal index*. It is always measured in kg/m². If the body mass index is greater than the normal, then the person is overweight, and conversely the person is underweight if the body mass index is low. A useful definition of overweight and obesity is given in Table 11.1.

The increase in body mass in obesity largely represents an accumulation of fat (Fig. 11.4). The fat content of the body may be measured in a number of ways. It can be measured by weighing an individual in air, and then again under water, making a correction for the buoyant effect of air in the lungs. This gives a measure of the body density, which can be used to calculate the percentage of fat. More simply, we can measure the *skinfold thickness* at different sites on

Table 11.1 A system for grading overweight and obesity.

Classification	BMI, kg/m²
Normal	18.5–24.9
Overweight	25.0 - 29.9
Obese:	> 30.0
Class I	30.0–34.9
Class II	35.0–39.9
Class III	> 40

From the International Obesity Task Force.

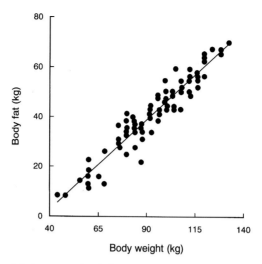

Fig. 11.4 Relationship between body fat content and body weight in a series of 104 women. Adapted from Webster *et al.* (1984).

the body using a caliper to 'pinch' the skin and underlying fat. The skinfolds at defined sites can be related to body fat content using published tables that are based on the comparison of these measurements, in large numbers of subjects, with the results from underwater weighing. Strictly it is *adipose tissue* rather than pure triacylglycerol which accumulates in obesity, in which there is also non-fat mass – adipose tissue cytoplasm, supporting connective tissue, blood vessels, etc. Thus, an obese subject will also have an increased non-fat component (fat-free mass).

11.4.2 How does obesity develop?

If an individual is overweight or obese, then clearly that individual must have been through a period when his or her intake of energy was consistently greater than his or her energy expenditure. (Note that this is true for everyone during the period of growth.) It does not necessarily follow that this is true *now*; an obese subject may be in energy balance, with a stable weight. Then we can ask the question: if energy intake was greater than energy expenditure, did this arise through (1) an elevated rate of energy intake, compared with people of normal and steady body weight; or (2) a diminished rate of energy expenditure (again, compared with people of normal and steady body weight)? The answer may not, of course, be the same for all obese subjects. This question is of interest because if the answer is (2) – i.e. diminished energy expenditure – then it implies that the individual will also have a particularly hard job losing excess calories, because he or she has a 'biologically' low metabolic rate; it also implies that we might look, in metabolic terms, for the cause of this oddity of metabolism.

This is a deceptively simple question that has taken many years to answer. The reason for the difficulty in answering it lies in the very precision of energy balance discussed earlier. In most people, as we have seen, energy intake and energy expenditure match each other to within a fraction of one percent over a reasonably long period. On the other hand, from day to day they may differ considerably. We must ask: what sort of a mismatch between energy intake and energy expenditure are we looking for?

Many people who are overweight have become so over a period of many years of gradual accumulation. Take as an example a person of height 1.8 m and body weight 100 kg, i.e. body mass index of 30.9 kg/m²; and suppose that he or she increased in weight from 70 kg (body mass index 21.6 kg/m²) over a period of 10 years. The gain is 30 kg of adipose tissue with an energy density of about 30 MJ/kg (as earlier), i.e. a total 'integrated mismatch' between energy intake and expenditure of $30 \times 30 = 900$ MJ, or 90 MJ per year, or about 250 kJ per day. A 'throughput' of energy is about 10 MJ/day (i.e. the amount we eat and expend), so this is an imbalance of about 2.5%. The task is therefore to measure both energy intake and energy expenditure to a degree of precision which will enable us to say whether one or the other is 2.5% outside normal values, which in themselves vary from person to person and which both vary enormously from day to day. This is an almost impossible experimental task. What is more, we have to do this *not* when the person comes to the clinic complaining of weighing 100 kg, but before that, during the phase of weight gain.

In fact, the question has been answered quite clearly in a slightly indirect way. The energy expenditure of obese subjects has been measured and compared with that of normal subjects (Table 11.2). *On average*, it is clear that obese subjects have higher rates of energy expenditure than subjects of normal weight. Now we see why this is an indirect answer: it is not even one of the results we were expecting. At first sight, an increased rate of energy expenditure should result in thinness rather than fatness. But remember that fat itself – i.e. the triacylglycerol in adipose tissue and other tissues – is not 'metabolically active'; energy expenditure occurs in the other components of the body, the fat-free or lean body mass. Fat-free mass is also increased in obese people; it represents the non-fat components of adipose tissue and other supporting tissues. The rate of energy expenditure is, in fact, closely related to the fat-free or lean body mass in people of all body weights, lean and obese (Fig. 11.5). Thus, we see that obese people have a high rate of energy expenditure because they

Table 11.2 Rates of energy expenditure (MJ/day) in subjects measured in an indirect calorimetry chamber.

	Total metabolic rate	Resting metabolic rate	Sleeping metabolic rate
Lean	8.44	6.12	5.67
Moderately obese	9.60	6.65	6.05
Obese	10.04	7.59	6.22

From Ravussin *et al.* (1982).

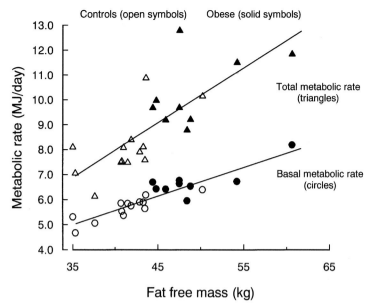

Fig. 11.5 Relationship between metabolic rate and fat free mass (FFM; a measure of lean body mass), in lean and obese women. The graph shows both *basal metabolic rate* (BMR) (circles), measured in a calorimeter, and *total metabolic rate* (TMR) (triangles), measured during normal life with double-labelled water (Box 11.3). Open symbols: lean subjects; solid symbols, obese. Note (1) the close relationship between BMR and FFM (or lean body mass) over a wide range (referred to in Section 11.3.2); (2) that the obese group have both greater FFM (i.e. lean tissue), and greater metabolic rate, than the lean. Regression lines for BMR and TMR against FFM are shown. Adapted from data in Prentice *et al.* (1986).

have accumulated excess lean body mass along with their excess fat. But, on the other hand, if they are now at a stable weight, the implication is that their rate of energy intake matches their rate of energy expenditure, and is therefore also greater than normal. Of course, these are not necessarily measurements made during the period of weight gain; but it is argued that if these people who are obese now have elevated rates of energy intake and energy expenditure, it seems highly unlikely that their obesity was brought about initially by a decreased rate of energy expenditure.

Thus, the message from such studies is clear: for the majority of obese people, the cause of the obesity is not a defect in energy expenditure but a rate of energy intake that is greater than normal. The same message is coming out of the single-gene defects discovered in markedly obese children: those discovered are all genes involved in the pathways of appetite regulation rather than of energy expenditure. Of course, if energy expenditure per unit of fat free mass is also lower than normal, perhaps because of lack of physical activity or because of subtle genetic changes affecting the basal metabolic rate, then the situation will be made worse.

Table 11.3 Health consequences of obesity.

	Possible metabolic cause
Adverse consequences	
Cardiovascular disease	Elevated LDL-cholesterol, decreased HDL-cholesterol and elevated triacylglycerol concentrations in serum; high blood pressure (see Box 10.1, insulin resistance and Box 9.6, atherogenic lipoprotein phenotype)
Hypertension (high blood pressure)	May result indirectly from insulin resistance
Type 2 diabetes mellitus	Insulin resistance
Gallstones	Increased cholesterol flux into bile (? related to insulin resistance and high insulin concentrations)
Reduced fertility (males), polycystic ovary syndrome (females)	Decreased androgens, increased oestrogen production in adipose tissue*
Breast and other cancers	Increased oestrogen production in adipose tissue*
Obstructive sleep apnoea (pausing breathing, usually during sleep)	Not thought to be metabolic: more a mechanical effect of excess fat. But serious nonetheless as it makes people sleepy during the day so that they may fall asleep driving. It has also been shown that obstructive sleep apnoea is a risk marker for coronary heart disease
Osteoarthritis in weight-bearing joints	Not metabolic: due to excess weight
Accidents and suicides	Not metabolic: obesity and depression are closely linked
Benefits	
Protection against post-menopausal osteoporosis	Increased oestrogen production in adipose tissue

Based on van Itallie (1985) and Garrow (1991).

*Increased oestrogen production occurs because adipose tissue contains the enzyme *aromatase*, which converts androgens (e.g. testosterone) into oestrogens.

11.4.3 Health implications of obesity

Obesity is associated with a number of adverse consequences for health. These are really outside the scope of this book except in so far as they have identifiable metabolic causes. Some are listed in Table 11.3. In the following, we will concentrate on the associated metabolic changes.

11.4.4 Metabolic changes in obesity

Many of the metabolic changes in obesity seem to stem from the associated insulin resistance. For instance, it was discussed in Section 10.2.3 how insulin resistance could, in a susceptible individual, lead to the development of Type 2 diabetes.

In addition, insulin resistance has effects on lipid metabolism, discussed in Box 10.1. The typical metabolic picture in obesity is of a tendency to elevation of LDL-cholesterol concentration, a depression of HDL-cholesterol and an elevation of plasma triacylglycerol concentration. Plasma non-esterified fatty acid concentrations also tend to be high, especially in the period after meals, both because there is more adipose tissue to release non-esterified fatty acids and because insulin resistance means that suppression after meals is less effective.

Why does insulin resistance arise in obesity? The answer is not entirely clear. Many changes in insulin action have been shown in animal models of obesity: a decrease in the number of insulin receptors on the cell surface, a decreased activity of the insulin receptor tyrosine kinase, and changes in intracellular metabolic pathways which render them less sensitive to insulin. To some extent there is a vicious spiral: for instance, insulin resistance leads to inappropriately elevated non-esterified fatty acid concentrations in the fed state and these impair muscle glucose utilisation by the glucose–fatty acid cycle discussed in Section 6.4.1.2.

Insulin resistance is a function not only of the total amount of body fat, but also of the way in which it is distributed. Different patterns of body fat distribution may be discerned: the fat may be concentrated around the abdomen and upper body, or around the hips and lower body. It is predominantly the former pattern that is associated with insulin resistance, and with increased risk of coronary heart disease. Nevertheless, the severely obese usually have plenty of fat in all regions, and insulin resistance to go with it. Upper body fat distribution reflects accumulation of adipose tissue within the abdomen as well as subcutaneous fat. Some of this intra-abdominal adipose tissue – associated with the mesentery and omentum which support the small intestine – releases its non-esterified fatty acids directly into the portal vein and thus to the liver. It has been suggested that an increased influx of fatty acids to the liver may have particular metabolic effects, some of which lead directly to the consequences of insulin resistance that were listed in Box 10.1.

11.5   Treatment of obesity

11.5.1   Dieting from the viewpoint of metabolic regulation

Obesity, as we have seen, results from an excess of energy intake over energy expenditure. If the obese or overweight person wants to lose weight, then the solution is simple and unarguable: energy expenditure must exceed energy intake for a suitable length of time. The only alternative is surgery to remove some excess fat. Of course, this message is simple in principle, but extraordinarily difficult to put into practice. Here, we shall consider why it is difficult, and also look at dieting from a metabolic viewpoint.

It was stressed in Section 8.3 that the body is able to adapt admirably well to starvation. Indeed, it has clearly been important throughout evolution to be able to minimise the impact of a period of partial or total lack of food. We should not, then, be surprised that dieting is difficult: it is a fight against mechanisms that have evolved over many millions of years precisely to minimise its effects. In our consideration of starvation, we saw the factors that bring about this protection. As food intake drops, the level of thyroid hormone falls and metabolic rate is lowered. Then, of course, food intake has to be reduced yet further to drop below the level of energy expenditure. Hunger mechanisms, outlined in Box 11.1, lead us to search for food – although it is said that the feelings of hunger disappear after a few days of total starvation, perhaps because ketone body concentrations rise and may suppress appetite. In addition, as weight loss occurs, the lean body mass will drop as well as the fat mass – and we have seen that this in itself will reduce daily energy expenditure (Fig. 11.5).

Equally dispiriting for the aspiring dieter is the pattern of weight loss. Over the first 24 hours or so of total starvation – longer if the food deprivation is partial – the liver glycogen store will be reduced almost to nothing. This is a store of around 100 g (Section 8.2.1). Since glycogen is stored with about three times its own weight of water, around 400 g will disappear over a period of a few days, or a week or so with partial food deprivation. Muscle glycogen will also be depleted – again, with its stored water – leading to further loss of perhaps 800 g. So more than 1 kg will be lost relatively quickly, leading the dieter to great hopes of a rapid transformation to skeletal proportions. But then, as we have seen, the body's strategy is to derive as much as possible of the necessary energy expenditure from fat, the store of which we have most. Suppose, after this initial period, that almost all the energy expenditure is derived from fat. A typical dieter's daily energy expenditure may be around 9 MJ. The energy density of adipose tissue is around 30MJ/kg, as we saw earlier. So 1 kg of adipose tissue will disappear every 3–4 days in total starvation; on a diet of 4 MJ per day, then weight would be lost at about 1 kg per week. The contrast is this: when we derive energy mainly from the hydrated glycogen stores, each MJ of energy expenditure represents loss of about 240 g weight; when we derive it mainly from fat in adipose tissue, each MJ used represents loss of about 33 g weight. So now psychological factors will intervene: weight loss, so promising at first (when it represented mainly water!) is now much less than hoped for, and for some there may be a tendency to resign oneself to a life of overweight and resume a 'normal' diet. Of course, the situation is not helped if the diet is relaxed for any reason: the first response to a resumption of normal food intake will be a rebuilding of the glycogen stores (with their associated water), so 1 kg or more will go on surprisingly quickly. Thus, the body's mechanisms which have evolved to minimise the effects of a period of food deprivation lead to difficulties for those who want to override them to *maximise* the effect of a period of food deprivation.

11.5.2 Pharmacological treatment of obesity

Various drugs have been used to help the process of weight loss. The mitochondrial uncoupler 2,4-dinitrophenol was used in the past; like the action of UCP1 in brown adipose tissue (Section 4.5.2), this allows metabolic energy to be dissipated as heat without generation of ATP. But there were some fatalities caused by rapid overheating. Thyroid hormone treatment has been used in an attempt to up-regulate energy expenditure, but excessive thyroid hormone levels are harmful to health (they raise blood pressure and cause tremor) and at lower levels, the body's own thyroid hormone secretion adjusts to compensate. At present only two drugs are licensed for the treatment of obesity. One, sibutramine, acts to raise concentrations of serotonin (5-hydroxytryptamine, a catecholamine-related neurotransmitter) in the brain, and this tends to reduce appetite. The other, tetrahydrolipstatin or orlistat, is an inhibitor of pancreatic lipase and, when taken with food, inhibits fat digestion in the small intestine. Therefore a proportion of dietary fat is excreted in the faeces, and not absorbed into the body. The extent to which fat digestion can be inhibited is limited by obvious unpleasant side effects. Both these treatments appear useful in helping obese people to lose weight but neither produces dramatic results.

Leptin, produced by recombinant DNA techniques, has been tested in humans and, at high doses, produces a modest effect of weight loss, but presumably the 'leptin resistance' seen in obesity renders it less effective than many people hoped when it was discovered.

The pharmaceutical companies are presently busy trying to exploit the enormous growth in knowledge of appetite regulation summarised in Box 11.1. In addition, there are attempts to increase energy expenditure, for instance by up-regulating the expression of the uncoupling proteins. We may certainly expect new developments in this field soon.

11.6   Further reading

Articles marked * all come from a Nature Insight section on Obesity in which there are also other good reviews: *Nature* 2000; 404: 631–677.

Body weight regulation and body composition
Jéquier, E. & Tappy, L. (1999) Regulation of body weight in humans. *Physiol Rev* 79: 451–480.
Ellis, K.J. (2000) Human body composition: in vivo methods. *Physiol Rev* 80: 649–680.

General on obesity prevalence, genetics and adverse effects on health
*Barsh, G.S., Farooqi, I.S. & O'Rahilly, S. (2000) Genetics of body-weight regulation. *Nature* 404: 644–651.
*Kopelman, P.G. (2000) Obesity as a medical problem. *Nature* 404: 635–643.

Metabolic aspects of energy metabolism and obesity

Levin, B.E., Dunn-Meynell, A.A. & Routh, V.H. (1999) Brain glucose sensing and body energy homeostasis: role in obesity and diabetes. *Am J Physiol Regul Integr Comp Physiol* 276: R1223–R1231.

Levine, J.A., Schleusner, S.J. & Jensen, M.D. (2000) Energy expenditure of nonexercise activity. *Am J Clin Nutr* 72: 1451–1454.

*Lowell, B.B. & Spiegelman, B.M. (2000) Towards a molecular understanding of adaptive thermogenesis. *Nature* 404: 652–660.

*Schwartz, M.W., Woods, S.C., Porte, D., Jr., Seeley, R.J. & Baskin, D.G. (2000) Central nervous system control of food intake. *Nature* 404: 661–671.

Chen, H.C. & Farese, R.V., Jr. (2001) Turning WAT into BAT gets rid of fat. *Nat Med* 7: 1102–1103.

Prevention and treatment of obesity

Tremblay, A. & Buemann, B. (1995) Exercise-training, macronutrient balance and body weight control. *Int J Obesity* 19: 79–86.

Booth, F.W., Gordon, S.E., Carlson, C.J. & Hamilton, M.T. (2000) Waging war on modern chronic diseases: primary prevention through exercise biology. *J Appl Physiol* 88: 774–787.

*Bray, G.A. & Tartaglia, L.A. (2000) Medicinal strategies in the treatment of obesity. *Nature* 404: 672–677.

Notes

1   One base-pair has been lost from the DNA of the leptin gene: therefore the sequence of amino acids is incorrect beyond that point and the protein is terminated prematurely.

2   *Fat-free mass* is the total body mass minus the mass of chemical fat; *lean body mass* is the total body mass minus the mass of adipose tissue. Although they are not quite the same, they measure the same thing.

References

Aarsland, A., Chinkes, D. & Wolfe, R.R. (1997) Hepatic and whole-body fat synthesis in humans during carbohydrate overfeeding. *Am J Clin Nutr* 65: 1774–1782.

Abumrad, N., Coburn, C. & Ibrahimi, A. (1999) Membrane proteins implicated in long-chain fatty acid uptake by mammalian cells: CD36, FATP and FABPm. *Biochim Biophys Acta* 1441: 4–13.

Acheson, K.J., Flatt, J.P. & Jéquier, E. (1982) Glycogen synthesis versus lipogenesis after a 500 gram carbohydrate meal in man. *Metabolism* 31: 1234–1240.

Acheson, K.J., Schutz, Y., Bessard, T., Ravussin, E., Jéquier, E. & Flatt, J.P. (1984) Nutritional influences on lipogenesis and thermogenesis after a carbohydrate meal. *Am J Physiol* 246: E62–E70.

Ainslie, P.N., Campbell, I.T., Frayn, K.N., Humphreys, S.M., Maclaren, D.P.M. & Reilly, T. (2002) Physiological and metabolic responses to a hill walk. *J Appl Physiol* 92: 179–187.

Ainsworth, B.E., Haskell, W.L., Leon, A.S. *et al.* (1992) Compendium of physical activities: classification of energy costs of human physical activities. *Med Sci Sports Ex* 25: 71–80.

Alberti, K.G. & Zimmet, P.Z. (1998) Definition, diagnosis and classification of diabetes mellitus and its complications. Part 1: diagnosis and classification of diabetes mellitus provisional report of a WHO consultation. *Diabetic Med* 15: 539–553.

Alberti, K.G.M.M., Boucher, B.J., Hitman, G.A. & Taylor, R. (1990) Diabetes mellitus. In: *The Metabolic and Molecular Basis of Acquired Disease* Vol. 1 (eds Cohen, R.D., Lewis, B., Alberti, K.G.M.M. & Denman, A.M.). London: Baillière Tindall, 765–840.

Alonso, M.D., Lomako, J., Lomako, W.M. & Whelan, W.J. (1995) A new look at the biogenesis of glycogen. *FASEB J* 9: 1126–1137.

Arner, P., Kriegholm, E., Engfeldt, P. & Bolinder, J (1990) Adrenergic regulation of lipolysis in situ at rest and during exercise. *J Clin Invest* 85: 893–898.

Åstrand, P.-O. & Rodahl, K. (1977) *Textbook of Work Physiology*, 2nd edn. New York: McGraw-Hill.

Bergström, J., Fürst, P., Norée, L.-O. & Vinnars, E. (1974) Intracellular free amino acid concentration in human muscle tissue. *J Appl Physiol* 36: 693–697.

Bergström, J., Hermansen, E., Hultman, E. & Saltin, B. (1967) Diet, muscle glycogen and physical performance. *Acta Physiol Scand* 71: 140–150.

Bergström, J. & Hultman, E. (1966) Muscle glycogen synthesis after exercise: an enhancing factor localized to the muscle cells in man. *Nature* 210: 309–310.

Bliss, M. (1983) *The Discovery of Insulin*. Edinburgh: Paul Harris.

Bloom, S.R., Vaughan, N.J.A. & Russell, R.C.G. (1974) Vagal control of glucagon release in man. *Lancet* II: 546–549.

Bollen, M., Keppens, S. & Stalmans, W. (1998) Specific features of glycogen metabolism in the liver. *Biochem J* 336: 19–31.

Brunicardi, F.C., Sun, Y.S., Druck, P., Goulet, R.J., Elahi, D. & Andersen, D.K. (1987) Splanchnic neural regulation of insulin and glucagon secretion in the isolated perfused human pancreas. *Am J Surg* 153: 34–40.

Buono, M.J. & Kolkhorst, F.W. (2001) Estimating ATP resynthesis during a marathon run: a method to introduce metabolism. *Adv Physiol Edu* 25: 142–143.

Burkitt, H.G., Young, B. & Heath, J.W. (1993) *Wheater's Functional Histology*, 3rd edn. Edinburgh: Churchill Livingstone.

Christensen, H.N. (1982) Interorgan amino acid nutrition. *Physiol Rev* 62: 1193–1233.

Cinti, S. (2001) The adipose organ: morphological perspectives of adipose tissues. *Proc Nutr Soc* 60: 319–328.

Cohen, P. (1999) The Croonian Lecture 1998. Identification of a protein kinase cascade of major importance in insulin signal transduction. *Philos Trans R Soc Lond B Biol Sci* 354: 485–495.

Considine, R.V., Sinha, M.K., Heiman, M.L. *et al.* (1996) Serum immunoreactive-leptin concentrations in normal-weight and obese humans. *N Engl J Med* 334: 292–295.

Coppack, S.W., Fisher, R.M., Gibbons, G.F. *et al.* (1990) Postprandial substrate deposition in human forearm and adipose tissues *in vivo*. *Clin Sci* 79: 339–348.

Cornish-Bowden, A. & Cárdenas, M.L. (1991) Hexokinase and 'glucokinase' in liver metabolism. *Trends Biochem Sci* 16: 281–282.

Costill, D.L., Coyle, E., Dalsky, G., Evans, W., Fink, W. & Hoopes, D. (1977) Effects of elevated plasma FFA and insulin on muscle glycogen usage during exercise. *J Appl Physiol* 43: 695–699.

Durrington, P.N. (1995) *Hyperlipidaemia: Diagnosis and Management*, 2nd edn. Oxford: Butterworth-Heinemann Ltd.

Dutta-Roy, A.K. (2000) Cellular uptake of long-chain fatty acids: role of membrane-associated fatty-acid-binding/transport proteins. *Cell Mol Life Sci* 57: 1360–1372.

Dyck, D.J., Putman, C.T., Heigenhauser, G.J.F., Hultman, E. & Spriet, L.L. (1993) Regulation of fat-carbohydrate interaction in skeletal muscle during intense aerobic cycling. *Am J Physiol* 265: E852–E859.

Elia, M. & Livesey, G. (1992) Energy expenditure and fuel selection in biological systems: the theory and practice of calculations based on indirect calorimetry and tracer methods. In: *Metabolic Control of Eating, Energy Expenditure and the Bioenergetics of Obesity. World Review of Nutrition and Dietetics* Vol. 70 (ed. Simopoulos, A.P.). Basel: Karger, 68–131.

Farooqi, I.S., Jebb, S.A., Langmack, G. *et al.* (1999) Effects of recombinant leptin therapy in a child with congenital leptin deficiency. *N Engl J Med* 341: 879–884.

Felber, J.-P., Acheson, K.J. & Tappy, L. (1993) *From Obesity to Diabetes.* Chichester: John Wiley.

Felig, P. (1975) Amino acid metabolism in man. *Annu Rev Biochem* 44: 933–955.

Felig, P., Pozefsky, T., Marliss, E. & Cahill, G.F. (1970) Alanine: key role in gluconeogenesis. *Science* 167: 1003–1004.

Fell, D. (1997) *Understanding the Control of Metabolism.* London: Portland Press.

Fery, F.D., Attellis, N.P. & Balasse, E.O. (1990) Mechanisms of starvation diabetes: study with double tracer and indirect calorimetry. *Am J Physiol* 259: E770–E777.

Fielding, P.E. & Fielding, C.J. (1996) Dynamics of lipoprotein transport in the human circulatory system. In: *Biochemistry of Lipids, Lipoproteins and Membranes* (eds Vance, D.E. & Vance, J.E.). Amsterdam: Elsevier Science BV, 495–516.

Frayn, K.N. (1982) Acute metabolic responses to injury. In: *Topical Reviews in Accident Surgery* Vol 2 (eds Tubbs, N. & London, P.S.). Bristol: John Wright, 47–66.

Frayn, K.N. (1986) Hormonal control of metabolism in trauma and sepsis. *Clin Endocrinol* 24: 577–599.

Frayn, K.N. (2003) Nutrition: Biochemical background. In: *Oxford Textbook of Medicine*, 4th edn (eds Warrell, D.A., Cox, T.M., Firth, J.D. & Benz, E.J.). Oxford: Oxford University Press, 1037–1043.

Frayn, K.N., Coppack, S.W., Humphreys, S.M., Clark, M.L. & Evans, R.D. (1993) Periprandial regulation of lipid metabolism in insulin-treated diabetes mellitus. *Metabolism* 42: 504–510.

Frayn, K.N., Williams, C.M. & Arner, P. (1996) Are increased plasma non-esterified fatty acid concentrations a risk marker for coronary heart disease and other chronic diseases? *Clin Sci* 90: 243–253.

Gardner, D.F., Kaplan, M.M., Stanley, C.A. & Utiger, R.D. (1979) Effect of tri-iodo-thyronine replacement on the metabolic and pituitary responses to starvation. *N Engl J Med* 300: 579–584.

Garrow, J. (1991) Importance of obesity. *Br Med J* 303: 704–706.

Garrow, J.S. (1988) *Obesity and Related Diseases.* Edinburgh: Churchill Livingstone.

Gerich, J., Davis, J., Lorenzi, M. *et al.* (1979) Hormonal mechanisms of recovery from insulin-induced hypoglycemia in man. *Am J Physiol* 236: E380–E385.

Goldspink, D.F. & Kelly, F.J. (1984) Protein turnover and growth in the whole body, liver and kidney of the rat from the foetus to senility. *Biochem J* 217: 507–516.

Goldspink, D.F., Lewis, S.E.M. & Kelly, F.J. (1984) Protein synthesis during the developmental growth of the small and large intestine of the rat. *Biochem J* 217: 527–534.

Gould, G.W. & Holman, G.D. (1993) The glucose transporter family: structure, function and tissue-specific expression. *Biochem J* 295: 329–341.

Griffiths, A.J., Humphreys, S.M., Clark, M.L., Fielding, B.A. & Frayn, K.N. (1994) Immediate metabolic availability of dietary fat in combination with carbohydrate. *Am J Clin Nutr* 59: 53–59.

Gurr, M.I., Harwood, J.L. & Frayn, K.N. (2002) *Lipid Biochemistry: An Introduction*, 5th edn. Oxford: Blackwell Science.

Harrison, D.E., Christie, M.R. & Gray, D.W.R. (1985) Properties of isolated human islets of Langerhans: insulin secretion, glucose oxidation and protein phosphorylation. *Diabetologia* 28: 99–103.

Hegsted, D.M., McGandy, R.B., Myers, M.L. & Stare, F.J. (1965) Quantitative effects of dietary fat on serum cholesterol in man. *Am J Clin Nutr* 17: 281–295.

Henry, C.J.K., Rivers, J.P.W. & Payne, P.R. (1988) Protein and energy metabolism in starvation reconsidered. *Eur J Clin Nutr* 42: 543–549.

Hirsch, D., Stahl, A. & Lodish, H.F. (1998) A family of fatty acid transporters conserved from mycobacterium to man. *Proc Natl Acad Sci USA* 95: 8625–8629.

Hitman, G.A. & Niven, M.J. (1989) Genes and diabetes mellitus. *Br Med Bull* 45: 191–205.

Hodgetts, V., Coppack, S.W., Frayn, K.N. & Hockaday, T.D.R. (1991) Factors controlling fat mobilization from human subcutaneous adipose tissue during exercise. *J Appl Physiol* 71: 445–451.

Holloszy, J.O, & Booth, F.W. (1976) Biochemical adaptations to endurance exercise. *Annu Rev Physiol* 38: 273–291.

Hue, L. & Rider, M.H. (1987) Role of fructose 2,6-bisphosphate in the control of glycolysis in mammalian tissues. *Biochem J* 245: 313–324.

Humphrey, C.S., Dykes, J.R.W. & Johnston, D. (1975a) Effects of truncal, selective, and highly selective vagotomy on glucose tolerance and insulin secretion in patients with duodenal ulcer. I. Effect of vagotomy on response to oral glucose. *Br Med J* 2: 112–114.

Humphrey, C.S., Dykes, J.R.W. & Johnston, D. (1975b) Effects of truncal, selective, and highly selective vagotomy on glucose tolerance and insulin secretion in patients with duodenal ulcer. II. Comparison of responses to oral and intravenous glucose. *Br Med J* 2: 114–116.

Hunt, S.M. & Groff, J.L. (1990) *Advanced Nutrition and Human Metabolism*. St Paul, MN: West Publishing Co.

Issekutz, B., Bortz, W.M., Miller, H.I. & Paul, P. (1967) Turnover rate of plasma FFA in humans and in dogs. *Metabolism* 16: 1001–1009.

Jones, D.A. & Round, J.M. (1990) *Skeletal Muscle in Health and Disease. A Textbook of Muscle Physiology*. Manchester: Manchester University Press.

Joost, H.-G., Bell, G.I., Best, J.D. *et al.* (2002) Nomenclature of the GLUT/SLC2A family of sugar/polyol transport facilitators. *Am J Physiol Endocrinol Metab* 282: E974–E976.

Karpe, F., Olivecrona, T., Walldius, G. & Hamsten, A. (1992) Lipoprotein lipase in plasma after an oral fat load: relation to free fatty acids. *J Lipid Res* 33: 975–984.

Kawaguchi, T., Takenoshita, M., Kabashima, T. & Uyeda, K. (2001) Glucose and cAMP regulate the L-type pyruvate kinase gene by phosphorylation/dephosphorylation of the carbohydrate response element binding protein. *Proc Natl Acad Sci USA* 98: 13710–13715.

King, R.F.G.J., Almond, D.J., Oxby, C.B., Holmfield, J.H.M. & McMahon, M.J. (1984) Calculation of short-term changes in body fat from measurement of respiratory gas exchange. *Metabolism* 33: 826–832.

Koo, S.H., Dutcher, A.K. & Towle, H.C. (2001) Glucose and insulin function through two distinct transcription factors to stimulate expression of lipogenic enzyme genes in liver. *J Biol Chem* 276: 9437–9445.

Leslie, R.D.G., Lazarus, N.R. & Vergani, D. (1989) Aetiology of insulin-dependent diabetes. *Br Med Bull* 45: 58–72.

Lewis, B. (1990) Hyperlipidaemia. In: *The Metabolic and Molecular Basis of Acquired Disease* Vol. 1 (eds Cohen, R.D., Lewis, B., Alberti, K.G.M.M. & Denman, A.M.). London: Baillière Tindall, 860–920.

Lewis, S.E.M., Kelly, F.J. & Goldspink, D.F. (1984) Pre- and post-natal growth and protein turnover in smooth muscle, heart and slow- and fast-twitch skeletal muscles of the rat. *Biochem J* 217: 517–526.

Malkova, D., Evans, R.D., Frayn, K.N., Humphreys, S.M., Jones, P.R. & Hardman, A.E. (2000) Prior exercise and postprandial substrate extraction across the human leg. *Am J Physiol Endocrinol Metab* 279: E1020–E1028.

Maughan, R., Gleeson, M. & Greenhaff, P.L. (1997) *Biochemistry of Exercise and Training*. Oxford: Oxford University Press.

McCullough, A.J., Miller, L.J., Service, F.J. & Go, V.L.W. (1983) Effect of graded intraduodenal glucose infusions on the release and physiological action of gastric inhibitory polypeptide. *J Clin Endocrinol Metab* 56: 234–241.

McGarry, J.D., Mannaerts, G.P. & Foster, D.W. (1977) A possible role for malonyl-CoA in the regulation of hepatic fatty acid oxidation and ketogenesis. *J Clin Invest* 60: 265–270.

McGivan, J.D. & Pastor-Anglada, M. (1994) Regulatory and molecular aspects of mammalian amino acid transport. *Biochem J* 299: 321–334.

Newsholme, E.A. & Challiss, R.A.J. (1992) Metabolic-control-logic: its application to thermogenesis, insulin sensitivity, and obesity. In: *Obesity* (eds Björntorp, P. & Brodoff, B.N.). Philadelphia: Lippincott, 145–161.

Newsholme, E.A. & Leech, A.R. (1983) *Biochemistry for the Medical Sciences*. Chichester: John Wiley.

Nilsson, L.H. & Hultman, E (1973) Liver glycogen in man – the effect of total starvation or a carbohydrate-poor diet followed by carbohydrate refeeding. *Scand J Clin Lab Invest* 32: 325–330.

Nordlie, R.C., Foster, J.D. & Lange, A.J. (1999) Regulation of glucose production by the liver. *Annu Rev Nutr* 19: 379–406.

O'Brien, R.M. & Granner, D.K. (1991) Regulation of gene expression by insulin. *Biochem J* 278: 609–619.

O'Brien, R.M. & Granner, D.K. (1996) Regulation of gene expression by insulin. *Physiol Rev* 76: 1109–1161.

Oliver, M.F. & Opie, L.H. (1994) Effects of glucose and fatty acids on myocardial ischaemia and arrhythmias. *Lancet* 343: 155–158.

Owen, O.E., Tappy, L., Mozzoli, M.A. & Smalley, K.J. (1990) Acute starvation. In: *The Metabolic and Molecular Basis of Acquired Disease* Vol. 1 (eds Cohen, R.D., Lewis, B., Alberti, K.G.M.M. & Denman, A.M.). London: Baillière Tindall, 550–570.

Palacín, M., Estévez, R., Bertran, J. & Zorzano, A. (1998) Molecular biology of mammalian plasma membrane amino acid transporters. *Physiol Rev* 78: 969–1054.

Pilkis, S.J. & Granner, D.K. (1992) Molecular physiology of the regulation of hepatic gluconeogenesis and glycolysis. *Annu Rev Physiol* 54: 885–909.

Prentice, A.M., Black, A.E., Coward, W.A. *et al.* (1986) High levels of energy expenditure in obese women. *Br Med J* 292: 983–987.

Randle, P.J., Garland, P.B., Hales, C.N. & Newsholme, E.A. (1963) The glucose fatty-acid cycle. Its role in insulin sensitivity and the metabolic disturbances of diabetes mellitus. *Lancet* 1: 785–789.

Rang, H.P. & Dale, M.M. (1991) *Pharmacology*. Edinburgh: Churchill Livingstone.

Ravussin, E., Burnand, B., Schutz, Y. & Jéquier, E. (1982) Twenty-four hour energy expenditure and resting metabolic rate in obese, moderately obese, and control subjects. *Am J Clin Nutr* 35: 566–573.

Reaven, G.M., Hollenbeck, C., Jeng, C.-Y., Wu, M.S. & Chen, Y.-D.I. (1988) Measurement of plasma glucose, free fatty acid, lactate, and insulin for 24 h in patients with NIDDM. *Diabetes* 37: 1020–1024.

Robertson, R.P. & Porte, D., Jr. (1973) Adrenergic modulation of basal insulin secretion in man. *Diabetes* 22: 1–8.

Romijn, J.A., Coyle, E.F., Sidossis, L.S. *et al.* (1993) Regulation of endogenous fat and carbohydrate metabolism in relation to exercise intensity and duration. *Am J Physiol* 265: E380–E391.

Ruderman, N.B. (1975) Muscle amino acid metabolism and gluconeogenesis. *Annu Rev Med* 26: 245–258.

Salway JG. (1999) *Metabolism at a Glance*, 2nd edn. Oxford: Blackwell Scientific Publications.

Schuit, F.C. (1997) Is GLUT2 required for glucose sensing? *Diabetologia* 40: 104–111.

Shepherd, P.R. & Kahn, B.B. (1999) Glucose transporters and insulin action. Implications for insulin resistance and diabetes mellitus. *N Engl J Med* 341: 248–257.

Sidossis, L.S. & Wolfe, R.R. (1996) Glucose and insulin-induced inhibition of fatty acid oxidation: the glucose-fatty acid cycle reversed. *Am J Physiol* 33: E733–E738.

Simons, L.A. (1986) Interrelations of lipids and lipoproteins with coronary artery disease mortality in 19 countries. *Am J Cardiol* 57: 5G–10G.

Snell, K. (1986) The duality of pathways for serine biosynthesis is a fallacy. *Trends Biochem Sci* 11: 241–243.

Snell, K. & Fell, D.A. (1990) Metabolic control analysis of mammalian serine metabolism. *Adv Enzyme Regul* 30: 13–32.

Söderlund, K., Greenhaff, P.L. & Hultman, E. (1992) Energy metabolism in type I and type II human muscle fibres during short term electrical stimulation at different frequencies. *Acta Physiol Scand* 144: 15–22.

Taylor, R., Price, T.B., Katz, L.D., Shulman, R.G. & Shulman, G.I. (1993) Direct measurement of change in muscle glycogen concentration after a mixed meal in normal subjects. *Am J Physiol* 265: E224–E229.

Thorens, B. (1993) Facilitated glucose transporters in epithelial cells. *Annu Rev Physiol* 55: 591–608.

Thorens, B. (1996) Glucose transporters in the regulation of intestinal, renal, and liver glucose fluxes. *Am J Physiol* 270: G541–553.

van der Vusse, G.J. & Reneman, R.S. (1996) Lipid metabolism in muscle. In: *Handbook of Physiology*, section 12 (eds Rowell, L.B. & Shepherd, J.T.). New York: American Physiological Society, 952–994.

van Itallie, T.B. (1985) Health implications of overweight and obesity in the United States. *Ann Intern Med* 103: 983–988.

Wallner, E.I., Wada, J., Tramonti, G., Lin, S. & Kanwar, Y.S. (2001) Status of glucose transporters in the mammalian kidney and renal development. *Renal Failure* 23: 301–310.

Webster, J.D., Hesp, R. & Garrow, J.S. (1984) The composition of excess weight in obese women estimated by body density, total body water and total body potassium. *Human Nutr: Clin Nutr* 38C: 299–306.

Wright, E.M. (1993) The intestinal Na^+/glucose cotransporter. *Annu Rev Physiol* 55: 575–589.

Index